MW01518293

INNATE IMMUNE SYSTEM OF SKIN AND ORAL MUCOSA

INNATE IMMUNE SYSTEM OF SKIN AND ORAL MUCOSA

Properties and Impact in Pharmaceutics, Cosmetics, and Personal Care Products

NAVA DAYAN AND **PHILIP W. WERTZ**

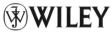

A JOHN WILEY & SONS, INC., PUBLICATION

Library of Congress Cataloging-in-Publication Data:

Innate immune system of skin and oral mucosa : properties and impact in
pharmaceutics, cosmetics, and personal care products / [edited] by Nava Dayan,
Philip W. Wertz.
    p. ; cm.
  Includes bibliographical references.
  ISBN 978-0-470-43777-3 (cloth)
  1. Skin–Immunology. 2. Natural immunity. 3. Mouth–Immunology. 4. Oral
mucosa. 5. Dermatologic agents–Immunology. 6. Cosmetics–Immunology. 7.
Toilet preparations–Immunology. I. Dayan, Nava. II. Wertz, Philip W.
  [DNLM: 1. Skin–immunology. 2. Cosmetics–adverse effects. 3. Immunity,
Innate–drug effects. 4. Mouth Mucosa–immunology. 5. Pharmaceutical
Preparations–adverse effects. WR 102]
  RL97.I56 2011
  616.5′079–dc22

                           2010045237

Printed in Singapore.

10 9 8 7 6 5 4 3 2 1

CONTENTS

PREFACE

Innate immunity is the ancient first line of protection against potential microbial or viral environmental insult. This insult and response to it can be modified by various environmental factors including pollution, radiation, or chemicals. Innate immunity is inherent to the natural biological makeup of the organism and does not depend upon prior exposure to specific antigens. The fact that it requires no memory to respond is both an advantage and a limitation. It is composed of the physiological and anatomical barriers, mechanical removal of invaders, beneficial flora, enzymes, low pH, a variety of lipids and peptides, and a number of cells that respond quickly, specifically but without the need of prior acquired memory. In recent years, scientists and research groups around the world started unraveling a few of the key components of the innate immunity in skin, oral mucosa, and other body surfaces or openings. Yet, there is no book that compiles this valuable information in one edition. The importance of this compilation lies in providing an overview of the available scientific findings, so one can acquire a general idea of the known components of this system. It may provide a key to the understanding of unsolved disorders. Part I of this book presents an overview emphasizing mechanisms for control of bacteria at the skin surface. This includes historical and ethical aspects of skin cleaning products. Over the past decade, there has been a great deal of interest in the antimicrobial peptides and their roles in innate immunity of the skin and oral mucosa, and more recently antimicrobial lipids have received some attention. Part II of the book includes chapters discussing antimicrobial peptides and lipids in innate immunity of skin and mucosa. Part III deals with cellular components of innate immunity and the link between innate and adaptive immunity. Part IV deals with stressors that can influence innate immunity. These include radiation and oxidative stress, cosmetic formulations, and aging. Finally, microbial challenges are discussed in Part V.

We hope this book will be of use to people working in the areas of dermatology, oral pathology, cosmetics, personal care, and pharmaceutics. It is especially hoped that it will stimulate thought leading to discussion and further research. It is felt that this book can serve as a valuable introduction to newcomers and a useful reference for more established investigators.

The contributors to this book were carefully selected as experts in their areas. They come from different disciplines in academia and industry. Working with them was a pleasure and a learning experience and we thank them sincerely. We also extend our appreciation to the publishers of this book for their patience, understanding, and cooperation.

We hope that you enjoy and benefit from this edition.

Nava Dayan
Philip W. Wertz

CONTRIBUTORS

Niroshana Anandasabapathy, Laboratory of Cellular Physiology and Immunology, The Rockefeller University, New York, NY

Chris D. Anderson, Department of Dermatology, Linköping University, Linkoping, Sweden

Shamim A. Ansari, Colgate-Palmolive Co., Technology Center, Piscataway, NJ

Carol L. Bratt, Dows Institute, University of Iowa, Iowa City, IA

Kim A. Brogden, Dows Institute, University of Iowa, Iowa City, IA

Karen E. Burke, Department of Dermatology, Mt. Sinai Medical Center, New York, NY

Whasun O. Chung, Department of Oral Biology, University of Washington, Seattle, WA

Deborah V. Dawson, Dows Institute, University of Iowa, Iowa City, IA

Nava Dayan, Lipo Chemicals Inc., Paterson, NJ

Anna Di Nardo, Department of Medicine, University of California San Diego, La Jolla, CA

Henrik Dommisch, Department of Oral Biology, University of Washington, Seattle, WA; Department of Periodontology, Operative and Preventive Dentistry, University of Bonn, Bonn, Germany

David R. Drake, Dows Institute for Dental Research, University of Iowa, Iowa City, IA

Peter M. Elias, Department of Dermatology, University of California San Francisco Medical Center, San Francisco, CA; Dermatology Service, VA Medical Center, San Francisco, CA

Martha N. Gardner, Massachusetts College of Pharmacy and Health Sciences, Boston, MA

Barbara Geusens, Department of Dermatology, Ghent University Hospital, Ghent, Belgium

Jennifer R. Hill, Dows Institute, University of Iowa, Iowa City, IA

Steven B. Hoath, Cincinnati Children's Hospital Medical Center, Department of Pediatrics, Division of Neonatology and Pulmonary Biology, Skin Sciences Institute, University of Cincinnati, Cincinnati, OH

Genji Imokawa, School of Bioscience and Biotechnology, Tokyo University of Technology, Tokyo, Japan

Jo Lambert, Department of Dermatology, Ghent University Hospital, Ghent, Belgium

Roger L. McMullen, International Specialty Products, Wayne, NJ

Ilse Mollet, Department of Dermatology, Ghent University Hospital, Ghent, Belgium

Neelam Muizzuddin, Estee Lauder Companies and SUNY Stony Brook, Melville, NY

Vivek Narendran, Cincinnati Children's Hospital Medical Center, Department of Pediatrics, Division of Neonatology and Pulmonary Biology, Skin Sciences Institute, University of Cincinnati, Cincinnati, OH

Rudranath Persaud, Safety Evaluation, L'Oreal USA, Inc., Clark, NJ

Thomas Re, Safety Evaluation, L'Oreal USA, Inc., Clark, NJ

Kenneth A. Richman, Massachusetts College of Pharmacy and Health Sciences, Boston, MA

Michael S. Roberts, Therapeutics Research Centre, Department of Medicine, Southern Clinical Division, Princess Alexandra Hospital, University of Queensland, Woolloongabba, Australia; School of Pharmacy & Medical Sciences, University of South Australia, North Terrace, Adelaide, Australia

Jennifer Tebbe-Grossman, Massachusetts College of Pharmacy and Health Sciences, Boston, MA

Sarah Terras, Department of Dermatology, Ghent University Hospital, Ghent, Belgium

Giuseppe Valacchi, Department of Biomedical Sciences, University of Siena, Siena, Italy

Marty O. Visscher, Cincinnati Children's Hospital Medical Center, Department of Pediatrics, Division of Neonatology and Pulmonary Biology, Skin Sciences Institute, University of Cincinnati, Cincinnati, OH

Zhenping Wang, Department of Medicine, University of California San Diego, La Jolla, CA

Philip W. Wertz, Dows Institute, University of Iowa, Iowa City, IA

PART I

OVERVIEW OF SKIN AND MUCOSAL INNATE IMMUNITY: HISTORY, ETHICS, AND SCIENCE

CHAPTER 1

GERM FREE: HYGIENE HISTORY AND CONSUMING ANTIMICROBIAL AND ANTISEPTIC PRODUCTS

Jennifer Tebbe-Grossman and Martha N. Gardner

Massachusetts College of Pharmacy and Health Sciences Boston, MA

1.1 INTRODUCTION

In our current society, cleanliness is a virtue. Our conventional wisdom is that washing our hands and body with personal care products is something we all should do to maintain our health—and social acceptability. However, what the "virtue" of cleanliness is—as well as the products that we use in order to become clean—has changed significantly over time. In fact, cleanliness has not always been viewed as a virtue. Europeans and Americans began to significantly identify cleanliness as a cornerstone of health and morality only in the mid-nineteenth century. From this period through the early to mid-twentieth century, public health efforts to implement infection control, cleanliness, and hygiene practices in hospitals, schools, workplaces, and the home developed. Relatedly, in the late nineteenth century, the medical and scientific community, as well as the general public, debated but eventually accepted antisepsis and the germ theory of disease. Marketed products emerged with promises to keep you clean, destroy germs, assure economic advancement and social desirability, assuage guilt, and uphold morality.

Beliefs about hygiene and cleanliness have varied over time and place. In Western Europe, from the classical Roman era through the nineteenth century, the use of public or private home baths, for instance, was alternately considered desirable for medicinal or social purposes or unacceptable because of concerns about immorality or health dangers [1,2]. Throughout this time period, the foundational theory of health and disease in Western civilization posited a balance of "humors" in the body that needed to be kept in equilibrium [3]. Many Europeans feared and generally avoided water, especially hot water, since they believed its moisture opened pores to bad air, poisons, and disequilibrium within the body [1]. With the appearance of the "Black

Innate Immune System of Skin and Oral Mucosa: Properties and Impact in Pharmaceutics, Cosmetics, and Personal Care Products, First Edition. Nava Dayan and Philip W. Wertz.
© 2011 John Wiley & Sons, Inc. Published 2011 by John Wiley & Sons, Inc.

Death" in Europe, many argued that using water made people easy targets for the plague's invasion through their moistened pores [4].

From the 1500s to the 1700s, the important factor in cleanliness "applied exclusively to the visible parts of the body" ([1], p. 226). Faces and hands were splashed with water in basins but more intimate parts of the body were not washed. As people began to understand the role of skin, its oils, and perspiration, white linen was perceived for some time as a way of cleansing the body. Those who could afford to changed and washed their linen ([4], p. 106). Perfumes also masked body odor while a variety of "objects of refinement"—gloves or handkerchiefs—"defended the user against external dirt" ([5], p.192). Not until the late seventeenth and early eighteenth centuries did the growing bourgeois classes come to think of cleanliness as hygiene in connection to a healthy body. It became acceptable to bathe (without soap) the whole body in warm water for its "purifying function." Personal hygiene soon became a moral and civilizing issue ([1], pp. 170, 193). By the mid-nineteenth century, historians Richard and Claudia Bushman argued that "cultural values" had "interlocked with social forces that gave cleanliness intense social importance." For the middle classes,

Dirty hands, greasy clothes, offensive odors, grime on the skin—all entered into complex judgments about the social position of the dirty person and actually about his or her moral worth ... Cleanliness indicated control, spiritual refinement, breeding; the unclean were vulgar, coarse, animalistic. (*Source*: Ref. 6, p.1228.)

Since the poor had little access to water, cleanliness became a class as well as a moral issue.

Cleanliness in the public environment posed additional problems. As people moved from rural to urban areas, population density greatly increased, and with it, poor sanitation. Urban streets and alleys were strewn with excrement, dead animals, and garbage. Water was scarce, filthy, and foul smelling. Working sewer systems were virtually nonexistent. Endemic and epidemic diseases flourished [7,8]. Within the context of beliefs that "miasmas" or filth and foul smelling air caused disease, nineteenth-century public health reformers focused on improving urban sanitation through such policies as garbage collection and disposal, well-engineered sewer systems, and indoor plumbing systems. The public effort to improve sanitation was a massive one. Water became an increasingly important element of everyday life in public and private places, and sewer systems and pipes for running water were built in short order during the late nineteenth and early twentieth centuries [9–12].

As sanitation improved and cleanliness became an accepted social value, soaps also improved. Early soaps, generally very harsh and used for household cleaning, were often made at home in small batches by boiling some combination of animal fat and alkali (e.g., plant or wood ashes). The so-called "toilet" soap for personal use did not appear to be more generally utilized until a natural vegetable oil was added in the early 1600s and the first soap companies began to form. Such alkaline and olive oil-based soap products as the Castile soap from Spain were favored by wealthier social classes that could afford to purchase the products. Men used toilet soaps for shaving while women saw them as luxurious and costly cosmetics. With the rise of a consumer-based economy in Europe and the United States in the late nineteenth century, people relied less on their "homemade soap or chunks of soap bought at the local dry goods store" and began to purchase "packaged" soap bars ([13], p. 54). Producing in ever greater volume, early soap companies marketed their products to schools and hospitals and sold them in general stores, drugstores, and later grocery stores.

As the soap industry would continue to grow, concerns about both soap's purity and skin irritation and its civilizing characteristics would recur in advertisements and public commentary. In 1885, the Reverend Henry Ward Beecher endorsed Pears soap declaring that "if Cleanliness is next to Godliness Soap must be considered as a Means of Grace and a Clergyman who recommends moral things should be willing to recommend Soap" ([6], p. 1218). During the nineteenth century, various technological and transportation changes allowed for soaps to be produced more cheaply and in greater volume, especially as companies sought "purity" in soap and experimented with various oils—olive, cottonseed, coconut, and palm [4, 14].

This chapter will look at hospital and home settings as places where health professionals and consumers pursued cleanliness as they came to connect cleanliness to health. Three historical moments emphasize how fears about dirt, infection, and the spread of disease related to efforts to develop and use cleanliness products. The first moment occurred in the nineteenth and early twentieth centuries primarily as a medical conflict emerged over the connection between cleanliness and disease. The second moment occurred with the discovery of such "miracle drugs" as sulfonamides and antibiotics (especially penicillin) in the 1940s. The third moment took place in the 1990s as fears about "new" or "emerging" bacteria and infections prompted new waves of hygiene products in the late twentieth and early twenty-first centuries.

1.2 HYGIENE BELIEFS AND PRODUCTS AS THE GERM THEORY EMERGES (NINETEENTH TO EARLY TWENTIETH CENTURIES)

1.2.1 Early Ideas and Realities Concerning Hand Washing in the Hospital

The struggle for physicians to understand the causes of maternal and infant mortality during childbirth was the first moment when physicians made the connection between cleanliness and disease. "Childbed fever" (also called "puerperal fever") was a serious problem from the seventeenth to mid-twentieth centuries, sometimes reaching epidemic proportions—especially among women who had physicians deliver their babies. Although most physicians rejected the idea that their practices could cause this disease, it is clear now that they in fact were the culprits. Hand washing and other cleanliness practices were not yet used, and physicians typically went from one bedside to another without changing their clothing or washing their hands. In some instances, puerperal fever could kill up to two-thirds of women during childbirth [15].

By the late eighteenth century, some physicians began to speculate on their involvement in this disease. Their speculation preceded scientific understanding of germ theory. Alexander Gordon, who practiced medicine in Aberdeen, Scotland, published in 1795, *A Treatise on the Epidemic Puerperal Fever of Aberdeen*. In it, he argued that women were "seized" by "a specific contagion" that was "delivered" by a physician or nurse "who had previously attended patients affected with the disease . . . " He acknowledged "I myself was the means of carrying the infection to a great number of women." ([16], p. 35). This prophetic idea did not immediately catch on, however. In 1843, prominent American physician Oliver Wendell Holmes published a paper, "The contagiousness of puerperal fever," in which he argued that *"the disease known as Puerperal Fever is so far contagious as to be frequently carried from patient to patient by physicians and nurses"* (author's italics) ([17], p. 131). He saw that the spread of the disease occurred "through the agency of the examining fingers." He suggested a variety of methods to prevent the spread of this disease including urging physicians and nurses to wash their hands in chlorinated water when treating obstetric patients. Although some physicians listened to Holmes' ideas, most challenged Holmes' conclusions about personal contagion and did not improve their hygiene as they treated patients [17].

Unaware of Holmes' research, Hungarian obstetrician Ignaz Semmelweis observed in 1847 that attending physicians and medical students at a teaching hospital in Vienna performed gynecological exams without washing their hands. Based on observation, Semmelweis mandated that physicians and surgeons scrub their hands with a brush and chlorinated lime solution before touching patients. The rate of death fell "from 20% to 1%" and was slightly lower than that of the midwife ward for the brief time that physicians followed the hand-washing regimen ([18], p. 1284). Historians have argued that he "sabotaged" his discovery by arrogantly ordering colleagues to change their habits rather than more effectively advocating for hand cleansing. His important assertion that the main cause for the deaths among the young women in the obstetrics ward was contaminated hands was not accepted [17,19,20].

Rather than an outright rejection of hand washing, many physicians who doubted the theories of Gordon, Holmes, and Semmelweis were unwilling to accept the idea that *physicians* spread disease by personal contact. Generally, physicians embraced the miasmic or "zymotic" theory. They believed that infection and disease in the hospital came from vapors or smells emanating from stagnant water, waste products, filth, garbage, or "specific organic poisons (zymes) coming from outside the body, or generated from within" ([21], p. 11). According to this logic, disease spread in a way similar to fermentation or putrification processes.

Concurrently, the influential English nurse Florence Nightingale described zymotic theories of disease in a variety of ways. She believed that "filth, disorder, and contaminated atmosphere were responsible for hospital fevers and infections" ([22], p. 92). Hospitals were places where diseases from many places converged. She explained, "the smallest transference of putrescing miasm from a locality where such miasm exists to the bedside of a lying-in patient is most dangerous" ([23], p. 29). She also believed that physicians had little help to offer hospital patients; instead, it was *nature* that cured. In hospitals, orderly conditions needed to be provided while nature took its course. She argued for competent nursing care, bandage changes, better sanitation and scrupulous cleanliness, improved design and organization of patient wards, ventilation, and better nutrition during patient hospitalization. As nursing scholar Elaine Larson has noted, Nightingale did not focus attention on hand washing, but rather supported hand washing within the "context of general hygiene" ([20], p. 97). Some hospitals and physicians implemented Nightingale's hygienic measures while others resisted them for some time.

While Louis Pasteur and Robert Koch gave pioneering ideas about disease coming from microbes in the late nineteenth century, Scottish physician Joseph Lister was the first to approach hospital sepsis and hygiene in relation to microbial origins. Lister used these new, unfamiliar ideas to understand infections in surgery, connecting the formation of wound pus to bacterial growth. Arguing that the contamination's source was the air, he researched the application of chemicals to infected wounds. He published his findings about antiseptic procedures in surgery in *The Lancet* in 1867 and initially urged spraying carbolic acid in the surgical arena. Later, because of toxic reactions to this practice, he recommended the application of such measures as the direct application of carbolic acid (phenol) on surgical incisions. His idea that bacterial growth needed to be combated in order to prevent infection coming from surgery was significant, even though his own understanding of the specifics was not complete. Lister himself did not especially emphasize hand washing immediately before surgery, for instance [24,25].

Lister's general idea that infection came from bacteria that could be prevented using antiseptic methods began to spread among physicians in Europe and the United States. Lister provided "the simple lesson that microorganisms existed, they were dangerous, and it was the surgeon's duty to keep them at bay" ([26], p. 105). Again, even though some physicians continued to dismiss claims that *they* could be responsible for passing infection from one patient to another, by 1876 Lister's ideas had gained enough traction for him to be a highly acclaimed speaker at the International Medical Congress that was held in Philadelphia during the centennial of the U.S. Declaration of Independence in 1876. Seated next to President Ulysses S. Grant at the Congress, Lister delivered a speech on antisepsis that lasted for two and a half hours and then continued for an hour of questions because of the high level of interest in the topic [27,28].

In the mid-1890s, one student of Lister, Malcolm Black, an obstetrician at the Glasgow Maternity hospital, implemented an "antiseptic ritual" for doctors and nurses: "washing hands with soap and water; then immersing them briefly in turpentine and methylated spirit, then in corrosive sublimate solution for one minute; finally, rinsing them in creolin solution to get rid of the corrosive solution, and lathering in Lysol solution for lubrication. The hands were dried in the air, not with a towel, and nail brushes were boiled and immersed in carbolic solution." ([26], p. 237). However, some physicians, including internationally acclaimed gynecological surgeon Lawson Tait, discounted Listerism especially in regard to gynecology, since he saw that "antiseptics seemed actually to harm the patients rather than relieve them" ([29], p. 130). Many other physicians had similar doubts and continued to believe that improvements in surgery were as much a consequence of better sanitation in general, improved nutrition, and better surgical skill [30].

Even so, antisepsis had gained a place at the table and became protocol in hospitals. In 1895, Albert Abrams, a widely read author and medical quack, satirized germ theory and antisepsis in medicine in his satirical pamphlet *Transactions of the*

Antiseptic Club. The pamphlet included a list of antiseptic protocols to be practiced by this fictional organization including daily baths "in antiseptic solutions," "to ensure absolute destruction of the germs" ([31], pp. 22–23). He claimed that "by the time [the physician] was sterilized the patient had recovered" because the antiseptic ritual was so elaborate ([31], p. 23). Such satire ridiculed these new rituals but also showed that Lister's ideas had come to be widely used in hospitals ([28], p. 121). As historian Roy Porter argued, Lister's antisepsis achievement was "in making routine an effective form of it, and thus making surgery safe" ([24], p. 370).

1.2.2   Early Hand Hygiene Products in the Hospital

As the acceptance of the value of cleanliness and antisepsis developed during the 1870s and 1880s, so too did the products. In Europe and the United States, surgeons, nurses, and hospital administrators implemented a variety of methods to ensure infection control. Medical and related journals published articles describing approaches and products. In some cases, these products assured cleanliness through *asepsis*—a thorough removal of dirt and germs. Some focused on *antisepsis*—using ingredients that killed germs. The comparative value of each of these methods was a part of the discussion of these products.

Green soap, a soft soap high in alkali and often sold in jelly-like form, was a popular product used in most hospitals. As the soap and hospital supply industries expanded, various entrepreneurial researchers used phenol derivatives from organic compounds to develop new soaps with antiseptic properties. These researchers used tars derived from coal and wood, cresol compounds and carbolic acid, which had microbe-killing properties, finding ways to combine these substances with various oils and other components to make effective, healthy, safe, and marketable soaps [32]. As they did so, they had to confront many difficulties in making such a product. Obtaining cleanliness without skin irritation was a difficult challenge. As a 1907 pharmacology textbook summarized, "most toilet soaps . . . are too strongly alkaline and often contain irritating essential oils; while many cheap kinds are made with animal fat which has not been properly purified" ([33], 417).

Soaps and solutions were developed including Synol, Listerine, and the Carrel–Dakin solution (later redeveloped as Zonite for use in homes). Robert Wood Johnson, a pharmacist from New York, focused his entrepreneurial attention on making antiseptic products for use during surgery and in hospitals with the help of his two brothers. Incorporated as Johnson & Johnson in 1887, this company's first products were antiseptic bandages and plasters that were soaked in phenol. By the early 1900s, the company also developed a liquid soap named "Synol soap" for the washing of surgeon's hands, and it became one of the standard-bearers for surgeons and physicians, the liquid property minimizing the dryness and corresponding skin cracking that occurred with the older "green soap" that many had used. Synol soap's main antiseptic ingredient was derived from wood tar [34,35].

The development of Synol soap actually occurred because of a felt need expressed to those at the Johnson & Johnson Company by physicians. As hospitals worked to become clean and sterile, especially during surgery, they found that the soap available was not up to the task. As one Virginia surgeon explained in 1900:

In my personal observation in several leading hospitals, where surgical cleanliness was often carried to the point of sterilizing iodoform and protecting the hands with rubber gloves, I have failed to note a single instance in which an effort was made to eliminate the possibility of infection from the soap-dish; on the contrary, the universal practice was to have an open jar or bowl of green soap on the washstand, into which the operator, assistants and nurses freely inserted hands soiled from routine work or septic from an operation just completed. (*Source*: Ref. 36.)

The liquid quality of Synol soap was touted as a great improvement on the soap sitting in a soap dish that many hands touched.

Synol soap was recommended and used by hospital and community physicians to cleanse hands and instruments. The cover of a 1915 issue of *Red Cross Notes*, a publication sent to physicians by the Johnson & Johnson Company, featured a bottle of Synol soap and a physician holding his hand above a basin. Indicating the public value placed on cleanliness at this time, the text in an insert asserted: "The modern surgeon is, or should be, the cleanest man that walks the earth," a claim that illustrated the value placed on cleanliness in the early twentieth century [37]. Articles throughout the publication continued to tout the lifesaving importance of cleanliness, especially that the doctors' hands should be "clean" as well as "soft and smooth" [38].

While a variety of antiseptic soaps were introduced into hospitals, many also found problems with them, questioning their effectiveness and noting their irritating qualities. In 1894, a West Virginia physician wrote an essay in the *Journal of the American Medical Association* (*JAMA*) where he acknowledged that "[d]isease is propagated by germs," but he insisted that "[a]ntiseptics have by no means the powers that have been attributed to them." The "so-called antiseptics" he insisted were unproven, and efforts to prevent exposure to germs in the sickroom would be a superior approach [39]. A 1919 study appearing in *JAMA* compared the various germicides used by physicians in hospitals and found that not all were reliable; the authors concluded that there needed to be standardized testing of these products to counteract the "wide usage of so-called germicides based on advertising literature and other unreliable data" ([40], p. 1635). Other physicians brought up the possibility of toxicity to both patients and physicians if antiseptics were used at high levels. One mentioned that carbolic acid could be a "dangerous poison" especially if "applied sufficiently to destroy microbes" [41,42]. These physicians were encountering problems that have recurred in many different times and places concerning antiseptic products: skin irritation, safety, and effectiveness.

Alongside such antiseptic products in the hospital stood Ivory soap, introduced by Procter & Gamble in 1879. This toilet soap was primarily introduced for the consumer market but was also used in hospitals. An 1894 ad for Ivory claimed that it was "the best for the [hospital] ward and the operating room as well as for the hospital kitchen and laundry" [43]. Procter & Gamble made a point of packaging small cakes of soap in order to prevent physicians, patients, and health care workers from having to use a bar someone else might have contaminated. By 1920, a typical Ivory ad in the trade magazine *Modern Hospital* boasted that "the majority of hospitals" in the United States used Ivory. Emphasis in Procter & Gamble's literature was on "aseptic" cleanliness, with advertisements highlighting the importance of the removal of infectious agents—which did not require antiseptic ingredients [44,45].

1.2.3 Early Consumer Hygiene Products

Germ-free cleanliness was a concept that generated interest much more broadly than in hospitals and health care settings; it also resonated strongly with the general public. As historian Nancy Tomes has shown, by the late nineteenth century, even before germ theory was understood, the sanitary movement for improved health was very much a domestic one as well as a medical one [46]. Ideas of cleanliness were centered on fresh air and clean water. A good mother should—and usually did—try to do all she could to protect her home and family from sickness. By the early twentieth century, voluntary public health campaigns to clean up the city and prevent the scourges of tuberculosis and other infectious diseases were everywhere [47–50]. This public concern for cleanliness and health was one on which soap companies capitalized.

As hygiene products emerged in the late nineteenth century, the public was also clearly engaged in considering "germs" and "microbes," thanks to attention given to the topic in popular media [51]. Nancy Tomes cites an 1874 editorial in the sanitarian that warned: "From the cellar, store-room, pantry, bedroom, sitting room and parlor . . . everywhere, a microscopic germ is propagating." ([48], p. 64). Such messages of dread fit in well with the omnipresent call for housewives to keep their houses clean and families safe. Americans were able to more easily clean themselves and their houses with the introduction and successful marketing of reasonably priced "antisepticonscious" and attractive white porcelain fixtures—the toilet, sink, bathtub—in the bathroom and later "sanitary" sinks in the kitchen and laundry room ([46], p. 64).

Antimicrobial products originally developed for physicians and patients made the leap from hospitals to the consumer market during this time period ([27], p. 13, [30]). Synol soap, the liquid antiseptic soap introduced in 1900 for physicians, was quite quickly marketed toward the general public as well. By the early twentieth century, New Jersey pharmacist Frederick Kilmer had become Johnson & Johnson's Scientific Director and was a tireless and dynamic promoter of the company's products. As Kilmer claimed in the *First Aid Manual*, a very popular early twentieth-century reference guide that Johnson & Johnson published for use in the home: "Medicated or antiseptic soaps are now being adopted by surgeons, dermatologists and others, to the exclusion of ordinary toilet soaps. This example is one which may be followed by the laity with good results." ([35], [52], pp. 19–20, 55–57). Such claims that what was good for the physicians would also be good for the public resonated throughout soap advertisements. Materials used in Synol soap would, Kilmer claimed, "exert double effect" of both cleaning and medicating against disease. In contrast, Kilmer decried the "cheap and unwholesome material" used in ordinary soaps. Kilmer's claim that antimicrobial soap was superior to ordinary soap for everyone has resonated in many instances throughout the twentieth century and into the twenty-first century [53].

Johnson & Johnson ran a concerted campaign to popularize this product alongside other antiseptic products for the home, using their much-touted effectiveness in the hospitals to illustrate how their product was superior to the merely sweet smelling toilet soaps bought by most consumers. Some ads dramatically focused on illnesses among children, reminding readers that "one-half of the entire population die before reaching the age of sixteen." Emphasizing that "Any physician will tell you that antiseptic cleanliness is the first and last operation performed, under any circumstances or conditions, as a means of prolonging life and warding off diseases of any nature," these Synol soap advertisements connected respect for the physician and fear of infant death with the appeal of their product [54,55]. In their trade magazine directed at druggists, *Red Cross Messenger*, the Johnson & Johnson Company referred to their widespread ad campaigns for Synol soap in popular magazines such as *Good Housekeeping*, pointing out to pharmacists that these ads included pictures of the trusted druggist's hands, filled up with Johnson & Johnson medicated hygiene products: "The housewives who come into your store, who pass your store, have seen these hands. They are ready to accept the proffered articles." Articles also mentioned the public consciousness of the importance of cleanliness for maintaining health. As *Red Cross Messenger* editor and Johnson & Johnson Scientific Director Frederick Kilmer went on to explain:

> Clean up time means much more than it did a few years ago to most people. Now they do not simply plan to clean-up for the sake of tidiness. They aim to protect their homes, to make them safe for their children. They know that dirt, darkness and disease are partners, and that they are striking a blow at disease when they attack dirt and darkness.

He concluded by reinforcing the druggists' role as "leader" to housewives in the cleanup movement [56].

Another antiseptic product was also marketed first for hospitals, and then the home. With previous antiseptics deemed either too mild or too toxic, the Carrel–Dakin solution was developed by a surgeon and a chemist in France during World War I when the number of wounded with fast-spreading infections overwhelmed field and recovery hospitals. The Carrel–Dakin solution, while unstable, was heralded by its makers as the "ideal antiseptic." The solution was "non-poisonous and non-irritating. It could be used constantly in the deepest wounds without harm, yet it would destroy bacteria with an effectiveness undreamed of heretofore. Man had beaten the germ at last." The Zonite Products Company began selling the "improved Carrel–Dakin solution" (made from "hypochloride of soda") as Zonite, distributing it to drugstores in the United States and marketing it as having "far greater germ-killing power than pure carbolic acid." The solution was "cheap," "easy to prepare," and "practical." Such advertisements indicated not only recognition of the possible problems with antiseptics, but also the felt value in using them to destroy dangerous microbes and to prevent life-threatening infection by eradicating the germs ([57], p. 11). In the 1924 advertisement, "Is there a greater war story than this?" Zonite Products offered the

"Zonite Handbook on the Use of Antiseptics in the Home" and urged the American consumer to use Zonite on scratches or cuts, as a mouthwash, or as a throat or nasal spray, to "prevent colds and more serious contagious diseases" and "pyorrhea, trench mouth, and infected gums" ([58], p. 355). Zonite was later widely marketed to women as a douche solution.

Although Synol soap and Zonite solution promoters worked hard to cross over from hospital to home with their products, another company was far more successful with its own antiseptic soap product. Lever Brothers' Lifebuoy's distinctly red bar of soap had a unique ingredient familiar to all those who knew of Lister's recommendations—carbolic acid derived from coal tar. Created as a product for the general consumer rather than for physicians in the hospital, Lifebuoy's advertisements claimed that it was "*more* than soap, yet costs no more." First sold by Lever Brothers, Inc., in the United Kingdom in 1895, its market soon broadened to the United States. Although some complained that Lifebuoy had a "medicinal" smell, its appeal to health was effective. In fact, in some cases, the company even emphasized the odor as a sign that the soap was actively combating infection and disease. Lifebuoy, ads claimed, "disinfects while cleansing" providing a "safeguard [to] your health" (Figure 1.1) [59]. Lever Brothers also issued an advertisement in 1919 featuring Lifebuoy as a "health soap" and the fact that the army required soldiers to carry soap as part of their equipment with "every man in the United States Army . . . compelled to use it" [60].

Lifebuoy's claims of health protection were not necessarily proven, however. Public health leader Harvey Wiley, in his 1914 comprehensive review of "Food, Beverages, and Toilet Accessories," described Lifebuoy as "a good soap," but said that its claims to "prevent infection," "save life," and "preserve health" were "unwarranted." Although Lifebuoy certainly had carbolic acid among its ingredients, its effectiveness in preventing infection was not clearly shown. Such a problem would emerge again and again over the next century with reference to antimicrobial products for the home: just because an antimicrobial ingredient was *in* a product did not necessarily mean that the amount was enough to effectively kill dangerous microbes. The addition of an antiseptic ingredient did not directly translate into an effective (or safe) product. Although public health leaders such as Wiley worked to regulate the sale of these products—and to educate the public about the inaccuracies of many of the advertisement claims—sales and ads continued [61]. Created in 1906, the Food and Drug Administration was the executive agency of the federal government that began to address regulation of products to ensure safety and efficacy in what had been a freewheeling marketplace [62].

While antiseptic soap makers continued to market their products with claims that their products fought infectious germs, the longtime soap and candle company Procter & Gamble committed to an especially strong national and successful advertising campaign for Ivory soap, which was not an antiseptic product. Turning to the many newly expanding popular magazines to market their product at a time when national brands were just coming into existence, this soap manufacturer was a leader. As the economy expanded and the country urbanized, national products and

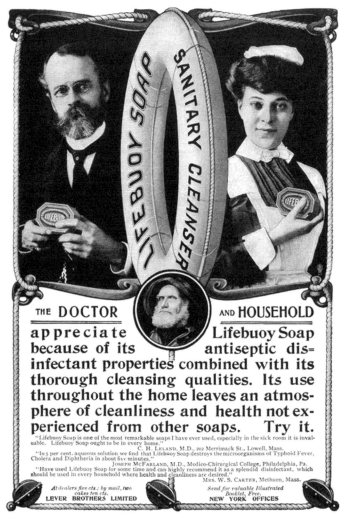

THE DOCTOR

AND HOUSEHOLD

appreciate Lifebuoy Soap because of its antiseptic dis=infectant properties combined with its thorough cleansing qualities. Its use throughout the home leaves an atmos-phere of cleanliness and health not ex-perienced from other soaps. Try it.

"Lifebuoy Soap is one of the most remarkable soaps I have ever used, especially in the sick room it is inval-uable. Lifebuoy Soap ought to be in every home."
C. H. LELAND, M.D., 202 Merrimack St., Lowell, Mass.
"In 5 per cent. aqueous solution we find that Lifebuoy Soap destroys the microorganisms of Typhoid Fever, Cholera and Diphtheria in about five minutes."
JOSEPH MCFARLAND, M.D., Medico-Chirurgical College, Philadelphia, Pa.
"Have used Lifebuoy Soap for some time and can highly recommend it as a splendid disinfectant, which should be used in every household where health and cleanliness are desired."
MRS. W. S. CARTER, Methuen, Mass.

At dealers five cts.; by mail, two cakes ten cts.
LEVER BROTHERS LIMITED

Send for valuable Illustrated Booklet, Free.
NEW YORK OFFICES

Figure 1.1 Introduced in the late nineteenth century, Lifebuoy soap was an early antimicrobial soap, containing carbolic acid, for use both by doctors and by housewives. Harper's monthly circa 1903.

modern life developed, and Victorian ways of the nineteenth century came to seem quaint. Ivory soap held a position similar to Camel cigarettes, Coca Cola, and numerous other brands that emerged in place of more localized products of the nineteenth century [63–65].

Concerns about infection prevailed even in the marketing of the non-antiseptic toilet soaps that dominated the market. For instance, one Ivory soap ad from 1890 explained, "Infection lurks in many cheap soaps. They are often made from the fat of diseased cattle." [66]. A "pure" soap—the word that would be the central focus for Ivory—was important to use in order to preserve health, according to this and many other ads. As this ad went on to recommend, consumers should "read the Scientific Reports of microscopical [sic] examinations of various soaps." As calls for hygiene took on scientific language and techniques at the turn of the century, the company hired a full-time chemist, carefully maintained the quality of their product, and advertised heavily on its 99.44% purity, as proven in laboratory tests. As a 1913 ad proclaimed, "an Ivory soap bath feels as good as it looks ... it is glowing, refreshing, healthy, in contrast to that cleanliness which is mere absence of dust and soil" [67,68]. Procter & Gamble's strategy proved effective [69,70].

Ivory soap also used the "purity" ideal to criticize the antiseptic soaps on the market. As one typical ad from 1893 claimed "the simpler the soap, the better." "[C] arbolic soap" and "tar soap" held no "positive virtue ... as is so generally supposed." Such additives, the ad implied, might in fact mask impurities [71]. At a time before these products were comprehensively regulated, Ivory makers tried to group the medicated soaps with the plethora of toiletry products whose advertisements included many outlandish claims. Another Ivory ad, this one praising its use in barbershops, warned that "[m]uch of the soap used by barbers is made of vile materials and strongly chemicalled." According to this rationale, contaminated and medicated soaps were similar—and both clearly inferior to "pure" Ivory [72].

But the makers of Ivory were not the only ones to question the health claims made by antiseptic soap makers; scientists of the time also did. One 1920 study that compared the effectiveness of 12 soaps chosen randomly from drugstore shelves concluded, "the cleansing properties of a soap are more important than its 'germicidal' or 'antiseptic' qualities." Bacteriologist John F. Norton explained that "more bacteria were found to be removed by the ordinary toilet soaps than by the special [germicidal] soaps" when he conducted a comparison of the amount of bacteria left on hands after hand washing in his University of Chicago laboratories. He also found that antiseptic soap remaining on the hands did not succeed in preventing bacteria from forming on the hands [73]. Even so, scientific claims by soap makers such as Lever Brothers continued in advertisements, with the medical value of their product's antiseptic ingredients being one main focus.

Soap advertisements also had a strong value-laden component, with "purity" indicating not only cleanliness, but also the superiority of those who used the right kind. Mothers of properly dressed, obedient—and almost universally white—children were "health doctors" in Lifebuoy advertisements, using Lifebuoy soap to preserve and protect their families [74]. Claiming "millions of mothers rely on Lifebuoy," these ads claimed that the soap "remove[d] germs and impurities from the skin, guarding against infection to which we are all constantly exposed—children especially." Ivory soap continued to make similar claims, and healthy, attractive (white) babies were a familiar part of Ivory ads as well.

Textbooks, public health leaders, and advertisements also emphasized cleanliness as a part of the prevailing social philosophy of the time, with racial superiority, upward social mobility, and public health morality all intertwined among the newly dominant white collar class. Children learned that they needed to practice personal hygiene from a variety of sources. President Theodore Roosevelt had written in 1907 that "our national health is physically our greatest asset. To prevent any possible deterioration of the American stock should be a national ambition" ([75], p. 11). This statement inspired a new emphasis on health education at all levels in U.S. schools. Students took required health courses with books that taught them about cleanliness and personal hygiene. One example of these is the New-World Health Series. The first book in the series, *Primer of Hygiene: Being A Simple Textbook on Personal Health and How to Keep It*, placed Roosevelt's statement about the "American stock" on its copyright page [75]. Other series also issued texts that emphasized personal cleanliness: "Health, Happiness, Success" (*Health Habits, Physiology and Hygiene*) or the "Malden Health Series" (*In Training for Health*). Students were warned that "clean skin gives the best protection" against "dirt and disease germs" and that "frequent use of soap and warm water is the best means of providing this protection" ([76], p. 11). The Cleanliness Institute, actually the publicity arm of the American Soap and Glycerine Producers, the trade organization of the soap industry, initiated many programs and advertising campaigns emphasizing the moral and social value of cleaning with soap [77–79].

But morality and proper upbringing were not enough by the 1920s; personal care product marketing also began to emphasize appearance and social propriety. Listerine was a leader in this new emphasis. Missouri physician Joseph Lawrence originally made the product in 1879 to be an antiseptic for use as a surgical wash, much like the Carrel–Dakin solution. But its unique ability to kill bacteria in the mouth led to its 1895 introduction as a mouthwash. The product's name made a direct connection to Joseph Lister and included four essential oils: menthol, thymol, methyl salicylate, and eucalyptol. First sold to the public over the counter in 1912, by 1920, ad text recommended that consumers wash their hands in Listerine in order to prevent the spread of colds (Figure 1.2) ([27], [80], p. 497). But the focus in advertisements was on killing mouth bacteria that created "halitosis" (a scientific sounding word the makers of Listerine coined to sell their product). These "halitosis" claims were the most memorable and enduring with numerous ads showing women who remained spinsters because of their bad breath and businessmen who failed for the same reason ([79], [81], pp. 28–34). Similarly, Lever Brothers introduced the abbreviation "BO" to refer to "body odor" in their Lifebuoy soap ads in the 1930s, emphasizing that their product was unique because of its "exclusive deodorizing ingredient" (carbolic acid) and claiming that "the crisp Lifebuoy scent" that bothered so many "rinses away," but "you're protected hours longer from 'BO'" [82]. At this time when white collar office jobs had become the new norm among the urban middle class, concerns about personal appearance and acceptability reached anxious heights and were a powerful seller. The socializing power of Lifebuoy soap could also be seen when the soap was introduced in Africa during the 1940s, first among whites and later among blacks as well. As historian Timothy Burke explained, Lifebuoy was sold "as a 'strong' soap for washing particularly dirty bodies" ([83], p. 151). Campaigns focused on the "Successful Man" associating "professional success within the colonial system and rigorous hygienic purification" and later in the postcolonial 1960s and 1970s on the theme "Keep Healthy ... Keep Clean ... Use Lifebuoy, the Health Soap," associating "the ability of men to work by securing continuous good health" ([83], p. 153).

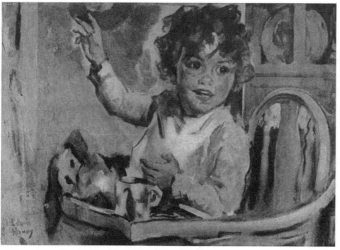

O careful mother ‚ ‚ *before baby's meals*
rid your hands *of germs*

If you could look at your hands under a micro-
scope you would hesitate to prepare or serve
baby's food, or give him a bath, without first
rinsing the hands with undiluted Listerine.

Because, breeding on them by millions, you
would see dangerous disease germs which are
easily transmitted to children by contact.

Certainly the use of Listerine on the hands
is a wise precaution.

Listerine, though delightful and safe to use
full strength, destroys such germs—all germs
—in a few seconds. Even the virulent Staphylococcus Aureus (pus) and Bacillus Typhosus
(typhoid), resistant as they are to antiseptic
action, yield to Listerine in 15 seconds in

Prevent a cold
*Rinsing the hands with
Listerine before every
meal, destroys the germs
ever-present on them.*

*Gargle full strength Lis-
terine every day. It inhibits development of sore
throat, and checks it
should it develop.*

counts ranging to 200,000,000.

We could not make this statement unless
prepared to prove it to the entire satisfaction

of the U. S. Government and the medical
profession.

Recognizing Listerine's germicidal power,
you can understand its marked success against
infections. You can realize now why it has
warded off millions of cases of cold and sore
throat why also it has checked millions of
other cases before they became serious. You
can appreciate why doctors have prescribed it
for half a century.

See that your family makes a habit of
gargling with undiluted Listerine at least twice
a day. It is a pleasant, safe, and effective aid
in maintaining health. Lambert Pharmacal
Company, St. Louis, Mo.

L I S T E R I N E enemy of sore throat
K*ills* 200,000,000 *germs in* 15 *seconds*

Figure 1.2 Listerine was not originally a mouthwash, instead it was used to wash hands in both the hospital and home. This 1930 advertisement for Listerine advocates mothers washing their hands in "undiluted" Listerine before bathing or feeding the baby in order to kill harmful germs [80]. Courtesy of Johnson and Johnson. (*See the color version of this figure in Color Plates section.*)

1.3 HYGIENE BELIEFS AND PRODUCTS IN THE AGE OF "MIRACLE DRUGS" (1940S–1960S): HEXACHLOROPHENE IN THE HOSPITAL FOR CONSUMERS

1.3.1 Beliefs

Before the 1940s, then, germicidal soap not only found a measure of popular appeal, but also endured challenges and competition. During the 1940s, biomedicine had gained a distinctive position of respect with public optimism at an unprecedented high about the ability of scientists to conquer disease. With rates of infant mortality and infectious disease at all-time lows, advances in medicine received a great deal of the credit for the nation's improved health, and physicians and their discoveries had come to be popular public phenomena. Scientist "microbe hunters" were gaining success in the fight to find "magic bullets" that could kill microbes. Most notably, penicillin emerged as a "wonder drug," to much fanfare, with articles illustrating its ability to cure disease appearing in *Life Magazine* and other popular periodicals [84,85]. Riding the wave of confidence and prestige that was the golden age in medicine, scientists and marketers found a public grateful for the curative powers of antibiotics and eager to use antimicrobials in other settings as well, including hygiene.

Clearly, until well into the first half of the twentieth century, hygiene, both personal and public, was the first and major defense in fighting infections. Despite breakthroughs in the discovery of the "germ theory of disease," there were no drugs or "magic bullets" existing that were safe and effective in fighting infection. With the discoveries of sulfonamides and antibiotics, physicians, scientists, and the general public were ready to believe that germs could finally be conquered. By 1984, Gwyn McFarlane, the author of a biography of Alexander Fleming, the scientist credited with the penicillin's discovery, argued that "penicillin therapy is probably the greatest single medical advance of all time" ([86], p. 102). Antibiotics were quickly incorporated into regular use in hospitals, especially by surgeons "who were now confident they could manage infection and were routinely carrying out more ambitious operations" ([86], p. 99). Many government and health experts believed that it was possible to soon eradicate all infectious diseases with these new drug weapons. In 1948, the U.S. Secretary of State, George C. Marshall, proposed at the Washington, DC meeting of the Fourth International Congress on Tropical Medicine and Malaria that a combination of higher crop yields and microbe control would allow for "all the earth's microscopic scourges to be eliminated" ([87], p. 30). In 1967, U.S. Surgeon General William H. Stewart argued that fear of infectious disease could be set aside and the national focus placed on addressing the complexities of chronic illnesses [87].

Unfortunately, as confidence grew that new drugs could conquer disease, the beginning of drug resistance emerged in hospital settings. Because of the belief in the curative powers of the new drugs, "good aseptic techniques were considered unnecessary and often ignored, but after a few years' use of penicillin in hospitals, outbreaks of penicillin-resistant *Staphylococcus aureus* were reported" ([88], p. 223). Early in the 1950s, hospital workers and the popular press reported about rising infection rates, especially from staphylococcal disease. Calls for more attention to hygiene and to the proper application of antiseptic and aseptic methods were made. Hospitals began to utilize bacteriologists as infection control experts. Concerns about the misuse, overuse, and general abuse of antibiotics rapidly grew at the same time as new antibiotic products were widely introduced ([86], [89]).

1.3.2 Hospital Products in the Age of Miracle Drugs

Scientist William S. Gump of the Givaudan-Delawanna, Inc. chemical company synthesized the chemical compound "hexachlorophene" in 1939, the most popular and effective germicide to be used in both hospital and consumer products until the early 1970s. The product soon gained great popularity as an effective ingredient in surgical scrubs. As one 1952 medical journal article account explained, hexachlorophene (also called G-11 and AT-7.) had become widely used in the surgical scrub because of its "greater germicidal action" compared to previous antiseptic soaps as well as a "lasting effect on the skin" and a "great reduction of the time" necessary for surgeons to scrub [90,91]. With its ability to kill infectious microbes, to decrease the amount of time necessary to clean hands, and to continue to effectively kill germs even after the initial hand wash, hexachlorophene quickly became a hospital staple.

But while the benefits of hexachlorophene seemed clear to some physicians, they did not go undisputed. Resonating with early twentieth-century concerns about the toxicity and effectiveness of antiseptic products, some voiced caution about hexachlorophene as well. For example, surgeon and researcher Philip B. Price from the University of Utah College of Medicine presented a paper to the American Surgical Association in 1951 about the introduction of "a quick washing with G-11 soap." Price first noted how the "popularity of G-11 soap has risen phenomenally." Within 4 years going from "scarcely . . . heard of" to "only the exceptional hospital [being] without it," the use of the product was quite astounding ([92], p. 476). In his laboratory research, he compared washing with G-11 to washing with a "conventional soap" (with Ivory as the sample) for 7 min using a brush and soap and water, using a towel to dry hands, and then rubbing hands with 70% ethanol for 3 min. Price concluded that G-11 was "overrated." He explained: "Used properly, they may have something to contribute to the perfection of surgical technic, but there is danger that their use may create a false sense of security." ([92], p. 481). He feared that the antibacterial quality might make physicians abandon or minimize the important scrubbing ritual.

When Price's article was published in the *Annals of Surgery*, the journal also published comments in response, mostly from physicians arguing in favor of using G-11. For instance, Dr. Russell Best, from Omaha, NE, wrote that his hospital had conducted studies with a hexachlorophene bar soap (Dial) and found that a "three-minute scrub without a brush and without the alcohol rinse was more efficient than a ten-minute scrub with plain soap using the brush and an alcohol rinse" ([92], p. 482). In his and other comments, physicians introduced the complexities involved both in the practice of hand washing in hospitals and in the variety of products that were used. Nurses, surgeons, and other surgeons all developed hand-washing techniques, attempting to find the most efficacious methods, with dispute over what methods and products were best ([92], p. 485).

Marketers of G-11's competitors certainly did not just stand by as the new germicidal soap gained a prominent place in the hospital market. Procter & Gamble was especially active in reaching out to physicians and hospitals, using messages of reliability and popularity to market their Ivory soap. Already in a 1926 ad in the magazine *Modern Hospital*, Procter & Gamble boasted that Ivory was used in "the majority of hospitals in this country" [93]. As hexachlorophene emerged as an alternative, touted as providing more effective infection control, Ivory peppered publications for the hospital with advertisements emphasizing the affordability and purity of Ivory. These ads also offered busy physicians free "Ivory Handy Pads," with preprinted instructions to give patients on acne care and bathing your baby among other things. Emphasis on physicians continued, with the slogan "more doctors advise Ivory soap than all other brands together" emerging in the 1940s [94].

Even so, the antimicrobial soaps were catching on and gaining dominance in the soap and washes used in hospitals [95]. By 1953, a summary on the use of products for surgeons appeared in the *American Journal of Public Health*, explaining

> Careful washing without a brush with these liquid antiseptic soaps has replaced the conventional 10-minute scrub with a brush in the surgical wash to prepare the surgeon's hands, as well as for use as a bacteriostatic wash in the preparation of the patient . . . . (*Source*: Ref. 96, p. 427.)

Beyond surgery, as staph infections became a problem in newborn nurseries, a hexachlorophene solution became the common protocol for the washing of babies as well [97,98].

1.3.3   Consumer Hygiene Products in the Age of Miracle Drugs

Among the general public, the dangers or infectious disease had faded in the 1940s, and so too had the need to be clean in order to maintain health. However, the desire for a clean appearance continued, and even came to be a greater focus for many Americans. Correspondingly, the elimination of germs and bacteria gained a certain cachet as an advertising tool. During this time period, germicidal chemicals derived synthetically—not just elements of natural products such as those used to develop the products of the early twentieth century—characterized the new soaps. Industry chemists researched and analyzed toilet soaps, working to develop effective germicides that would combine well with other soap ingredients. One central figure was Eric Jungermann of the Armour and Company. In an introduction to one article that appeared in the *Journal of the American Oil Chemists' Society*, Jungermann looked back at the flaws in pre-World War II antiseptic soaps. He commented that these products typically used "certain cresol derivatives" that "tended to impart a strong characteristic odor to soaps, which limited their use in the consumer toilet soap market" ([32], p. 345). These cosmetic flaws were coupled with the questionable effectiveness of the products, problems confronted by the scientists who worked to develop synthetic chemicals that would effectively be used in soap.

Soon after the initial invention and patenting of the compound, inventor William Gump called for its use beyond the hospital. Just like Listerine, Lifebuoy, and Synol soap before it, this product began as a surgical wash but Gump now touted the home market in 1945 in the trade journal *Soap and Sanitary Chemicals*. "Why should not every person be using this germ-killing soap every time he washes his hands, for bathing, for shaving, for laundering, and on other occasions? . . . There is every reason why, in the interests of general health, in the reduction of contagion and epidemics, a germicidal, non-toxic, and non-irritating chemical should become an ingredient of a large part of the soap made in this country." [99]. Dial soap was the first and most successful consumer product to use this ingredient. Armour and Company, a meatpacking company located in Chicago, first marketed Dial soap in 1948, including hexachlorophene in the soap. With a desire to use by-products from their meat processing, soap was a product they had been making since 1888, but Dial soap was a major innovation for them, and their first full foray into the soap market. Dial has had an enduring position in the hygiene market ever since, largely due to hexachlorophene.

Advertisements for Dial soap emphasized the effectiveness of the product in killing a particular kind of bacteria—the kind that made human perspiration stink (Figure 1.3). Germ killing in this important instance was primarily to deodorize. Already by 1953, Dial had gained the #1 position in the soap market. As an initial ad from 1949 explained, Dial was "the first active, really effective deodorant soap in all history" because it "removes skin bacteria that *cause* perspiration odor because Dial and only Dial contains AT-7" (another iteration of hexachlorophene). Advertisements in magazines, newspapers, and on television included visuals of germs, removed from the body surface and Petri dishes with microbes, both before and after the application of Dial soap. Ivory continued to emphasize beauty and babies, and they also used their "More Doctors Advise Ivory than any other soap" in ads in popular magazines, but they could not hold onto their top position in the market.

Hexachlorophene had no proven connection to actual disease protection and health as it was used in Dial soap [100]. Similar to Lifebuoy in the early twentieth century, its makers could accurately claim that their product had an antibacterial ingredient, but its effectiveness was not clearly proven in the real-world context. However, the visual and intuitive power of their ads succeeded admirably in selling the product. Not many consumers wanted to leave their children at risk, or to let perspiration bacteria freely grow on their skin. As industry analysts observed at the time, antibacterial products overtook the soap market, with a majority of soap bars becoming antibacterial during the 1960s. Jungermann characterized them as "the most rapidly growing segment of the toilet bar market," and other commentators observed that their success occurred even though this type of soap was typically more expensive than other toilet soaps [101,102]. Among scientists, the choice of antimicrobial soap was seen a good one, because it appeared that over time the use of the product would significantly reduce the number of germs resident on the skin. Gump and others emphasized that this type of soap could therefore move people toward the "germ-free" safety touted by physicians and public health experts at the time.

However, such germ killing came at a cost. Risks associated with hexachlorophene ultimately affected its use as well, leading to its removal from the consumer market and its restriction in the hospital setting. Presciently, an analyst from Procter & Gamble mentioned in a 1968 analysis of the "toilet bar [soap] market," by the 1940s, that the number of ingredients used in soaps had grown exponentially, and he warned that antibacterial substances in particular had the possibility of adversely "affecting health" because "by their very nature they must be biologically active" ([102], p. 508). As it became a commonplace ingredient in numerous products, hexachlorophene's dangers were not seen at first. One physician commented in a letter to the journal *Pediatrics* that appeared after a child died from hexachlorophene poisoning from accidental ingestion, "Perhaps we are all guilty of becoming too familiar with hexachlorophene in soaps, deodorants, and even in at least one brand of toothpaste so as to breed carelessness." [103]. Another physician expressed surprise that the chemical could be poisonous, commenting that "[i]n our hospital and presumably others, we use individual 150 cc. bottles of Phisohex to bathe each newborn and the unused portion is sent home with the mother" [104]. This physician

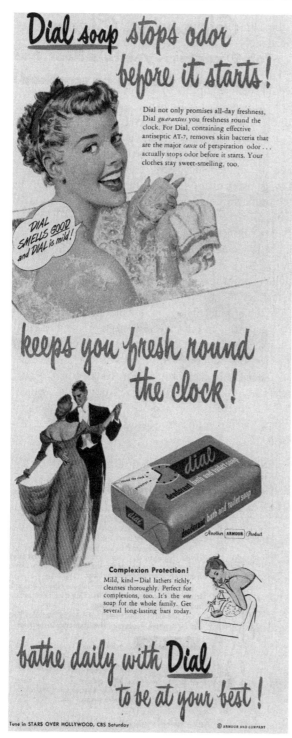

Figure 1.3   Dial soap was introduced in 1948. This 1955 magazine advertisement illustrates how its germ-killing ability was focused on the germs that caused body odor. Courtesy of Henkel of America, Inc. (*See the color version of this figure in Color Plates section.*)

was not alone; 2 years later, the Director of the Bureau of Drugs at the FDA reported to the American Academy of Pediatrics that these practices were "commonplace" and that there was "a 20-year history of widespread use" of the chemical ([105], p. 430).

Following a pattern that would become familiar to those studying antimicrobial products in soap, the use of hexachlorophene as a wash in hospitals had developed "in the absence of specific safety and efficacy protocols" ([105], p. 430). By the early 1970s, it had become clear that the chemical was creating neurological damage in infants, and the death of 39 infants in France. Although in the hospital setting the use of this antimicrobial agent had in fact proved successful in preventing infection, at least in higher concentrations it was also harmful—harmful enough for the FDA to step in and restrict its use. Hexachlorophene could only be used with a prescription by 1972, and even then at lower concentrations than had been standard [106]. As the *New York Times* explained, four million pounds of hexachlorophene were used each week in cosmetic and medical products; the FDA restrictions forced producers to alter their products significantly [107].

The makers of Dial doubted the proof that their product caused any harm, with producers of hexachlorophene calling the ban "hysterical" and a "tragedy" for consumers who could benefit from the product. They insisted that the concentration level used in their product was not harmful, and that overall, proper rinsing negated any damaging effects. Their protests did not stop the ban on consumer products, but it did indicate the appeal of antibacterial products, even in light of health concerns. Armour quickly found a replacement for hexachlorophene in triclocarban, a new antibacterial synthetic chemical [108]. With Dial still "outsell[ing] all the others combined," they did not abandon their marketing approach, but rather only changed the chemical used [109]. A germ killer protecting consumers from body odor had strong, resounding cultural appeal.

1.4 HYGIENE BELIEFS AND PRODUCTS IN THE AGE OF GERM PHOBIA AND ENVIRONMENTAL CONCERN

1.4.1 Beliefs, 1990s–Present

Even so, the optimism of the post-World War II era when hexachlorophene was synthesized now had become more complex. An innocence had been lost with the emergence of recalcitrant infections, with resistance to miracle products, and with the potential toxicity of the antibacterial products. As product designers, public health leaders, health care workers, and the public navigated these complicated waters, antimicrobial products took on contradictory meanings [110,111].

1.4.2 Antibacterial Beliefs and Products for the Hospital, 1990s–Present

In recent years, the general public has grown increasingly concerned about the rate of health care-associated infections (HCAIs). The 2009 *WHO Guidelines on Hand*

Hygiene in Health Care warned that "HCAI concerns 5–15% of hospitalized patients and can affect 9–37% of those admitted to intensive care units (ICUs)" ([112], p. 6). Also, in 2009, the U.S. Centers for Disease Control (CDC) reported approximately 1.7 million health care-associated infections and 99,000 associated deaths and cited HCAI as "one of the top 10 leading causes of death in the United States" [113–115]. The public has learned about the rise of infections in health care facilities and such new drug-resistant germs as methicillin-resistant *S. aureus* (MRSA) and *Clostridium difficile*, from such news articles as "Deadly bacteria found to be more common," "The lab coat is on the hook in the fight against germs," and "Nothing to sneeze at: doctors' neckties seen as flu risk" [116–118]. They have also found warnings from science writers who have authored books for a general public audience: Jessica Snyder Sachs, *Good Germs, Bad Germs: Health and Survival in a Bacterial World*, or Madeline Drexler, *Secret Agents: The Menace of Emerging Infections* [119,120]. In addition, the public can find on local bookstore shelves a number of "self-help" books marketed for patients and their families: *How to Survive Your Hospital Stay: The Complete Guide to Getting the Care You Need—and Avoiding Problems You Don't* (2002) or *Critical Conditions: The Essential Hospital Guide to Get Your Loved One Out Alive* (2008) [121,122]. The comedy, *Scrubs*, which some argue as actually the most accurate portrayal of the hospital on television, addressed hospital infection in a story arc that carried through two episodes. As a scene with patients and health care workers interacting unfolds, one of the comedy's surgeons explains to another doctor: "Do you know the number one cause of death in a hospital? Infection! And do you know how quickly infection can spread in a hospital . . . infection can start with a simple sneeze, and then a handshake, perhaps an accidental collision, and a simple touch on the shoulder . . . and just like that, you have a patient in trouble." Green-painted "germs" travel from person to person as the surgeon explains the process of infection [123].

One of the major culprits for health care infections has been identified as the hands of health providers and other health workers. In 2000, the CDC asserted that hygiene, especially hand washing, is "the most important tool in the health care worker's arsenal for preventing infection" ([124] [125], p. 15). Atul Gawande, a 2006 MacArthur fellow and Research Director of the Center for Surgery and Public Health at the Brigham and Women's Hospital in Boston, wrote about the "hand-washing" problem in *The New England Journal of Medicine* in 2004. On a tour of the Brigham and Women's Hospital with its infectious disease specialist, he learned that the biggest problem in infection control was "getting clinicians like me to do the one thing that consistently halts the spread of most infections: wash our hands" ([126], p. 1283). The news media has widely discussed this hygiene problem, especially during the last 20 years, assigning blame to surgeons, nurses, and all other health care workers [127]. While the television comedy *Scrubs* directly addressed the problem of hospital infections, in general the public found little evidence that health professionals take hand washing seriously when they watched hospital-based television entertainment programs. The popular dramatic series *ER*, for instance, was examined by researchers "to measure the frequency of mistakes in hand hygiene" ([128], p. 131). They found that "appropriate hand washing is never done, and this is also true for most other preventive recommendations" ([128], p. 131).

In the United States, national guidelines for hand washing were first published by the CDC in the 1980s. In the mid-1990s, the CDC/Healthcare Infection Control Practices Advisory Committee (HICPAC) discussed how hands should be washed and recommended that either an antimicrobial soap or a waterless antiseptic agent be used. In 2002, HICPAC defined alcohol-based hand rubbing, where available, as the standard of care for hand hygiene practices in health care settings with hand washing reserved for particular situations only. Some of these situations included medication handling or food preparation in which case the guidelines state that an alcohol-based hand rub or plain or antimicrobial soap and water could be chosen. Following extensive review of the literature reviewing evidence on hand hygiene, the 2009 *WHO Guidelines on Hand Hygiene in Health Care* based their consensus recommendations on the 2002 HICPAC findings ([112], p. 9). Significant evidence exists that health care workers with contaminated hands play an important role in transmitting health care-associated infections ([112], 12–24 [130]), ([114], pp. 12–24). Yet, halfway through the first decade of the twenty-first century, hand-washing adherence among health care workers, including doctors and nurses, was not high with "mean baseline rates ranging from 5% to 81% and an overall average of about 40% as determined by the CDC" ([129], p. 37 [130]).

Health care workers have reported a variety of reasons for low compliance in hand washing: workload and time constraints, access to sinks, skin irritations, ignorance about the problem, personal habits, insufficient staffing, and "patient acuity" ([131], [132, p. 69]). Numerous hand hygiene campaigns have been launched since the 1990s where governments and private institutions have joined forces in national and international contexts. In the two decades since, the campaigns goals have been to achieve significant progress in compliance especially among physicians. The "Clean Care is Safer Care" challenge of the Global Patient Safety Challenges element of the WHO Patient Safety Program was launched in 2005 with a major focus on reducing HCAIs. The challenge issued the "My 5 Moments for Hand Hygiene" approach ("before touching a patient, before clean/aseptic procedure, after body fluid exposure risk, after touching a patient, and after touching patient surroundings") to engage health care workers in proper hand washing [132]. In many health care institutions, patients and health care workers can find a poster illustrating the five moments. The CDC along with the Clean Hands Coalition participated in the "Clean Hands Save Lives" campaign in the mid-2000s, issuing various posters (Figure 1.4). Some showed such images as antibiotic-resistant pathogens on health care workers' hands or clinical care equipment, MRSA pathogens, or the moments during patient care when health care workers needed to be especially conscientious about hand hygiene [133].

Various incentive programs that have included gift cards, movie passes, and pizza parties have been instituted. Brigham and Women's Hospital in Boston reported reaching a compliance hand-washing rate of 80% when it offered movie passes for units "that kept their rates high." Unfortunately, the hospital found that there was a dramatic decrease in rates when the movie pass incentive was removed [134]. Nonetheless, the hospital continued its hand hygiene efforts with a partnership between the Infection Control Department and the Nursing Quality Safety and Care Improvement Committee in a "Be Patient Ready" campaign that

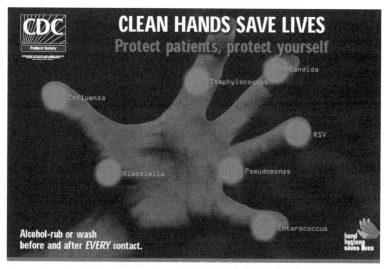

Figure 1.4   In 2005, the Centers for Disease Control first offered this poster on its web site to promote hand hygiene in health care facilities. The promotion stated that the poster "showed bugs that can lead to infection and may be found on unclean health care worker's hands [133]." In some ways, the poster can be compared to illustrations that appeared in the popular press in the early part of the twentieth century warning the public about how germs could be spread. Source: "Clean Hands Save Lives." 2005. Division of Healthcare Quality Promotion. Centers for Disease Control and Prevention. (*See the color version of this figure in Color Plates section.*)

included such strategies as the distribution of pins worn by health professionals that allowed patients "to ask their care providers a crucial question: "Did you wash your hands?" ([135], p. 2). In 2009, the hospital reported that their overall efforts had increased hand-washing compliance from 75% to 93% [136]. Massachusetts General Hospital developed an extensive hand hygiene strategy, organizing a multidisciplinary STOP ("Stop the Transmission of Pathogens") Task Force aimed at collaboratively involving hospital employees, patients, and visitors. The program "Clean Because We Care" included such strategies as the recruitment of volunteer "Champions" (including nurses, physicians, and housekeeping staff) trained as "peer leaders" across areas of the hospital. The "Champions" devised various positive motivational strategies from contests, poems, to "homemade" posters (Figure 1.5). The hospital introduced incentives that included coupons that could be used in hospital food outlets and the linking of an above 90% hospital-wide compliance hand hygiene compliance rate to the employees' annual bonus [137]. Staff in the same day surgery unit created a "Cal Stat Rap" (posted on YouTube) that depicted staff dancing and a nurse rapping while demonstrating proper hand hygiene with an alcohol-based hand sanitizer [138]. In early 2009, MGH reported compliance rates among its health care workers that "increased from 8% to 93% 'before contact' with the patient or patient's environment, and from 47% to 96% 'after contact'" [139].

Other hospitals have tried to test if health care workers are actually using hand sanitizer dispensers—Brigham and Women's Hospital used Purell and Massachusetts General Hospital used Cal Stat alcohol-based rub hand sanitizers in their compliance

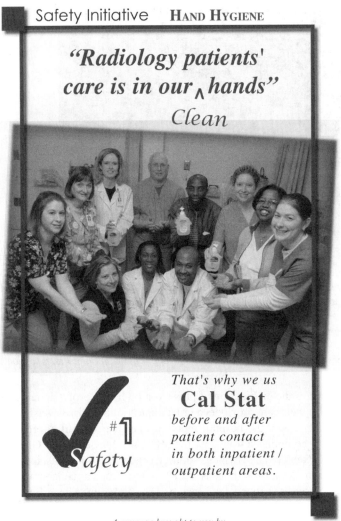

Safety Initiative   HAND HYGIENE

"Radiology patients'
care is in our ∧ hands"
Clean

That's why we us
Cal Stat
before and after
patient contact
in both inpatient /
outpatient areas.

#**1**
Safety

A message brought to you by
The **STOP** (**S**top **T**ransmission **O**f **P**athogens) **TASK FORCE**
The multidisciplinary group behind the MGH Hand Hygiene Program

Figure 1.5   "Radiology patients' care is in our [clean] hands." The Radiology Department's poster is an example of the multidisciplinary Hand Hygiene STOP Initiative begun in 2004 at the Massachusetts General Hospital to improve hand hygiene. Health care workers volunteered to develop and appear in posters that were made several times a year and posted in various inpatient health care units. Source: "Radiology patients' care is in our [clean] hands." 2006. Department of Radiology, Stop the Transmission of Pathogens Task Force (STOP), and Infection Control Unit, Massachusetts General Hospital.

campaigns. Believing that many "nontechnology" compliance strategies have been unsuccessful or have created an "adversarial relationship between the doctor and patient," the University of Miami–Jackson Health System Center for Patient Safety in 2009 piloted a "surveillance" system that tracks if health care workers are washing their hands when treating patients in hospital rooms and uses an audible warning system to remind them to do so [140]. Research continues to be conducted in efforts to assess the success rate of health professionals adopting the use of various alcohol-based hand rubs in health care settings [141].

Hospitals now provide foam soap or alcohol hand rubbing dispensers throughout their facilities, including corridors and outside the entrances to patient rooms. On May 5, 2009, in conjunction with the release of the new guidelines about hand hygiene in health care, the WHO launched a new global initiative "Save Lives: Clean Your Hands" reinforcing the 2005 initiative in its effort to "protect the patient, the health care worker and the health care environment against harmful germs and thus reduce HCAI. It aims to engage a wide range of health care facilities across the world to move countries from pledging to action at the point of care." [142]. The World Health Organization's multimodal hygiene improvement strategy was designed to provide a "suite of tools to support health care facilities to prepare effective Action Plans to improve hand hygiene, regardless of their starting point" [142].

The major change in encouraging hand hygiene in health care settings for American health care workers in the twenty-first century has been the introduction of alcohol-based hand rubbing. This practice has been widely used in Europe in health care settings in the twentieth century [144]. In the United States, in the 1930s, the surgeon Philip B. Price had recommended the use of 70% alcohol for contaminated hands even though soaps remained widely preferred by health care workers ([92], p. 482). Various studies have shown that alcohol solutions for hand washing work better than using plain soap and water and can be as effective or more effective than using an antimicrobial soap [145]. With alcohol-based hand rubbing recommended in most situations for health care workers in health care settings in the United States since the publication of WHO guidelines in 2002, many companies manufacturing alcohol-based hand sanitizers have increased promotion of their products. One of these companies was GOJO, which developed GOJO Hand Sanitizer to sell to rubber factory workers during Word War II. The company designed a portion-limiting soap dispenser in 1952 when they realized that many companies did not purchase their sanitizing product because of the expense of employees using too much of the sanitizer. They introduced Purell Instant Hand Sanitizer as a product that could kill germs on health care workers' hands in emergency situations in 1988. GOJO was the same company that initially introduced a consumer product line called Purell in 1997 [146].

GOJO stressed the fear of germs in their marketing and educational materials directed to health care facilities and health care workers:

> Hand hygiene is the simplest and most effective way of reducing the threat of hospital acquired infection. The responsibility to reduce HAI's is quite literally in the hands of everyone working in the hospital environment—from the cleaner to the consultant. GOJO has developed its PURELL alcohol based hand rub range to provide a convenient and flexible way to kill germs on hands. (*Source*: Ref. 147.)

GOJO had clearly responded to health care institutions' fears of infections spreading in the hospital especially as the press continued its coverage of this problem. In an article in the *New York Times*, "In hospitals, simple reminders reduce deadly infections," a health professional was featured in a photograph pumping a hand sanitizer dispenser before entering a patient's room. GOJO and its emerging competitors marketed the kind of dispenser shown. What the photograph also showed, however, was another fear of how germs might spread because a person had to "touch" the dispensing apparatus in order to get the product on the hands [148]. GOJO responded to this concern with the development of a "touch-free, trouble-free dispensing system" in foam or gel. A supply company advertising the new dispenser on its web site warned that "when people want to get their hands clean, the last thing they need is to touch a dirty dispenser.... The future of hand hygiene is touch-free." The web site proclaimed that the CDC "recommended the use of alcohol-based hand sanitizers to help prevent the spread of germs in hospitals, offices, and schools" and cited a study asserting that health care workers "sanitized their hands 20% more often when Purell was provided in a touch-free dispenser." Other companies of course competitively followed with the development and marketing of their own version of this new type of dispenser [149]. The press has reported, generally in articles focusing on the need for infection prevention in hospitals, that with dispensers appearing everywhere in hospital settings, hand hygiene among workers has seen significant improvement [150].

In 2009, the *WHO Guidelines on Hand Hygiene in Health Care* also revisited the discussion of "state-of-the-art" surgical hand preparation reviewing the history of different practices in the past from Joseph Lister's contributions to disinfection in surgery through Dr. Philip B. Price's recommendations for a 7 min soap, water, and brush hand washing followed by 70% ethanol for 3 min after drying the hands with a towel ([112], p. 154 [151]). The WHO's review of current surgical hand washing noted that many surgeons in the United States use a 3 or 5 min hand scrub with a disposable sponge (rather than a brush) and use chlorhexidine- or povidone–iodine-containing soaps whose "most active agents (in order of decreasing activity) are chlorhexidine gluconate, iodophors, triclosan, and plain soap" ([112], p. 55). The report noted the worldwide ban on hexachlorophene "because of its high rate of dermal absorption and subsequent toxic effects" and problems with triclosan (a prevalent antibacterial chemical first used in the 1970s), that it is "mainly bacteriostatic, inactive against *P. aeruginosa*, and has been associated with water pollution in lakes" ([112], p. 55). The WHO Guidelines noted that neither hexachlorophene or triclosan are any "longer commonly used in operating rooms because other products such as chlorhexidine or povidone–iodine provide similar efficacy at lower levels of toxicity, faster mode of action, or broader spectrum of activity" ([112], p. 55). In reviewing recent research on a variety of products for surgical preparation, the WHO concluded that "the antibacterial efficacy of products containing high concentrations of alcohol by far surpasses that of any medicated soap presently available" and "preference should be given to alcohol-based products" ([112], p. 57).

The WHO also acknowledged that cultural factors come into play when assessing whether hospitals in the United States or worldwide might adopt the alcohol-based preference: "...some surgeons consider the time taken for surgical handscrub as a ritual for the preparation of the intervention and a switch from handscrub to handrub must be prepared with caution." ([112], p. 57). Just as in the late nineteenth century when physicians were reluctant to accept the idea that they could be spreading infection because they were not washing their hands, in the early twenty-first-century United States, physicians are often bound to their traditions and resistant to change—even if such change might be efficacious.

1.4.3   Consumer Hygiene Products in the Age of Germ Panic

Antimicrobial soaps have again gained a prominent position in the consumer market, with their germ-killing qualities a major selling point. During this more recent time period, the chemical triclosan has become a very common ingredient in hygiene and cleaning products in the home. At the time when hexachlorophene was banned by the FDA, this new antimicrobial was developed alongside triclocarban [152]. First used as a surgical scrub in the early 1970s, the 1990s saw the emergence of almost countless soaps and other products featuring triclosan. Between 1992 and 1999 alone, "over 700 consumer products with antibacterial properties, the vast majority of them containing triclosan, have entered the consumer market" ([153], p. 2).

Concurrently, concerns about emerging infections—begun by AIDS, epitomized by the 1995 movie *Outbreak*, and confirmed by news of panic-inducing new infectious diseases ranging from the Ebola virus to avian flu—caught the public's imagination and created a culture of fear. Fewer hygiene-related advertisements appeared in popularly read magazines between 1960 and 1980 than had the two decades earlier, but there was a "resurgence" between 1985 and 2000 [154]. Historian Nancy Tomes labels both the 1900–1940 era and the 1985–2000 era as periods of "germ panic" when there "was a consciousness of the germs" ([110], p. 192 [155]). Anxiety associated with globalism, especially global travel, heightened in the aftermath of the 9/11 attack on the World Trade Center in New York city, the anthrax scare, and smallpox and the fear of bioterrorism all have exacerbated this "germ panic" [156–159]. Popular self-help books epitomized germ phobia: *The Germ Freak's Guide to Outwitting Colds and Flu: Guerilla Tactics to Keep Yourself Healthy at Home, at Work and in the World*; *Don't Touch that Doorknob! How Germs Can Zap You and How You Can Zap Back*; *Where the Germs Are: A Scientific Safari*; and *A Field Guide to Germs* [160–163]. The fear of drug resistance and "revenge of the superbugs," increasingly reported in the press ("Microbes, microbes everywhere"; "Extreme hygiene: kill all the bacteria!"; and "An arsenal of sanitizers for a nation of germophobes"), created a demand for antibacterial products, and at the same time, tangible concerns about the dangers of these products [164–166].

Marketers responded to both new "germaphobic" concerns and other emerging cultural trends. In 1979, liquid soaps or washes were introduced into the consumer market. Tapping into consumer fear about what kinds of germs might be left on bar soaps after each use and the problem of soap dishes that did not sufficiently drain water from the bar between uses, companies developed liquid soap that would dispense separately for each use. Despite many doubts about its viability as a product, liquid soap quickly became a "personal care market success story" [167]. *Chain Drug Review* noted that the liquid soap category was already a $300 million market in 1993 [168]. Companies producing body washes and bar and liquid soaps reached out to traditionally female consumer groups as well other consumer target audiences with new offerings and by 1998 total sales were reported at $2.2 billion. Products were aimed specifically at men with Old Spice Hair & Body Wash or Dial Corporation's

Dial For Men Body Wash; at preteen and teen boys with "hypermasculine guideposts such as Instinct from Axe, Swagger by Old Spice, and Magnetic Attraction Enhancing Body Wash by Dial"; or at children, with comic character soap containers from Looney Tunes to Sponge Bob lining the drugstore or supermarket shelves. Companies also developed soaps featuring new and often exotic fragrances; exfoliants with "improved moisturizing and skin care benefits"; "natural" components from "shea butter" to fruits, flowers, spices, or nuts that make "anti-aging" and wrinkle prevention claims; or aromatherapy ingredients to reduce stress [169,170]. According to industrial researchers, introduction of these new products represented consumer desires for luxury, well-being, and good health, and for some, concerns about environmental ecology [171,172].

Liquid hand soaps often included antibacterials as major selling points. Softsoap and Dial antibacterial liquid hand soaps were introduced in the late 1980s. Both products were marketed for their added "active ingredients." Softsoap's brand manager in 1988 noted that "consumers, because of AIDS-inspired fears, are more concerned with personal hygiene and safety." As these two products geared up their marketing campaigns, a household products analyst at the advertising agency Kidder, Peabody & Co. argued that "as germs and viruses become more topical, companies are anxious to position their products as germ killers" ([173], p. 48). In 2002, of the top 10 selling liquid/hand soaps, 9 of them contained triclosan [174]. Dial launched a "Healthy You Complete Hand Washing Program" to support its liquid soap, identifying it as a "public health campaign" and offering physicians "starter kits" and educational materials to distribute in their offices. Softsoap's liquid soaps with triclosan were consistently among the top sellers ([167], p. 24).

The appeal of new germ-fighting chemicals extended beyond hand soap to household cleaning products and consumer goods. House cleaning products saw an 80% increase in market growth from 1987 to 1992, bolstered especially by the disinfectant category, which emphasized "safe, effective, germ-killing properties" ([175], p. 40). With the development of a process of bonding triclosan into products, numerous other antimicrobial consumer goods came on the market, all using familiar visual images and verbal cues about germs. Microban products include toilet paper, cutting boards, baby toys, shower liners, towels, clothes washers, sports equipment, and shoes, to name just a few. Although there is no scientific proof that the addition of triclosan to these products actually reduces infection, the intuitive appeal of a bacteria-killing ingredient has become a prevalent marketing tool ([176], [217]).

Research and development experts also noted that in the early 1990s, "green" companies began marketing such household products as dishwashing soap and toilet bowl cleaners. Their marketing emphasized that "things can be over-disinfected, and a sterile lifestyle is not necessarily a good thing." However, by 1992 these "environment-friendly" products had only generated a "modest 4% of the market" ([175], p. 40).

The category of "hand sanitizers" as personal cleanliness products that could clean hands without water gained increased consumer attention at the turn of the twenty-first century. In the 2002 *Chain Drug Store* list of best selling liquid soaps, the only product not containing triclosan was Purell, which called itself an "instant hand sanitizer" promising, as soaps with or without triclosan have done since the early twentieth century, to kill "99.99% of the most common germs that may cause illness."

The primary cleansing ingredient in Purell was the necessary over 60% ethanol with a small amount of isopropyl alcohol. Some versions of the product, for example, "Purell with Aloe" or "Purell Icy Blue Mint," also included "moisturizing" ingredients to prevent skin irritation with frequent daily use [177].

The company, GOJO, as previously noted, had earlier sold their products to the food service and health care facilities market, including hospitals [178]. One of the company's spokesmen noted that the company had received a "flood of calls from health care professionals eager to have the product for their personal use." GOJO launched it in the general consumer market in 1997 [179,180]. In an interview that year with *New Republic* journalist Hanna Rosin, the Purell spokesman Paul Alper defined the Purell target audience as "on the go" people. Rosin argued that this meant

an updated Norman Rockwell America: women who want to clean up between diaper changes, or after trips to a fast food joint. Men traveling with kids on weekends to the ballpark or picnics or fishing trips. Or, he adds as an aside, professionals eating a sandwich at their desk who can't get to a bathroom to wash their hands, or who are sitting in the window seat of the plane, or who shake lots of hands. Tipper Gore even plugged the product during her frenzy of hand pumping during the last election. (*Source*: Ref. 179, p. 29.)

With the introduction of Purell as a new product, drugstores, supermarkets, and other places that sold hand or body washing products had to address the issue of how to categorize Purell—as a liquid hand soap or in the separate category of hand sanitizer [181,182]. Other new liquid products were quickly developed to compete with Purell by such companies as Dial, Colgate-Palmolive, Unilever, and Lysol with names that generally indicated their germ-fighting capabilities: Germ-X Ultimate Antibacterial Foaming Hand Soap, Germ-X Hand Sanitizer, Lysol Healthy Touch, Vicks Early Defense, Cleanwell, Soapopular, Germ Blaster, or Sani Hands for Kids [183,184].

Companies have also used "educational" approaches in marketing these new hygiene products directly to the public as they did in partnering with the Cleanliness Institute in the 1920s. They have created pamphlets, posters, and stickers. They have issued "fact sheets" on their web sites referring to hand-washing messages or campaigns promoted by the CDC or the WHO, and in some cases they have partnered with infection control organizations promoting hand washing. In 2006, the ad goodness bloy posted that the J. Walter Thompson agency, hired by Johnson & Johnson promoted it through a "guerilla campaign" where stickers were placed on magazine covers in physician waiting rooms with such warnings as "Thumbed Through By Sick People Since October 2005" [185]. Companies assured consumers that they have "boosted" production of their products in response to each new flu scare, with SARS in 2003 and with flu vaccine shortages due to factory contamination closings in 2004 [186].

In 2002, Dial Corporation also addressed the fear of germs when it began a "branding campaign" with the theme "You're not as clean as you think." One ad used humor in showing two men unknowingly using the same towel to dry themselves after each separately left their gym's sauna [187]. Additional methods used by hygiene companies to attract consumer attention have included sampling the product in selected markets; newspaper inserts; coupons; special programs in stores selling the product such as front aisle displays; radio or television commercials; product placement in television drama, comedy, or reality show story lines; or medical journal advertising and direct mail campaigns to health professionals introducing a company's brand message [188,189].

In April of 2009, a strain of H1N1 influenza virus was first globally reported in Veracruz, Mexico. The World Health Organization and the Centers for Disease Control identified the new influenza outbreak as a pandemic in June 2009. Companies making hand sanitizers, from the small pocket-size to the table- or wall-mounted dispensers, increased their product manufacturing and marketing as public and government concerns about the outbreak incidence of H1N1 heightened with students returning to schools in the autumn of 2009 [190]. Most parents found a hand sanitizer included on the list of school supplies that children needed for the first day of classes.

Johnson & Johnson introduced its "Imagine a Touchable World" Campaign. The Purell web site included the claim that its product was the "#1 Doctor Recommended Hand Sanitizer." The web site also featured "Know the Facts," "Testimonials," and "In the News" pages. Emphasis was placed on how to fight the new H1N1 ("swine flu") epidemic. "In the News" noted that no hand sanitizer could "prevent" the flu but noted CDC recommendations about practicing good hand hygiene by washing with soap and water or using an alcohol-based sanitizer when soap and water may not be available [191].

Bath & Body Works also launched a new campaign for antibacterial products with its "Spread Love, Not Germs" collection that included a foaming hand soap, a deep cleansing hand soap, and a foaming hand sanitizer in such fragrances as sweet pea, soft musk, and fresh raspberry ([190], p. B1). While this new collection contained triclosan, another line of hand soap and hand sanitizer products offered for sale at Bath and Body Works developed by Cleanwell promised to "say goodbye to germs naturally" without the consumer having to choose between safety and efficacy" [193]. Vi-Jon Inc., the maker of the Germ-X product line, started promotion of new benzalkonium chloride-containing sanitizers with their "portable 1-ounce purse spray and individual wipes, to make sanitizing on the go more convenient." Vi-Jon's spokeswoman addressed the issue of assumed fears of H1N1 with their goal to "ensure that we are doing everything possible to have products on the shelf for those consumers as that extra peace of mind" ([194], p. B8). The Canadian-based MGS Soapopular, Inc. company also marketed its benzalkonium chloride-containing product line as "Alcohol-Free Hand Sanitizers, Soft Foam that's Rinse Free, Fragrance Free, and Dye Free, 99.9% effective against a broad spectrum of Bacteria, Germs and Viruses while Protecting The Skin" [195]. In a press release, Environmental Solutions International asserted that its Kids Smart and Silky Foaming Hand Sanitizer was "an answer for parents trying to keep their kids healthy and safe." It was as effective as an alcohol-based product but not "flammable or poisonous," especially "when put in or on the wrong hands" [196]. All of these hand sanitizers, including those containing the ingredient benzalkonium chloride that recent research in lab studies linked to the development of antibiotic resistance, shot up in sales [197]. As companies expanded their marketing campaigns, Nielsen Co. reported a near doubling of hand sanitizer sales from October 2008 to October 2009 [198,199].

Numerous news articles offered suggestions for what ordinary people could do to avoid the H1N1 flu [200,201]. Some reported new research on the effectiveness of hand-washing campaigns and generally included recommendations for washing hands or using a hand sanitizer in public and private settings [202,203]. Others dealt with consumers' fears of germ exposure. A *Wall Street Journal* article, "Where the worst germs lurk," reported on ongoing research at the University of Arizona sponsored by disinfectant producers as Clorox and Procter & Gamble that warned readers of the dangers of surface germs in offices and homes, on such surfaces as the computer mouse and keyboard, phones, elevator buttons, purses, wallets, cutting boards, and toothbrush holders. A press release issued by Clorox emphasized that the Arizona researchers had recommended "frequent" hand washing and the "daily" use of disinfectant wipes on surfaces as a way to "kill germs" while a *Wall Street Journal* reporter noted in her article that the lead Arizona researcher stressed that "more research is needed on the link between surface germs and disease, since it is irresponsible to say who will get sick" [204,205].

As the public attempted to be responsible and ward off disease, consumer groups raised concerns about what exactly are the known and unknown ingredients contained in the many new hygiene products introduced in the marketplace [206]. Industry groups were aware of these public fears. In early 2010, the Soap and Detergent Association implemented a "consumer product ingredient communication initiative" whose aim was to respond to consumer questions by recommending that product manufacturers offer more ingredient information through posting fuller ingredient contents on the label, through web sites, toll-free numbers, the mail, or "other non-electronic means" [207]. With the competition increasing in the personal and home cleaning products industry, especially with the introduction of new products that claim to be "natural" or "organic," industry groups organized to issue their own standards and guidelines for what can be considered a "natural" product. The Natural Products Association, made up of both manufacturers and retailers, in late 2009, introduced a seal placed on products for the consumer to see that certifies certain criteria have been met [208]. Legislators and environmental advocacy groups argued that these voluntary efforts of product manufacturers were not sufficient. Senator Al Franken introduced a bill in the U.S. Senate in late 2009 that would force producers of household cleaning products to "fully disclose all ingredients on their product labels" [209]. Advocates of consumer and environmental safety hired the law firm "Earthjustice" to use a 1971 state law to bring a suit to a New York State Court with the hopes that a victory would force manufacturers to disclose all product ingredients. Both the U.S. congressional proposal and the New York State Court case indicated consumer advocates wanted full disclosure rather than labels or other sources of information that could be "too selective and vague" [210].

Many commentators have focused on the potential harms of such antibacterial products as those with triclosan and benzalkonium chloride and the attitudes behind the promotion of them. As one commentator in the *New York Times* noted in 2004, "The fantasy of a germ-free home is not only absurd, but it is also largely pointless." Noting that there was no need for such a home in most instances and also that the products had not been proven to effectively create such an environment, this commentator reminded her readers that each person is home to "hundreds of trillions of bacteria" [211,212]. *Why Dirt is Good*, a book aimed at a general public audience by the immunologist Mary Ruebush, posited "The 5 Cardinal Rules for a Strong Immune System" with Rule #3 stating "Don't Encourage Superbugs: Avoid Anti-microbics Whenever Possible" [213]. The public health community also questioned the focus on the chemical solution used instead of the more basic but reliable focus on consistent hand washing. Public health professionals in general cautioned that such products might give consumers a false sense of security that would make them wash their hands for a shorter period of time [214].

Along with the possibility that consumers might be less careful about washing their hands, scientists have found that triclosan had become a potential environmental threat, with the chemical found in groundwater [215,216]. Public health leaders and concerned members of the public also cite concerns that its inclusion in so many products would potentially cause antibacterial resistance. Although hygiene products companies continue to deny such possibilities and tout their ability to kill potentially dangerous germs, the safety of triclosan and other antibacterials remained unclear [217,218].

And even if triclosan was found to be completely safe, there is no clear proof that it is efficacious as an ingredient in consumer products. The Association for Professionals in Infection Control released a public statement in 1997 warning that antimicrobial products had "no proven infection prevention benefit" [219,220]. A 2008 comprehensive meta-analysis of all the studies conducted on hand washing since 1960 found no greater efficacy for antibacterial products over soaps without any such ingredient. Others also noted that the greater public health problem in terms of infection prevention went back to the very basics: not everyone washes their hands. The same people who bought toilet paper with Microban often neglected to wash their hands after using the toilet. This curious short circuit is a common difficulty in our culture: the desire to be safe, but the neglect of simple preventive measures [221]. Like soaps touting germ-killing properties in earlier periods, both the efficacy and safety of these antibacterial products do not live up to advertising claims. Killing germs, it seems, is more an advertising gimmick than an effective public health measure in our current culture.

Such a disconnect between efficacy and marketing claims is clearly not a new problem. From carbolic acid in the nineteenth century all the way through to antibacterial soap and alcohol-based hand sanitizers now, germ-killing products have often been popular but not always necessary, effective, or safe. In addition, adherence to proper use of hygiene products has been difficult and often spotty. Perhaps, the high incidence of life-threatening MRSA and *C. difficile* infections and the pandemic H1N1 flu virus have increased public consciousness and initiated a new era of personal hygiene adherence. Hand sanitizer dispensers now proliferate in all kinds of settings. Public health campaign signs in restrooms urging the general public to sing the "Happy Birthday" song twice as they scrub their hands are posted along with the more accustomed signs reminding employees to wash before returning to work. On the other hand, perhaps product advertising and press coverage of these disease occurrences have simply generated a new era of "germ phobia." What is most important is that hygiene agents must be safe and beneficial and not result in misuse or overuse, causing rather than preventing disease. Whatever new sanitizing and sterilizing agents are discovered, manufactured, promoted, and used in the future, their worth ultimately rests upon the human factor.

REFERENCES

1. Vigarello G. *Concepts of Cleanliness: Changing Attitudes in France Since the Middle Ages.* Cambridge: Cambridge University Press, 1988.
2. Williams MT. *Washing "the Great Unwashed": Public Baths in Urban America, 1840–1920.* Columbus, OH: Ohio State University Press, 1991.
3. Brandt AM, Gardner M. The golden age of medicine? In: Cooter R, Pickstone J, editors. *Medicine in the Twentieth Century.* Amsterdam: Harwood Academic Publishers, 2000. pp. 2–37.
4. Ashenberg K. *The Dirt on Clean: An Unsanitized History.* New York: North Point Press, 2007. pp. 94–95.
5. Smith V. *Clean: A History of Personal Hygiene and Purity.* Oxford: Oxford University Press, 2007.
6. Bushman RL, Bushman CL. The early history of cleanliness in America. *J. Am. Hist.* 1988;74: 1213–1238.
7. Goubert JP. *The Conquest of Water.* Princeton, NJ: Princeton University Press, 1986.
8. Johnson S. *The Ghost Map: The Story of London's Most Terrifying Epidemic—and How It Changed Science, Cities, and the Modern World.* New York: Riverhead Books, 2006.
9. Rosen G. *A History of Pubic Health,* expanded ed. Baltimore, MD: Johns Hopkins University Press, 1993.
10. Leavitt JW. *Typhoid Mary: Captive to the Public's Health.* Boston, MA: Beacon Press, 1997.
11. Melosi MV. *The Sanitary City: Urban Infrastructure in America from Colonial Times to the Present.* Baltimore, MD: The Johns Hopkins University Press, 2000.
12. Campkin B, Cox R, editors. *Dirt: New Geographies of Cleanliness and Contamination.* London: I.B. Tauris, 2007.
13. Sivulka J. *Stronger Than Dirt: A Cultural History of Advertising Personal Hygiene in America, 1875–1940.* New York: Humanity Books, 2001.
14. Hunt JA. A short history of soap. *Pharm. J.* 1999;263(7076):985–989.
15. Loudon I. *The Tragedy of Childbed Fever.* New York: Oxford University Press, 2000.
16. Gordon A. *A Treatise on the Epidemic Puerperal Fever of Aberdeen.* London. Published as an appendix in Campbell W. *A Treatise on the Epidemic Puerperal Fever.* Edinburgh: Bell and Bradfute, 1822.
17. Holmes OW. *Medical Essays 1842–1882.* Boston: Houghton, Mifflin and Company, 1883.
18. Gawande AA. On washing hands. *New Engl. J. Med.* 2004;350:1283–1286.
19. Nuland S. *The Doctors' Plague: Germs, Childbed Fever, and the Strange Story of Ignac Semmelweis.* New York: W.W. Norton & Company, 2003.
20. Larson E. Innovations in health care: antisepsis as a case study. *Am. J. Public Health* 1989; 79(1):92–99.
21. Crellin JK. Internal antisepsis or the dawn of chemotherapy? *J. Hist. Med. Allied Sci.* 1981;36(1):9–18.
22. Rosenberg CE. Florence Nightingale on contagion: the hospital as moral universe. In: Rosenberg CE, editor. *Explaining Epidemics and Other Studies in the History of Medicine.* New York: Cambridge University Press, 1992.
23. Nightingale F. *Introductory Notes on Lying-In Institutions.* London: Longmans, Green, and Company, 1871.
24. Porter R. *The Greatest Benefit to Mankind: A Medical History of Humanity.* New York: W.W. Norton & Company, 1997.
25. Risse GB. *Mending Bodies, Saving Souls: A History of Hospitals.* New York: Oxford University Press, 1999.
26. Crowther MA, Dupree MW. *Medical Lives in the Age of Surgical Revolution.* London: Cambridge University Press, 2009.

27. Morgenstern L. Gargling with lister. *J. Am. Coll. Surg.* 2007;204:495–497.
28. Block SS. *Disinfection, Sterilization and Preservation*, 5th ed. Philadelphia, PA: Lippincott, Williams & Wilkins, 2001.
29. Greenwood A. Lawson Tait and opposition to germ theory: defining science in surgical practice. *J. Hist. Med. Allied Sci.* 1998;53:99–131.
30. Hamilton D. The nineteenth-century surgical revolution—antisepsis or better nutrition? *Bull. Hist. Med.* 1982;56:30–40. Some also speculated that the emergence of anesthesia during surgery helped to decrease mortality after surgery.
31. Abrams A. *Transactions of the Antiseptic Club.* New York: E.B. Treat, 1895. pp. 22–23.
32. Jungermann E. Soap bacteriostats. *J. Am. Oil Chem. Soc.* 1968;45:345.
33. Wilcox RW. *Pharmacology and Therapeutics*, 7th revised ed. Philadelphia, PA: P. Blakiston's Son & Co., 1907. p. 417.
34. Gurowitz M.Synol soap. Kilmer house: the story behind Johnson & Johnson and its people (blog). http://www.kilmerhouse.com/?p=230 (accessed June 23, 2009).
35. For a general history of Johnson & Johnson, see Foster LG. *A Company That Cares: One Hundred Year Illustrated History of Johnson & Johnson.* New Brunswick, NJ: Johnson & Johnson, 1986.
36. McGuire S. An aseptic soap-container. *JAMA* 1900;XXXV(2):112.
37. *Red Cross Notes* 1915;VII(4):cover.
38. The doctor's hands. *Red Cross Notes* 1914;VII(3):97.
39. Ulrich CF. Cleanliness the chief antiseptic. *JAMA* 1894;XXIII:305–307.
40. Post WE, Nicoll HK. The comparative efficiency of some common germicides. *JAMA* 1919; LV(19):1635–1639.
41. See Corson H. Ántiseptic. *JAMA* 1891; 765–770.
42. Greenley TB. Asepsis versus antisepsis in obstetrics as a preventive of puerperal septicemia. *JAMA* 1890;XV(6):197–203 (quote from p. 202).
43. Ivory Soap Advertising Collection, Procter & Gamble Company, 1891. http://sirismm.si.edu/archivcenter/ivorysoap/ivory_0207910169.jpg (accessed July 3, 2009).
44. See Ivory soap ads in Modern Hospital September 19, 1926. http://sirismm.si.edu/archivcenter/ivorysoap/ivory_0207910551.jpg (accessed July 3, 2009).
45. See Century Magazine May 1913, 68. http://sirismm.si.edu/archivcenter/ivorysoap/ivory_0207910852.jpg (accessed July 3, 2009).
46. Tomes N. *The Gospel of Germs: Men, Women, and the Microbe in American Life.* Cambridge, MA: Harvard University Press, 1998.
47. Teller M. *The Tuberculosis Movement.* Westwood, CT: Greenwood Press, 1988.
48. Hays JN. *The Burdens of Disease: Epidemics and Human Response in Western History.* New Jersey: Rutgers University Press, 1998.
49. Tomes N. Moralizing the microbe: the germ theory and the moral construction of behavior in the late-nineteenth-century antituberculosis movement. In: Brandt AM, Rozin P, editors. *Morality and Health.* New York: Routledge, 1997:271–295.
50. Markel H. *When Germs Travel: Six Major Epidemics That Have Invaded America and the Fears They Have Unleashed.* New York: Vintage Books, 2005.
51. See Hansen B. New images of a new medicine: visual evidence for widespread popularity of therapeutic discoveries in America after 1885. *Bull. Hist. Med.* 1999;73(4):629–678.
52. Kilmer FB. *Johnson's First Aid Manual*, 3rd ed. New Brunswick, NJ: Johnson & Johnson, 1903.
53. Company history: Johnson & Johnson. http://www.fundinguniverse.com/company-histories/Johnson-amp;-Johnson-Company-History.html (accessed June 5, 2009).
54. Death rate of children . . . Synol soap (advertisement). *New York Times* September 13, 1913, 7.
55. See also The sick room . . . Synol soap (advertisement). *New York Times* October 27, 1913, 4. (Synol Soap has been the principal antiseptic toilet soap in sick rooms and hospitals for many years. When one of the family is suffering from a contagious disease, Synol should be used freely, not only upon the body of the body of the sufferer, but the whole family should use it in order to keep the disease from spreading. It is the soap that physicians prescribe and use upon themselves to avoid infection.)
56. Kilmer FB. Let us introduce you to your hands. *Red Cross Messenger* 1917;IX(5):132–133.
57. Dr. Carrel favors antiseptics in war. New York Times November 28, 1915, 11.

58. Is there a greater war story than this? (advertisement), 1924. Jones ER. *Those Were the Good Old Days: A Happy Look at American Advertising, 1880–1930*. New York: Simon and Schuster, 1971. p. 355.

59. The doctor and household appreciate Lifebuoy soap (advertisement). *Harpers Monthly*, circa 1903. MagazineArt.Org web site http://www.magazineart.org/main.php/v/ads/personalitems/soap/Lifebuoy Soap-1900sA.jpg.html (accessed July 13, 2009).

60. Lifebuoy soap advertisement, 1919. J. Walter Thompson Archives, John W. Hartman Center for Sales, Advertising, and Marketing History, Duke University Rare Book and Special Collections Library found in Sivulka's *Stronger Than Dirt*, p. 14.

61. Wiley H. *1001 Tests of Foods, Beverages and Toilet Accessories, Good and Otherwise: Why They Are So*. New York: Hearst's International Library Co., 1914. p. 213.

62. Kilmer described the National Pure Food and Drugs Act of 1906 that created the FDA as "the country's first attempt at curbing the mounting abuses in the mass production of foods, drugs, medicines and liquors." See Foster's *A Company That Cares*, pp. 62–65.

63. Wiebe R. *The Search for Order, 1877–1920*. New York: Hill and Wang, 1967.

64. Strasser S. *Satisfaction Guaranteed: The Making of the American Mass Market*. New York: Pantheon Books, 1989.

65. Marchand R. *Advertising the American Dream: Making Way for Modernity, 1920–1940*. Berkeley, CA: University of California Press, 1985.

66. Ivory Soap Advertising Collection, Procter & Gamble Company, 1890. http://www.americanhistory. si.edu/archives/ivory/results.asp (FileName: 0207910127.jpg).

67. Ivory Soap Advertising Collection, Procter & Gamble Company, 1890. http://www.americanhistory. si.edu/archives/ivory/results.asp (FileName: 0207910422.jpg) (accessed June 23, 2009).

68. See also The Procter & Gamble Company (Company History, Funding Universe). http://www. fundinguniverse.com/company-histories/The-Procter-amp;-Gamble-Company-Company-History.html.

69. See Editors of Advertising Age. *Procter & Gamble: The House That Ivory Built*. Chicago, IL: NYC Business Books, 1989.

70. Dyer D, Dalzell F, Olegario R. *Rising Tide: Lessons from 165 Years of Brand Building at Procter & Gamble*. Boston, MA: Harvard Business School Press, 2004. pp. 23–42.

71. Ivory Soap Advertising Collection, Procter & Gamble Company, 1893 (http://americanhistory.si.edu/ archives/ivory/results.asp (FileName: 0207910186.jpg) (accessed June 23, 2009).

72. Christian Herald December 9, 1891. http://www.americanhistory.si.edu/archives/ivory/image.asp? index=0207910122.jpg (accessed June 23, 2009).

73. Norton JF. Soaps in relation to their use for hand-washing. *JAMA* 1920;75(5):305.

74. Contagion: The Spread of Eugenics Throughout American Popular Culture in the 1920s, by John F. McClymer. http://www1.assumption.edu/users/McClymer/his394/contagion.html (accessed June 9, 2009).

75. Ritchie JW, Caldwell JS. *Primer of Hygiene, New World Health Series: Book One*. New York: World Book Company, 1910.

76. Burkard WE, Chambers RL. *Health Habits, Physiology and Hygiene, Book Two*. Chicago: Lyons and Carnahan, 1925–1930.

77. Business and finance: Cleanliness Institute. *Time Magazine* December 23, 1929.

78. Vinikas V. *Soft Soap and Hard Sell: American Hygiene in an Age of Advertisement*. Ames, IO: Iowa State University Press, 1992. pp. 85–94.

79. Hoy S. *Chasing Dirt: The American Pursuit of Cleanliness*. New York: Oxford University Press, 1996.

80. O Careful mother [advertisement for Listerine] (1930) Medicine and Madison Avenue On-Line Project - Ad # MM0645, John W. Hartman Center for Sales, Advertising & Marketing History, Rare Book, Manuscript, and Special Collections Library, Duke University, Durham, North Carolina. http:// library.duke.edu./digitalcollections/mma/ (accessed March 12, 2009).

81. Marchand R. *Advertising the American Dream: Making Way for Modernity, 1920–1940*. Berkeley, CA: University of California Press, 1985. pp. 18–20.

82. It's nice to be liked (advertisement in *McCall's* August 1940). Reprinted in Vinikas's *Soft Soap and Hard Sell: American Hygiene in an Age of Advertisement*, p. 103.

83. Burke T. *Lifebuoy Men, Lux Women: Commodification, Consumption, and Cleanliness in Modern Zimbabwe*. Durham, NC: Duke University Press, 1996.

84. Advertisement for penicillin production from Life Magazine August 14, 1944. http://www .sciencemuseum.org.uk/broughttolife/objects/display.aspx?id=6086.
85. See Bud R. *Penicillin: Triumph and Tragedy.* New York: Oxford University Press, 2007. pp. 54–74.
86. McFarlane G. *Alexander Fleming: The Man and the Myth.* Cambridge, MA: Harvard University Press, 1984. p. 268. (Quoted in Parascandola J. The introduction of antibiotics into therapeutics. In: Leavitt JW, Numbers R, editors. *Sickness and Health in America: Readings in the History of Medicine and Pubic Health.* Madison, WI: University of Wisconsin Press, 1995.
87. Garrett L. *The Coming Plague: Newly Emerging Diseases in a World Out of Balance,* New York: Penguin, 1995.
88. Ayliffe GAJ, English MP. *Hospital Infection: From Miasmas to MRSA.* London: Cambridge University Press, 2003. p. 223.
89. Hillier K. Babies and bacteria: phage typing, bacteriologists, and the birth of infection control. *Bull. Hist. Med.* 2006;80:745, 759–760.
90. Cleland H. Hexachlorophene (G11) in the surgical scrub: a brushless surgical wash. *Can. Med. J.* 1952;66:464.
91. See also Seastone CV. Observations on the use of G-11 in the surgical scrub. *Surg. Gynecol. Obstet.* 1947;84:355–360.
92. Price PB. Fallacy of a current surgical fad—the three-minute preoperative scrub with hexachlorophene soap. *Ann. Surg.* 1951;134(3):476–482.
93. Procter & Gamble Co. Hospital approval since 1879. Modern Hospital 1926. Ivory Soap Advertising Collection, 1883–1998. Smithsonian Institution, National Museum of American History, Archives Center. http://sirismm.si.edu/archivcenter/ivorysoap/ivory_0207910551.jpg.
94. See Procter & Gamble Co., Ivory Soap Advertising Collection, 1883–1998. Smithsonian Institution, National Museum of American History, Archives Center.
95. See Canzonetti AJ, Dalley MM. Bacteriologic survey of scrub technics with special emphasis on phisoderm with 3 per cent hexachlorophene. *Ann. Surg.* 1952;135(2):228–233.
96. Maglio MM, Hannegan JM. Powdered antiseptic industrial cleaners. *AJPH* 1953;43:426–432.
97. Feteky FR, Buchbinder L, Shaffer SL, Goldberg S, Price HP, Pyle LA. Control of an outbreak of staphylococcal infections among mothers and infants in a suburban hospital. *AJPH* 1958;48: 298–310.
98. Farfar JO. The normal baby: routine care. *BMJ* 1971;7:28–32.
99. Gump WS. Development of a germicidal soap, parts I and II. *Soap and Sanitary Chemicals* March–April 1945, 36–39, 51, 85.
100. See Brody JE. Hexachlorophene: what price deodorant? *New York Times* December 12, 1971, E12.
101. Herrick AB, Jungermann E. The new toilet soaps. *J. Am. Oil Chem. Soc.* 1969;46:202–203.
102. Krause CC. Recent developments in the toilet-bar market. *J. Am. Oil Chem. Soc.* 1968;45:506–509.
103. Coleman AB. Letter to the editor. *Pediatrics* 1966;37(6):1031.
104. Stotzer DA. Letter to the editor. *Pediatrics* 1966;37(6):1030–1031.
105. Lockhart D, Simmons HE. Hexachlorophene decisions at the FDA. *Pediatrics* 1973;51(2):430–434.
106. Lyons RD. F.D.A. curbs use of germicide tied to infant deaths. *New York Times* September 23, 1972, 65.
107. Sloane L. Germicide used in cosmetics with sales set a $250 million. *New York Times* September 23, 1972, 25.
108. Dougherty PH. Advertising: Dial and the ban. *New York Times* September 26, 1972, 74.
109. Dougherty, quoting from the spokesman from Foot, Cone and Belding, the ad agency hired by Armour to market Dial.
110. Tomes N. The making of a germ panic, then and now. *AJPH* 2000;90(2):191–198.
111. Garrett L. *Betrayal of Trust: The Collapse of Global Public Health.* New York: Hyperion, 2000. pp. 1–15.
112. World Health Organization. *WHO Guidelines on Hand Hygiene in Health Care: First Global Patient Safety Challenge; Clean Care is Safer Care.* Geneva, Switzerland: WHO Press, 2009.
113. Healthcare-associated infections (HAIs). Centers for Disease Control and Prevention web site http://www.cdc.gov/ncidod/dhqp/hai.html (updated July 16, 2009; accessed August 12, 2009).
114. Archibald LK, Jarvis WR. Epidemic healthcare-associated infections. In Jarvis WR, editors. *Bennett & Brachman's Hospital Infections,* 5th ed. Philadelphia, PA: Lippincott, Williams & Wilkins, 2007. pp. 483–505.

115. Klevens RM, et al. Estimating health care-associated infections and deaths in U.S. hospitals, 2002. *Public Health Rep.* 2007;122(2):160–166.
116. Sack K.Deadly bacteria found to be more common. *New York Times* October 17, 2007. http://www .nytimes.com/2007/10/17/health/17infect.html?scp=1&sq=deadly%20bacteria%20found%20to% 20be%20more%20common&st=cse (accessed May 24, 2009).
117. Vinciguerra T. The lab coat is on the hook in the fight against germs. *New York Times* July 25, 2009, W2.
118. Smith R. Nothing to sneeze at: doctors' neckties see as flu risk. *The Wall Street Journal* November 19, 2009. http://online.wsj.com/article/SB125859205137154753.html (accessed November 20, 2009).
119. Drexler M. *Secret Agents: The Menace of Emerging Infections*. Washington, DC: Joseph Henry Press, 2002.
120. Sachs JS. *Good Germs, Bad Germs: Health and Survival in a Bacterial World*. New York: Hill and Wang, 2007.
121. Van Kanegan G, Boyette M. *How to Survive Your Hospital Stay*. New York: Simon and Schuster, 2003.
122. Ehrenclou M. *Critical Conditions: The Essential Hospital Guide to Get Your Loved One Out Alive*. Santa Monica, CA: Lemon Grove Press, 2008.
123. Scrubs, My Cabbage. Season 5, Episode 12. http://www.youtube.com/watch?v=9wyYHdfjokw& NR=1 (accessed June 12, 2009).
124. Why is handwashing important? Centers for Disease Control and Prevention Media Relations web site http://www.cdc.gov/od/oc/media/pressrel/r2k0306c.htm (accessed July 15, 2009).
125. Delaney LR, Gundeman RB. Hand hygiene. *Radiology* 2008;246(1):15.
126. Gawande A. On washing hands. *New Engl. J. Med.* 2004;350(13):1283–1286.
127. Yoffe E. Doctors are reminded, "wash up!" *New York Times* November 9, 1999. http://www.nytimes. com/1999/11/09/health/doctors-are-reminded-wash-up.html?scp=1&sq=doctors%20are% 20reminded,%20'wash%20up!&st=cse (accessed April 12, 2009).
128. Rosales SP, Hernandez MV, Huertas M. Infection control in ER: how hand-washing is avoided even in fiction. *Lancet Infect. Dis.* 2005;5:131–132.
129. Pittet D, Allegranzi B, Sax H. Hand hygiene. In: Jarvis WR, editor. *Bennett & Brachman's Hospital Infections*, 5th ed. Philadelphia, PA: Lippincott, Williams & Wilkins, 2007: 34–44.
130. Haas JP, Larson EL. Compliance with hand hygiene. *Am. J. Nurs.* 2008;108:8.
131. Dedrick RE, Sinkowitz-Cochran RL, Cunningham C, Muder RR, Perreiah P, Cardo DM, Jernigan JA. Hand Hygiene Practices After Brief Encounters with Patients: An Important Opportunity for Prevention. *Infection Control and Hospital Epidemiology*. 2007; 28:3:341–245.
132. WHO. Launch of the global patient safety challenge: clean care is safer care. October 13, 2005. http:// www.who.int/patientsafety/events/05/global_challenge/en/index.html (accessed July 16, 2009).
133. Clean Hands Save Lives, Department of Health and Human Services, Centers for Disease Control and Prevention web site http://www.cdc.gov/cleanhands/ (last modified February 18, 2008; (accessed July 16, 2009).
134. Demarco P. Your life is in their (clean) hands: handwashing can save patients' lives, but hospital workers still don't do it enough. The Boston Globe july 13, 2004, E1. (accessed February 12, 2010).
135. Ask me if I wash my hands. *BWH Bulletin: For and about the people of Brigham and Women's Hospital* June 19, 2009:2.
136. Our Commitment to Quality. Infection Prevention-Hand Hygiene web site http://www .brighamand womens.org/Quality/hygiene.aspx (accessed February 12, 2010).
137. Hooper DC. Making strides in hand hygiene compliance: to 90% and beyond. http://www. macoalition.org/Initiatives/docs/MassGeneralHospitalPresentation.pdf (accessed February 12, 2009).
138. Mucci K. Nurses rap about hand hygiene in Mass General Campaign. June 10, 2009. http://www .healthleadersmedia.com/content/234327/topic/WS_HLM2_QUA/Nurses-Rap-About-Hand-Hygiene-in-Mass-General-Campaign.html#%23 (accessed February 12, 2010).
139. Massachusetts General Hospital Quality and Safety Improvement Stories, 2011. http://qualityand safety.massgeneral.org/improvement/story.aspx?id=3 (accessed February 25, 2011).
140. Swedberg C. Patient-safety center tests RFID-enabled hand sanitizers. *RFID Journal August* 17, 2009. http://www.rfidjournal.com/article/view/5142 (accessed August 18, 2009).

141. Mody L, Saint S, Kaufman S, Kowalski C, Drein SL. Adoption of alcohol-based handrub by United States hospitals: a national survey. *Infect. Control Hosp. Epidemiol.* 2008;29(2):1177–1180.

142. Clean Care is Safer Care: Tools and resources. http://www.who.int/gpsc/background/en/index.html (accessed July 15, 2009).

143. Clean Care is Safer Care: Clean Your Hands: WHO's global annual compaign. http://www.who.int/gpsc/5may/en/ (accessed July 15, 2009).

144. Weinstein R. Hand hygiene—of reason and ritual (editorial). *Ann. Intern. Med.* 2004;141(1):65–66.

145. Rotter M, Koller W, Wewalka G, Werner HP, Ayliffe GAJ, Babb Jr., Arguments for alcoholic hand disinfection. *J. Hosp. Infect.* 2001;48:S4–S8.

146. GOJO Hygiene and Health Skin Company: History. http://www.gojo.com/company/index.asp (accessed April 2, 2009).

147. Purell hygienic and surgical hand rubs: reducing the threat of healthcare associated infection. www.supplychain.nhs.uk/.../purell_and_purell85_040709.pd (accessed July 25, 2009).

148. Hartocollis A. In hospitals, simple reminders reduce deadly infections. *New York Times* May 19, 2008. http://www.nytimes.com/2008/05/19/nyregion/19hospital.html (accessed July 25, 2009).

149. Parish Maintenance Supply web site http://www.parish-supply.com/industrial_sweeper_specifications.htm (accessed July 25, 2009).

150. Simon S. Ten steps to preventing infection in hospitals. *Wall Street Journal* October 27, 2009. http://online.wsj.com/article/SB10001424052970204488304574428950126681432.html (accessed October 27, 2009).

151. Price PB. The bacteriology of normal skin: a new quantitative test applied to a study of the bacterial flora and the disinfectant action of mechanical cleansing. *J. Infect. Dis.* 1938;63:301–318.

152. Makin SA, Lowry MR. Deodorant ingredients. In: Laden K, editor. *Antiperspirants and Deodorants*, 2nd ed. New York: Marcel Dekker, 1999:169–214.

153. Schweizer HP. Triclosan: a widely used biocide and its link to antibiotics. *FEMS Microbiol. Lett.* 2001;202(1):1–7.

154. Aiello A, Larson EL. An analysis of 6 decades of hygiene-related advertising: 1940–2000. *Am. J. Infect. Control* 2001;29(6):383–388.

155. Engel J. *The epidemic: a global history of AIDS.* New York: HarperCollins, 2006.

156. Rosner D, Markowitz G. *Are We Ready? Public Health Since 9/11.* Berkeley, California: University of California Press, 2006.

157. Kawamura LM. Have germs, will travel. *New York Times* June 2, 2007. http://www.nytimes.com/2007/06/02/opinion/02kawamura.html?_r=1&sq=have%20germs,%20will%20travel&st=cse& adxnnl=1&scp=1&adxnnlx=1250190229- + OuDgfnKN3VaHdnkIHIpbA. (accessed July 15, 2009).

158. Gandy M, Zumla A, editors. *The Return of the White Plague: Global Poverty and the 'New' Tuberculosis.* London: Verso, 2003.

159. Stephens B. Global view: swine-flu hysteria. *Wall Street Journal* May 5, 2009. http://online.wsj.com/article/SB124147910689984999.html (accessed August 14, 2009).

160. Janse A, Gerba C. *The Germ Freak's Guide to Outwitting Colds and Flu: Guerilla Tactics to Keep Yourself Healthy at Home, at Work and in the World.* Deerfield Beach, FL: Health Communications, Inc., 2005.

161. Brown J. *Don't Touch That Doorknob! How Germs Can Zap You and How You Can Zap Back.* New York: Warner Books, 2001.

162. Bakalar N. *Where the Germs Are: A Scientific Safari.* Hoboken, NJ: Wiley, 2003.

163. Biddle, W. *A Field Guide to Germs.* Hartswell, ME: Anchor Publishing, 2002.

164. Conry J. Microbes, microbes everywhere. *Boston Globe* March 10, 2005, H1, H5.

165. Kolata G. Extreme hygiene: kill all the bacteria! *New York Times* January 7, 2001: week in Review 1, 3.

166. Cortese A. An arsenal of sanitizers for a nation of germaphobes. *New York Times* February 27, 2005. http://query.nytimes.com/gst/fullpage.html?res=9C02E7DD143DF934A15751C0A9639C8B63. (accessed July 15, 2009).

167. Kleinman M. New life in the handsoap market: a new generation of products drives re-invigoration of $960 billion industry (Handsoap). *Soap Cosmet.* 2003;79(2):22–24.

168. Lever enters liquid soap arena. *Chain Drug Review*, April 26, 1993; 15(13):144.

169. Soap undergoing a metamorphosis. *Chain Drug Review* September 11, 2006; 28(15):50.

170. When it comes to soap, liquid is preferred (skin care) (sales of liquid soap increases). *Chain Drug Review* March 19, 2007:50.

171. The soap and other detergents manufacturing industry: trends and characteristics. Center for Competitive Analysis of the University of Missouri Outreach and Extension, University of Missouri, St. Louis, St. Louis, MO, May 2000:1–15.

172. Hoffman J. Masculinity in a spray can. *New York Times* January 31, 2010. http://www.nytimes.com/ 2010/01/31/fashion/31smell.html?ref=fashion (accessed January 31, 2010).

173. Freeman L, Walley W. It's germ warfare: liquid soaps try new tactic. *Advertising Age* October 31, 1988:46, 48.

174. Soap (liquid/hand soap) (sales data). *Chain Drug Review* June 24, 2002:254.

175. Ratcliffe M. Germ warfare. *Super Marketing* November 20, 1992, 40. http://query.nytimes.com/gst/ fullpage.html?res=9E04EED9133CF93AA35752C1A9629C8B63&sec=health (accessed June 12, 2009).

176. Microban Antimicrobial Product Protection. http://www.microban.com/americas/english/products (accessed July 28, 2009).

177. Purell. Product Protection. http://www.purell.com/page.jhtml?id=/purell/products/prd_hand_ sanitizer.inc (accessed July 24, 2009).

178. GOJO. http://www.gojo.com/company/timeline.asp (accessed July 24, 2009).

179. Rosin, H. Don't touch this: America's obsession with germs. *New Republic*. November 10, 1997: 24–31.

180. Sorkin AR, Saul S. Johnson & Johnson is close to deal for Pfizer unit. *New York Times* June 26, 2006. http://www.nytimes.com/2006/06/26/business/26pfizer.html (accessed July 24, 2009).

181. Soap (liquid/hand soap). *Chain Drug Review* June 24, 2002:254.

182. A case for common definitions. *Chain Drug Review* September 8, 1997:2.

183. Soap (hand sanitizers). *MMR* 2009;26(7):109.

184. Soap (liquid/hand). *MMR* 2009;26(7):110.

185. Purell adgoodness: the best and sometimes the worst around the globe blog, thumbed through by sick people since October 2005. Posted 2006. http://www.frederiksamuel.com/blog/index.php? s=thumbed+through+by+sick+people+&x=7&y=7 (accessed July 25, 2009).

186. Hopkins J. Alternative flu treatments expect big sales. *USA Today* October 7, 2004:B1.

187. Macarthur K. Clean break: dialing for dollars is a dirty business. *Advertising Age* January 14, 2002:3.

188. Sloan P. Lotions join war against bacteria. *Advertising Age* June 23, 1997:4.

189. Stelter B. Product placements, deftly woven into the story line. *New York Times* March 2, 2009. http:// www.nytimes.com/2009/03/02/business/media/02adco.html?scp=1&sq=product%20placements, %20deftly%20woven&st=cse (accessed July 30, 2009).

190. Steel E. Soap makers, others hitch ads to swine flu. *Wall Street Journal* April 30, 2009:B1.

191. In the News. Purell http://www.purell.com/page.jhtml?id=/purell/include/news.inc (accessed August 18, 2009).

192. Abelson J. Antiviral marketing. *Boston Globe* August 13, 2009:B1.

193. Cleanwell web site http://www.cleanwelltoday.com/ (accessed August 13, 2009).

194. Abelson J. Antiviral marketing: amid fears flu is headed back to school, too, germ fighters fill store shelves. Boston Globe August 13, 2009:B1, B8.

195. Soapopular Brand. http://www.soapyusa.com/ (accessed August 19, 2009).

196. Kids Hand Sanitizer arrives just in time for cold and flu season. September 14, 2009. http://www. businesswire.com/portal/site/home/permalink/?ndmViewId=news_view&newsId=20090914006037 &newsLang=en (accessed January 24, 2010).

197. McCay PH, Ocampo-Sosa AA, Fleming GTA. Effect of subinhibitory concentrations of benzalkonium chloride on the competitiveness of *Pseudomonas aeruginosa* grown in continuous culture. *Microbiology* 2010;156:30–38.

198. Danner P. Cleaning up with sanitizer. *San Antonio Express-News* December 17, 2009. http:// 74.125.113.132/search?q=cache:OgvVLCuDdeIJ:www.mysanantonio.com/business/Cleaning_up_ with_sanitizer.html+cleaning+up+with+sanitizer+%2Bpatrick+danner&cd=1&hl=en&t= clnk&gl=us (accessed December 18. 2009).

199. See also Steel E. Soap makers, others hitch ads to swine flu. *Wall Street Journal* April 30, 2009. http://online.wsj.com/article/SB124104831476470887.html (accessed April 30, 2009).

200. Franklin D.The consumer: hand sanitizers, good or bad? *New York Times* March 21, 2006. http://www.nytimes.com/2006/03/21/health/21cons.html?_r=1&scp=1&sq=hand%20sanitizers,%20good%20or%20bad?&st=cse (accessed May 26, 2009).

201. Forman J. Health answers: is the growing use of hand sanitizers changing the normal ecology of our hands, making it easier for the MRSA bacteria to grow? *Boston Globe* July 27, 2009:G7.

202. Parker-Pope. T. With soap and water or sanitizer, a cleaning that can stave off the flu. *The New York Times* September 15, 2009. http://www.nytimes.com/2009/09/15/science/15well.html?scp=1&sq=with%20soap%20and%20water%20or%20sanitizer&st=cse (accessed September 15, 2009).

203. Cooney E. Did you wash your hands? *Boston Globe* October 19, 2009. http://www.boston.com/news/health/articles/2009/10/19/did_you_wash_your_hands/ (accessed October 19, 2009).

204. Germs working overtime—especially at women's desks. http://files.shareholder.com/downloads/CLX/0x0x122195/dda4b770-cc99-4976-9b3d-fcbb2d2faa3e/CLX_News_2007_2_14_Brand_News.pdf (accessed January 24, 2010).

205. Landro L.Where the worst germs lurk. *Wall Street Journal* September 29, 2009. http://online.wsj.com/article/SB10001424052748703787204574440983321928144.html (accessed September 20, 2009).

206. King Jr. JC. The ABC's of H1N1. *New York Times* August 2, 2009. http://www.nytimes.com/2009/08/02/opinion/02king.html?scp=4&sq=children%20and%20hand%20sanitizers&st=cse (accessed August 10, 2009).

207. Consumer Product Ingredient Communication Initiative: Guidance for Participating Companies. Soap and Detergent Association web site http://www.cleaning101.com/ (accessed February 12, 2010).

208. Athavaley A. Defining 'natural' cleaners. *Wall Street Journal* February 11, 2010:D2.

209. Croman J. Franken seeks ingredient labeling for household cleansers. September 29, 2009. Organic Consumers Association web site http://www.organicconsumers.org/articles/article_19250.cfm (accessed February 12, 2010).

210. Peltz J. Cleanser makers told to come clean. *Boston Globe* February 5, 2010:B9.

211. Roach M. Germs, germs everywhere. Are you worried? Get over it. *New York Times*, November 9, 2004. http://www.nytimes.com/2004/11/09/health/09essa.html?r=1&scp=1&sq=germs,%20germs%20are%20everywhere&st=cse (accessed March 7, 2011).

212. Cortese A. An arsenal of sanitizers for a nation of germophobes. *New York Times*, February 27, 2005. http://www.nytimes.com/2005/02/27/business/yourmoney/27germ.html (accessed March 7, 2011).

213. Ruebush M. *Why Dirt Is Good: 5 Ways to Make Germs Your Friend.* New York: Kaplan Publishing, 2010.

214. Bialik C. Kills 99.9% of germs—under some lab conditions. *Wall Street Journal* December 16, 2009. http://online.wsj.com/article/SB126092257189692937.html (accessed December 20, 2009).

215. Singer H, Müller S, Tixier C, Pillonel L. Triclosan: occurrence and fate of a widely used biocide in the aquatic environment: field measurements in wastewater treatment plants, surface waters, and lake sediments. *Environ. Sci. Technol.* 2002;36(23):4998–5004.

216. Chalew TEA, Halden RU. Environmental exposure of aquatic and terrestrial biota to triclosan and triclocarban. *J. Am. Water Resour. Assoc.* 2009;45(1):4–13.

217. Levy SB. Antibacterial household products: a cause for concern. *Emerg. Infect. Dis.* 2001; 7(3):512–515.

218. Aiello AE, Larson EL, Levy SB. Consumer antibacterial soaps: effective or just risky? *Clin. Infect. Dis.* 2007;45(5):S137–S147.

219. Aiello AE, Coulborn RM, Perez V, Larson EL. Effect of hand hygiene on infectious disease risk in the community setting: a meta-analysis. *AJPH* 2008;98(8):1372–1381.

220. The use of antimicrobial household products: APIC 1997 Guidelines Committee Position Statement. APIC News 1997;6:13.

221. Bakalar N. Many don't wash hands after using the bathroom. *New York Times* September 27, 2005. http://www.nytimes.com/2005/09/27/health/27wash.html?scp=1&sq=don't%20wash%20hands&st=cse. (accessed June 20, 2009).

CHAPTER 2

ETHICAL RESPONSIBILITIES IN FORMULATING, MARKETING, AND USING ANTIMICROBIAL PERSONAL PRODUCTS

Kenneth A. Richman

Massachusetts College of Pharmacy and Health Sciences, Boston, MA

Antimicrobial personal care products such as antibacterial hand soaps have become widely used in the United States and other industrialized countries. They are attractive because we value cleanliness and because some microorganisms pose serious threats to human health. However, use, misuse, and overuse of antibacterial products have been blamed for contributing to the rise of dangerous antibiotic-resistant infectious agents such as methicillin-resistant *Staphylococcus aureus* (MRSA) and have been associated with endocrine disruption and toxic by-products.

This chapter discusses these issues from the perspective of philosophical ethics. Relevant ethical questions include the following: Who (if anyone) is to blame for any ill effects of antimicrobial products? Do consumers have a responsibility to avoid using antimicrobial products? Is it morally wrong to market antimicrobial products to consumers? What are the responsibilities of scientists in the face of inflammatory news stories and Internet sites denouncing antimicrobials? Should antimicrobial products be controlled more strictly? How should we act in the face of uncertainty about whether projected harms from these products will come about? Good answers to these questions will depend on facts about the world, but these questions are not just about plain facts. As questions of ethics, they concern how things ought to be, not simply how things are.

The chapter begins with a discussion of some of the scientific background relevant to the impact of antimicrobial products. Next, the concepts of ethics, aesthetics, and health are explored to shed light on the values relevant to our duties in this area. It is argued that aesthetic values should not be allowed to distract us from our ethical duties. After identifying some of the responsibilities of individuals and corporations, it is argued that the issue is best understood in the context of public

Innate Immune System of Skin and Oral Mucosa: Properties and Impact in Pharmaceutics, Cosmetics, and Personal Care Products, First Edition. Nava Dayan and Philip W. Wertz.

health. As with much in philosophy, the goal is not so much to come to specific answers as to map the terrain on which answers must lie. In the process, concepts and conflicts become clarified so that the significance of questions, policies, and disagreements comes into view and work toward solutions can become more productive and ethically responsible.

2.1   BACKGROUND: ANTIMICROBIAL PRODUCTS

Antimicrobial ingredients have been added to a variety of personal and home care products, including hand soaps, dishwashing liquids, antiperspirants, toothpastes, and clothing fabrics. They have also been added to plastics used for shower curtains and other bathroom accessories and even to computer keyboards.

For a variety of historical, cultural, and scientific reasons, there appear to be three options for antimicrobial agents in personal products. Triclocarbans can be effective on body odor, but are effective only on resident skin (Gram-positive) flora. Parachlorometaxylenol (PCMX), sold in the United Kingdom and India as Dettol, also prevents body odor, but has a distinctive smell that limits its use for personal care products. Triclosan is effective against Gram-negative bacteria, which makes it more effective against the microbes that pose greater threats to individuals. Triclosan is oil soluble and can be incorporated into a variety of formulations.

Other antimicrobial agents are less appropriate for personal care products. Alcohol is effective on a variety of microbes, including viruses, but is not attractive for international marketing because Muslims won't use it. Iodine is a slow but persistent antimicrobial, but poses aesthetic challenges because it stains skin and clothing. Chlorhexadine was developed after the relevant FDA regulations took effect, and so missed being included in the grandfather clause allowing the use of established ingredients. In addition, chlorhexadine is cationic, so it could be used only in liquids and may be irritating when used in personal product applications. Quaternary ammonium compounds (quats) are good for surfaces, but are also cationic, which limits their applications.

Triclosan is therefore the ingredient of choice for antimicrobial personal care products. It is the active ingredient in a wide variety of antimicrobial products, including Odor Eaters socks, liquid soaps, underarm deodorants, toothpastes, and hard plastics such as toilet paper dispensers.

Although home use of personal care products applied to the skin is of greatest relevance to this book, some of the most significant uses of triclosan have been in medical devices. For instance, catheters with antimicrobial properties have been shown to reduce patients' need for antibiotics. Studies by Bayston et al. [1] on antimicrobial-impregnated catheters for continuous ambulatory peritoneal dialysis and by Cadieux et al. [2] on ureteral stents suggest that triclosan can help reduce the need for antibiotic treatment. This can reduce cost, risk of drug interactions, and length of hospital stays, and can reduce the overall amounts of antimicrobials (including antibiotic medications) released into the environment.

The scientific claims about triclosan have been the subject of controversy. Much of this controversy seems to arise from different reactions to accepted facts.

For instance, it is accepted that triclosan reacts with water to form chloroform [3]. Some find this to be categorically unacceptable; others judge the quantity of chloroform to be insignificant. Because it is oil soluble, triclosan sticks to naturally occurring lipids on our skin. To some this looks like a wonderful added protection; others worry about weak residual activity that may lead to the rise of resistant strains of bacteria. Measurable levels of triclosan have been found in human urine, milk, sea mammals, estuary waters, and so on. While some activists claim that this portends an environmental disaster, many scientists are simply impressed by the ability of modern instruments to measure the presence of any substance at such tiny concentrations (less than one hundredth of a microgram per liter in some cases).

Triclosan works by targeting a specific enzyme in bacteria, and bacteria have been found with mutations that resist triclosan's antibacterial mechanism [4]. On the other hand, industry insiders tell that when bacteria common today are compared with collections of historical strains of bacteria, little or no difference is found in resistance to triclosan.

Lack of information about triclosan has also elicited diverse reactions. In 2000, the American Medical Association's Council on Scientific Affairs called for further investigation to examine the concerns that triclosan may be responsible for the emergence of antibiotic-resistant bacteria [5]. Favero [6] argues just 2 years later (and citing very little research done in the interim) that there is no good evidence for the claim that triclosan use leads to resistant bacterial strains and that, therefore, "Although there may be an overuse of germicides in these [health care and home] settings the consequence is a cost issue and not one that involves the development of antibiotic resistant microorganisms" ([6], p. 72S). Fiss et al. [3] call for caution and more investigation on the potentially hazardous by-products of triclosan, such as chloroform.

Given the controversy, it is reasonable to ask whether using these products provides much benefit over regular soaps. Some investigations have concluded that antimicrobial soaps with triclosan make a significant difference when it comes to removing bacteria from the skin [7]. On the other hand, it is widely accepted that antimicrobial soaps do not offer a clear hygiene advantage over traditional products in realistic household practice:

> Generally, plain soaps *do not kill* microorganisms, but rather wash them off with the soap, with the help of friction and rubbing. As a result, the majority of microorganisms picked up in daily life are removed. Handwashing with plain soap and water for 15 seconds reduces skin bacterial counts by 50 to 90%, and washing for 30 seconds reduces counts by 90 to 99%. For general home use—when household members are healthy—plain soaps are adequate for removing microbes. (*Source*: Ref. 8, p. 101.)

It should also be noted that not all bacteria on our hands are unwelcome and that antimicrobial soaps do not target disease germs over desirable normal resident flora.

The science of antimicrobials and the skin will be covered properly elsewhere in this book. The scientific issues raised here are meant to provide a minimal basis for the discussion that follows.

2.2 ETHICS, AESTHETICS, AND HEALTH

The goal of this chapter is to explore the ethical issues and values relevant to the development, marketing, and use of antimicrobial personal care products. In this context, it can be difficult to sort through the relationships among three concepts: ethics, aesthetics, and health. These areas are related but should not be confused.

Defining health can be a complex affair (cf. Ref. 9). For our purposes here, let us take health as a biomedical concept. We will assume that it is possible to determine an individual's health status on the basis of observable quantifiable criteria (e.g., blood tests) and that the criteria themselves can be identified on the basis of universal, validated facts. This is a limited, idealized notion of health. It ignores facts about how disease concepts have evolved through history, and may not leave room for mental health per se. However, objectivity, universality, and being based in observable, scientifically measurable variables are all aspects of our modern Western notion of health, at least of health of the body physiologically [10].

Having a healthy body may be valuable in a variety of ways and for a variety of reasons. This does not mean that health is a value concept in itself. In contrast, ethics and aesthetics deal directly with values.

Ethical values help us to determine what is good and bad in behavior. Ethics helps us to identify which actions are permissible, impermissible, obligatory, better, or worse. Some people believe that there is no objective basis for ethics and that no claim about the moral value of an action is better justified than any other. A less repugnant view is that there is a range of acceptable ethical claims. Most people would agree that while there is not just one permissible way to live life, not anything goes. Some actions are just not OK, and would never be acceptable even if an entire community or culture agreed that it was acceptable. The atrocities committed by the Nazis or the Khmer Rouge can be used as examples. The point is that even if everyone in the world decided that sending people to life-threatening forced labor in concentration camps or killing fields was ethically permissible, they would still be wrong. Ethics is not (or not *just*) about culture, politics, or what people believe.

It is possible to believe that an action is morally wrong without being able to say why it is wrong. Even when people tend to agree that some action is wrong, such as randomly killing people or torturing animals, folks will disagree, sometimes intensely, over why. The reasons we give for the judgment that some action is morally wrong can be significant in assessing whether we got the particular case correct, and in the implications of our judgment for other relevant cases. For instance, a utilitarian might say that truth telling is morally required because lying tends to cause unhappiness, whereas others might say that truth telling is morally required because lying is simply a bad thing to do. (Although some distinguish between ethics and morals, I do not find that a useful distinction; here 'ethical' and 'moral' are used with the same meaning.)

In addition to getting the value-related reasons right, it is also important to get the facts right. Descartes believed that vivisection, the dissection of animals while they are still alive, was ethically permissible because animals could feel no pain. Now that we have a different understanding of what it means to feel pain, someone might say that Descartes's position on this ethical issue was wrong not on the basis of the ethical values involved, but because he got his facts wrong. In applied ethics, facts and values must come together to support any claim about what is right or wrong.

It is also possible to believe that an action is morally wrong and not be motivated to avoid that action. (Some philosophers disagree with this claim.) This is particularly true when the action is like lowering one's carbon footprint or avoiding the overuse of antibacterial skin products. The impact of these actions is incremental. The real threat is from many millions of people, not just from little old me, so we may not have a sense that we are doing anything too terribly wrong when we go against our values on these items.

Aesthetics is the system of values concerning beauty and art. Philosophers working in the field of aesthetics might, for example, examine what gives da Vinci's Mona Lisa greater artistic value than my photograph of that famous painting. Some who work in the practical arts of applying cosmetics and beauty treatments call themselves aestheticians. As with ethics, philosophers have debated whether aesthetic values depend on universal facts or on social/cultural contingencies. Here, cultural relativism seems less objectionable. As with ideals of ethics and health, Western ideals of female beauty have famously changed, and have included the curves depicted by Rubens and the straight lines of Twiggy. Putting aside the ways in which ideals of beauty can be used to harm women, the fact that there are such ideals and that they change is not in itself morally bad. The same can be said of other aesthetic values.

Values concerning personal cleanliness, style, and hygiene fall under the umbrella of aesthetics. Certainly, we are in the sway of contingent cultural forces in our views of beauty; as Tebbe-Grossman and Gardner (Chapter 1) show, the same can be said of our views on personal hygiene. There does not seem to be anything terribly objectionable about this fact. Being aware of it can help us to understand our choices and to make changes when we find that our aesthetic values conflict with health or ethics.

Aesthetic judgments can be connected to health judgments. For instance, we often judge healthy-looking people to be beautiful. A 1976 magazine advertisement for Ivory soap's "Nominate the Ivory Girl" campaign had a bold invitation: "Ivory girls of America . . . Show off your healthy looking skin!" [11]. Lovelock, famous for the Gaia hypothesis, wrote

> Another of our instincts which probably favours survival is that which associates fitness and due proportion with beauty in individuals. (*Source*: Ref. 12, p. 143.)[1]

Lovelock suggests that we connect healthy traits with beauty because this lends a selective advantage.

But we know that aesthetic values and health can diverge. We can look back with regret on the dark "San Tropez tan" valued in the 1970s or on returning trends toward overly thin fashion models. I doubt that anyone really viewed the bound

---

[1] Lovelock even connects beauty with scientific truth, not only in quoting Keats ("Beauty is truth, truth beauty. . .") but also by suggesting that, perhaps, ". . .beauty also is associated with lowered entropy, reduced uncertainty, and less vagueness" ([12], p. 143).

female feet historically considered beautiful in certain Asian cultures to be healthy (except insofar as they might attract wealthy suitors and increase the likelihood of survival and reproduction in particular communities). Aesthetics and health are connected, but not necessarily so. It is quite possible, even likely, for us to find aesthetically valuable something that is quite unhealthy. The ideal of ridding our skin of bacteria is probably an example.

Like aesthetics, ethics has often been connected with health in Western consciousness:

> . . . societies have throughout history developed complex and sophisticated explanations for the causes and prevalence of disease. Embedded in these explanatory frames are deeply held, if often unstated, sensibilities about right and wrong, good and bad, responsibility and danger. (*Source*: Ref. 13, p. 1.)

Illness has been blamed on evil spirits, sexual immorality, or general lack of virtue (cf. Ref. 14). This nexus of ethical and medical ideas rings of blaming the victim, a theme that has been weakened but not extinguished by modern explanations of disease and illness.

Ethics can also diverge from health. In general, we have a duty to protect our health and those of other human beings. However, there may be times when we have an ethical obligation to act in unhealthy ways. Protesters on hunger strike put their health in danger to meet what they see as their ethical obligations. So do those who volunteer for wars they see as justified. There are times when we accept a patient's choice to refuse care and be allowed to die even when this means that his/her health will decline faster than it otherwise would.

Even if we do not treat health as valuable in itself like ethical and aesthetic values, we do value health. Health contributes to happiness and human life, both of which can be described as intrinsically valuable.

When it comes to determining how we may or must act, ethics is by definition the guide. We might wonder what we should do in order to reach some goal—in order to make ourselves more beautiful or healthier, for example. But we can still ask whether these are the right goals to pursue. Any answer to the simple question "What should we do?" is an ethical judgment. This means that aesthetic values may not be used as an excuse for what is immoral. Demand from the public is not a good excuse for providing an unsafe or ineffective product. We might even say that the personal care products industry has a responsibility to use its influence on popular ideals of hygiene in ways that balance the interests of all stakeholders.

2.3   RESPONSIBILITIES OF INDIVIDUALS AND ORGANIZATIONS

Individuals (whether scientists, marketing executives, or consumers) have ethical responsibilities. These will overlap with the responsibilities of corporations, such as companies developing and marketing personal care products. Individuals may have duties based on relationships (e.g., kinship relationships) that corporations do not have; corporations may have duties to shareholders and other stakeholders that individuals do not have. What are some responsibilities relevant to developing and marketing antimicrobial products? Let us consider some responsibilities we might have to other humans, to ourselves, to other species, and even to the Earth itself.

2.3.1 Responsibilities to Other Humans and Ourselves

The great enlightenment philosopher Immanuel Kant famously wrote that we have a duty to *treat humanity, whether in ourselves or in others, always as an end in itself and never as a means only* [15]. Humanity has inherent value, and we have a responsibility to preserve and promote what is inherently valuable. We also have a responsibility not to use people for our own purposes without at the same time treating them with dignity and respect. For instance, I may not persuade consumers to use a product that I know is bad for them simply so that I can make a profit. As Kant makes clear, if other humans are valuable in themselves, then, as a human, so am I. Each of us therefore has a responsibility to look after ourselves.

Two important ways of thinking can be distinguished here. On one, there are certain actions (such as using people) that are simply impermissible. This approach, called deontology, does not emphasize the consequences of an action, but focuses on the action itself. A contrasting approach holds that the consequences of an action are what count ethically. On this approach, called consequentialism, the type of action does not matter so much as whether net harm or net benefit results from the action. The most common consequentialist theory is utilitarianism. Utilitarianism holds that the morally relevant consequences of an action are happiness and unhappiness. While Kant and other deontologists emphasize treating people with respect or dignity, utilitarians emphasize maximizing happiness (pleasure) or well-being.

Even if we do not accept a responsibility to promote the well-being of our fellow humans, we at least have a responsibility to avoid harming them. J. S. Mill's "harm principle" [16] states that individual liberties should be limited only by our duty not to harm others. Developing, distributing, or using a product that has detrimental effects, such as contributing to the emergence of treatment-resistant pathogenic microorganisms, could be construed as a violation of the harm principle, which is akin to what bioethicists call the principle of nonmaleficence (*primum non nocere*: first do no harm).

Uncertainty complicates the matter. We cannot predict the future with certainty. Even where we can quantify the risk as a percent chance of a specific harm, how do we assess responsibility for what might not happen or, once it has happened, what might not have happened? That is, determining the therapeutic window in the face of uncertainty is especially challenging.

2.3.2 Responsibilities to Future Humans: Intergenerational Justice

In addition to responsibilities to other human beings alive now, we may also have responsibility to people who do not yet exist. Psychologically, we tend to take events less seriously when they are remote in time. This, no doubt, affects behaviors such as overeating and smoking—a nicotine hit now is more important to the smoker than lung cancer later. This is not only because the cancer is only a probabilistic event but also because of the ways in which we "discount" the future. Some philosophers and economists have suggested that benefits and harms far in the future should not count as much in the risk/benefit analysis as those we would enjoy or suffer soon (cf. Ref. 17 for a discussion).

This raises issues of *intergenerational justice*. Justice is about the distribution of benefits and burdens. Questions about taxation and social services are questions about justice. A fair distribution is just, an unfair distribution unjust. Parfit rejects the idea of discounting future events, "The moral importance of future events does *not* decline at n percent per year. A mere difference in timing is in itself morally neutral" ([18], p. 31).

> Consider predicted deaths from escaped radiation. According to a discount rate of 5 percent, one death next year counts for more than a billion deaths in 400 years. Compared with the single death, the billion deaths are less important to prevent. (*Source*: Ref. 18, p. 32.)

This "indefensible" ([18], p. 33) result shows us that discounting for the future is unreasonable. Application to the present topic is clear: if we should find that there are bad effects of triclosan but that they will not occur for a long time, the time delay will not in itself be a reason to think that we need not take the effects seriously.

2.3.3   Responsibilities to Other Species

The actual effects of triclosan on other species are controversial, but as we survey the responsibilities that may be relevant to the marketing and use of antimicrobials, we should not ignore the fact that humans are not the only ones exposed.

Humans are affected by what happens to animals in many ways. I worry when my cat is ill, and farm animals can spread disease among humans. Some of our responsibilities to humans will require that we tend to the welfare of animals. But do we have responsibilities to help or not to harm the animals just for themselves, independently of effects on people? Philosophers call this the question of *moral standing*. If something has moral standing, it counts—we are responsible for considering it in our deliberations about what to do.

Some traditions deny that any nonhuman animals have moral standing. This can be defended on the basis that only humans were made in the image of God or on the basis that moral standing requires self-awareness and the ability to choose freely what to do.[2] Others will say that all sentient animals have moral standing because they have interests that can be harmed (cf. Ref. 19). The utilitarian Peter Singer has argued that animal pains and pleasures count in utilitarian calculations, and that

---

[2] "It has always been a firmly held concept in the fields of law, ethics, and government that for every right we enjoy, there is a corresponding duty which we must fulfill" ([31], p. 26). "We know that animals can never be held to a set of legal *duties*—like not killing each other—because . . . their behavior is governed solely by instinct; they cannot distinguish right from wrong; they have no moral sense as humans do" ([31], p. 27).

failing to count these pains and pleasures is "speciesism pure and simple, and it is as indefensible as the most blatant racism" ([20], p. 6).

This is obviously related to the issue of animal rights. As Tom Beauchamp puts it:

> Animals have moral standing; that is, they have properties (including the ability to feel pain) that qualify them for the protections of morality. It follows from this that humans have moral obligations toward animals, and because rights are logically correlative to obligations, animals have rights. (*Source*: Ref. 21, p. 113.)

I will not defend any claim about the moral standing of animals. However, if we do have responsibilities toward animals, then the same issues of intergenerational justice apply—we are responsible to both future animals and present ones.

2.3.4   Responsibilities to Mother Earth

The moral status of animals falls under the general category of environmental ethics, but environmental ethics also addresses the question of whether the concept of moral standing applies to the environment as a whole. As with questions about the status of animals, much of the discussion in this area addresses anthropocentrism and what it might mean to reject it.

Merchant argued that "Each part contributes equal value to the healthy functioning of the whole. All living things, as integral parts of a viable ecosystem, thus have rights." ([22], p. 293). As Beauchamp suggested, rights and responsibilities are linked. If each part of the ecosystem has rights, then we have responsibilities to respect these rights (not to violate them).

Another approach has been to shift the level at which we consider the environment and its components. We have become accustomed to thinking of the moral world as made up of individual people or perhaps people and animals. However, some have argued that there is another, more (or equally) significant level—that of the environment, nature, or the Earth as a whole. The most famous version of this approach is called the Gaia hypothesis: "The Gaia hypothesis implies that the stable state of our planet includes man as a part of, or partner in, a very democratic entity" ([12], p. 145). One version of the Gaia hypothesis holds that the Earth itself has moral standing, and we have responsibilities to respect the stability and integrity of the Earth [23].

2.3.5   Legal Liability as a Conceptual Framework for How These Responsibilities Might Be Applied

Law is not ethics. However, some laws are intended to reflect ethical values, and concepts and categories from law can be helpful in thinking about moral responsibility. Here, let us consider the ways in which structures from the U.S. products liability law can be helpful in thinking about responsibility for the harmful effects of one's actions.

Product liability is treated somewhat differently from state to state. In some instances, the governing concept is *negligence*. Negligence is breach of duty to use reasonable care. In the present context, there is a duty to use reasonable care in design and manufacture of products. As negligence is not so much concerned with consequences as with what the responsible party did or did not do, this is a deontological concept. We have a duty to take reasonable care, and have done something wrong if we do not do so.[3] Note that taking reasonable care involves being in the right mental state. We must think about the potential dangers or effects of our product as designed, think about what might reasonably go wrong in the manufacturing process to meet the design, and take appropriate steps to avoid harming others. If things happen to go wrong anyway, one is not guilty of negligence.

A different standard that applies in some legal settings is *strict liability*. Strict liability is a consequentialist concept. Under strict liability, it does not matter what one was thinking or how carefully the design and manufacture of a product were undertaken. If harm occurred, there is responsibility.[4]

The kinds of damages discussed in the context of triclosan invoke catastrophic events such as unstoppable deadly infections and the extinction of species whose reproductive systems have been disrupted (think along the lines of Rachel Carson's *Silent Spring* [24]). Thus, the type of liability taken on in various jurisdictions may have enormous consequences for those designing, manufacturing, and selling antimicrobial products, both from ethical and from legal standpoints.

No one would like to see triclosan or antimicrobials as a whole become the next DDT or DES. Both of these promised net benefits (control of pests such as malarial mosquitoes for DDT; preventing miscarriage for DES), but both were promoted long after it was known that the specific uses caused more harm than benefit [24,25]. Citing scientific studies and government reports, some objectors suggest that we may be there already with triclosan (see, for example, a web site titled "What's Lurking in Your Soap? The Trouble with Triclosan" [26]).

Some parties claim that triclosan has already been proven to be very dangerous indeed. If this is so, then some players in the personal care products industry have acted reprehensibly and may face serious consequences. One alternative is that the scientific record shows the net effects of triclosan to be more or less neutral. In that case, consumers may have spent more than needed to get the same results, but this would not make this case different from so many others, especially with luxury products. Creating perception of need for products that do not add to our well-being is an accepted part of the game in what is sometimes called "late capitalism."

---

[3] In law, there is no negligence unless there are damages. This is obviously a consequentialist aspect of the legal concept of negligence. A deontologist might say that failure to take reasonable precautions is a bad thing to do even when no damage results.

[4] In addition to negligence and strict liability, American product liability law can invoke implied warranties of merchantability (that the product is fit for the ordinary purposes of that type of product, meets industry standards, etc.) and fitness (fitness applies when a product is sold for a specific intended purpose and applies only to those who regularly deal in the type of product).

But what if we allow that the long-term cost–benefit ratio for triclosan is really unknown? As the legal concept of negligence points out, we expect responsible parties to take reasonable precautions. Relevant questions should be asked, tests run, and answers sought. The reasonableness required to avoid negligence requires care and thoughtfulness, but it does not require omniscience.

Some level of risk is acceptable, but consumers do not expect personal care products to increase their risk above the level of their ordinary activities. This background level of risk (which is called "minimal risk" in research ethics) could be used as part of a standard of reasonableness in this context. However, when presented with claims about risk, consumers often put their everyday risks out of mind and assume that any risk at all is an increase over what they started with. This is similar to concerns raised about measurable amounts of lead in lipstick when the actual exposure from lipstick use is lower than for many things we happily ingest [27]. Public reaction is not always a good indication of whether a product is actually acceptable.

Of course, the discussion is not solely about the actual risks of using the product. If the risk level is unknown, industry must concern itself with the risk that there will turn out to be risk. This metarisk must be considered. Industry players need to consider the likelihood that a product will turn out to have bad effects, and how to balance different scenarios, such as a very small likelihood of causing great harm and a greater likelihood of causing a small harm.

In a different context, Robert F. Card has rejected what he calls "the zero probability argument." According to this argument,

> Persons should not perform an action unless it is true that there is a zero probability that their action (or their contribution to an action) will issue in immoral results. The zero probability argument leads to absurd results because the mere possibility of contributing to immoral results exists with virtually anything a human being does ... More specifically, the mere possibility of contributing to wrongdoing applies to many acts performed by a medical professional (e.g., dispensing cold and sinus medicines that might be abused in various ways) and would suggest that such professionals should stop assisting patients in general. This is unacceptable; it is simply unreasonable to withhold medication because of the *mere possibility* that this may contribute to an immoral result. (*Source*: Ref. 28, p. 11.)

There is always some level of concern that we are wrong about the safety of some substance or practice. (This is the basis of some memorable jokes is in Woody Allen's *Sleeper*.) It is unreasonable to expect industry to withhold any product that has a nonzero chance of having ill effects.

But what if reasonable care is taken and we turn out to be unlucky? We can be responsible for bad results without being blameworthy for the action that led to these results. If I make a legitimate mistake despite taking reasonable precautions, or if the brakes on my car fail despite regular maintenance, I can be responsible for making restitution even though I did nothing culpable. This is the idea captured by the legal concept of strict liability. Unlike negligence, strict liability does not require a *mens rea* (guilty mind).

We can see how the ethical considerations depend not only on the facts of how people act but also on the scientific facts. Negligence is illegal and immoral. It is also imprudent because reasonable care helps to avoid financial losses and other harms. On the other hand, a corporation could be found responsible under strict liability even when we would not say that there was wrongdoing. The latter case may simply be bad luck.

2.4   A PRISONER'S DILEMMA

Stories about increasingly dangerous microorganisms such as MRSA are likely increasing consumers' sense that they need antibacterial products to protect themselves even when those very products are blamed for the emergence of these "bugs." This creates what philosophers have called a prisoner's dilemma.[5] If it turns out that widespread use of these products actually does have very bad consequences, then the group as a whole would do best if everyone stopped. However, it seems to be in my interest for everyone *else* to stop using these products while I continue. That way I get the protection without the damage. I know that others also recognize this fact, but I don't want to be without whatever advantage the others get from using the product.

Where the interests of individuals are or appear to be in conflict with the interests of the group as a whole, responsible conduct becomes a social matter. That is, it makes sense in such cases to limit the choices that individuals have in order to promote the interests of the group and thus the (average) well-being of individuals in the group. This is when we start thinking not about the ethics of individuals but of policy.

2.5   A PUBLIC HEALTH APPROACH

A move to the level of public health can be described as a move away from an ethics of responsibility to a communitarian ethics. Communitarian approaches avoid blaming individual components of the community. Communitarians tend to question the concept of individual choice as the basis of ethics and ethical analysis. For our purposes, we can treat communitarian approaches as simply an alternate level of examination that is more fitting for some topics than for others.

Public health ethics recognizes that

> ... the world of harms is not exhausted by self-imposed and other-imposed injuries. There is a third and very large set of problems that affects the community as a whole and that results primarily from inadequate safeguards over the practices of the common life.

---

[5] The name derives from the classic formulation of the dilemma, in which two prisoners are separated and must decide independently whether to confess to a crime where the consequences for each depend on what the other does.

Economists and others often refer to this class of harms as "summing up problems" or "choice-in-the-small" rather than "choice-in-the-large." (*Source*: Ref. 29, p. 66.)

If there are ill effects from triclosan-containing products, they result from the sum of many small choices that may seem to have little impact in themselves. The public health/communitarian level of approach is required here because looking for actions that make one individual is responsible for harming another gives us no traction on the issue.[6]

The goals of public health policies and campaigns include changes in behaviors and attitudes. These can be pursued by education (e.g., via public service announcements) or by imposing paternalistic restrictions (such as seatbelt laws). The basic assumption is that there are some goods for which it is permissible to limit the freedom of individuals.

2.5.1 Public Health and the Case Against Antimicrobials

The above considerations provide material for some arguments in favor of regulating or banning triclosan in personal care products for everyday home use. For instance, a case could be made that the likelihood that there will turn out to be substantial harm from continued widespread use of triclosan-containing products is too high to allow continued use without restrictions. The assessment of this likelihood would no doubt be contentious. So would the determination that this degree of likelihood, if low or moderate, is unacceptable. It is hard to imagine anyone, particularly policy makers whose deliberations are subject to public scrutiny, offering sufficiently clear and effective justifications for these types of determinations.

If we accept that antimicrobials are not necessary for adequate personal hygiene in households where the people are generally healthy, we might claim that the ways in which many antimicrobial products are marketed are deceptive and, as Favero suggests, merely take consumer's money for no benefit. This, too, would be a difficult claim to support given what we allow in the marketing of other products.

We might, however, use a determination that triclosan confers no benefit to support a version of the zero probability argument that sidesteps Card's objections: even a small chance of harm is unacceptable in an ingredient offering no benefit at all. This looks like the strongest position for changes in the way triclosan is regulated. This argument, if found to be based on fact, could support limiting access to triclosan-containing products to licensed health clinics or to consumers by prescription only.

---

[6] "Strengthening the public health includes not only the practical task of improving aggregate welfare, it also involves the task of reacquainting the American public with its republican and communitarian heritage, and encouraging citizens to share in reasonable and practical group schemes to promote a wider welfare, of which their own welfare is only a part" ([29], p. 67).

2.5.2   Public Health and the Case for Antimicrobials

The theory that some diseases are caused by microorganisms has not been around forever, and neither has the idea that hand washing and other hygiene practices can help limit the spread of disease. Lever Brothers' campaign for Lifebuoy following the cholera epidemic of the 1890s was an early effort to tout the health-related benefits of soap. Part of the campaign was to link the otherwise off-putting smell of the soap to its effectiveness as a health aid: "The mild carbolic odour you note in Lifebuoy Soap is the sign of its splendid protective qualities" [30]. Sweeter smelling soaps may have been just as good for the consumer's health, but the medicinal smell offered an observable indication that Lifebuoy did something significant.

The effectiveness of providing external confirmation of the health benefits of washing provides the basis of a significant argument in support of promoting antimicrobials for home use. The argument was offered by an industry insider who asked not to be named. It is a pretty good argument, but one those in the personal care products industry will not stand behind. It goes like this: Without the claims (and, where necessary, the stink to back up these claims), people won't practice good hygiene. People need to be reminded that hygiene is important; antimicrobial products remind people. This is why we need the products. Promoting these products is promoting basic hygiene and therefore makes the community healthier. These effects could be obtained from regular soap, but that's just not how consumers behave. Therefore, the benefits of triclosan-containing personal care products are substantial and outweigh some risk of harm.

Again, the success of this argument depends on facts. In this case, the relevant facts are about consumer behavior and the balance between benefits and potential for harm. This argument also raises the question of whether consumers could be educated to practice good hygiene without looking (or sniffing) for active ingredients.

2.6   CONCLUSIONS

Our discussion has identified several values relevant to the development and marketing of products containing triclosan. First, we saw that while aesthetics involves values, these values are not the ultimate guides for actions in the way that ethics is. We can ask whether it is right to pursue beauty; it makes no sense to ask whether it is right to do what is right. Next, we discussed the types of things that can be held to have moral standing. These included, on various theories, people, future people, animals, all elements of the natural environment, and the natural environment as a whole. Following this discussion, we looked at the legal concepts of negligence and strict liability, which allow us to distinguish between being guilty of failing to take appropriate precautions (negligence) and simply being responsible for the results of one's actions (strict liability). Obviously, these values and concepts are relevant to many issues affecting many industries. Triclosan-containing personal care products just happen to be the items most relevant to this book.

For those who believe that widespread use of antimicrobials is dangerous, a prisoner's dilemma arises in which the interests of individuals seem to conflict with the interests of the group. In this type of circumstance, it makes sense to move from a discussion of the rights and responsibilities of individuals to a discussion of policy and public health. The strongest argument in favor of restricting the use of triclosan depends on two claims: that it offers no benefit and that it has some chance of causing harm. The strongest argument against restricting use is that even if triclosan itself adds no direct benefit, substantial benefit accrues when having these products on the market improves consumer hygiene behavior by reminding us that cleanliness can prevent illness. This argument depends on the assumption that there is no better way to get the same behavioral results from the public. We may not ever be able to assess the truth of these claims to the satisfaction of all parties. As a philosopher, I am not in a position to answer them at all. My job is done if the questions have now been more clearly articulated.

ACKNOWLEDGMENTS

For significant assistance with this chapter, I am indebted to Nava Dayan, Nicolette Nagamatsu, and an industry insider who wishes to remain anonymous.

REFERENCES

1. Bayston R, Fisher LE, Weber K. An antimicrobial modified silicone peritoneal catheter with activity against both Gram-positive and Gram-negative bacteria. *Biomaterials* 2009;30:3167–3173.
2. Cadieux PA, Chew BH, Nott L, Seney S, Elwood CN, Wignall GR, Goneau LW, Denstedt JD. Use of triclosan-eluting ureteral stents in patients with long-term stents. *J. Endourol.* 2009;23:1187–1194.
3. Fiss EM, Rule KL, Vikesland PJ. Formation of chloroform and other chlorinated byproducts by chlorination of triclosan-containing antibacterial products. *Environ. Sci. Technol.* 2007;41:2387–2394.
4. Schweizer HP. Triclosan: a widely used biocide and its link to antibiotics. *FEMS Microbiol. Lett.* 2001;202:1–7.
5. Tan L, Nielsen NH, Young DC, Trizna Z, Council on Scientific Affairs, American Medical Association. Use of antimicrobial agents in consumer products. *Arch. Dermatol.* 2002;138:1082–1086.
6. Favero MS. Products containing biocides: perceptions and realities. *Symp. Ser. Soc. Appl. Microbiol.* 2002;(31):72S–77S.
7. Fischler GE, Fuls JL, Dail EW, Duran MH, Rodgers ND, Waggoner AL. Effect of hand wash agents on controlling the transmission of pathogenic bacteria from hands to food. *J. Food Prot.* 2007;70:2873–2877.
8. Aiello AE, Larson EL, Sedlak R. *Against Disease: The Impact of Hygiene and Cleanliness on Health.* Washington, DC: The Soap and Detergent Association, 2007.
9. Richman KA. *Ethics and the Metaphysics of Medicine: Reflections on Health and Beneficence.* Cambridge, MA: MIT Press, 2004.
10. Szasz TS. The myth of mental illness. *Am. Psychol.* 1960;15:113–118.
11. Proctor & Gamble. Pure Fun: Ivory History, 2009. http://www.ivory.com/purefun_history.htm (accessed December 2009).
12. Lovelock J. *Gaia: A New Look at Life on Earth.* New York: Oxford University Press, 1979. p. 143.
13. Brandt AM, Rozin P. Introduction. In: Brandt AM, Rozin P, editors, *Morality and Health.* New York: Routledge, 1997. pp. 1–11.

14. Engelhardt HT. The disease of masturbation: values and the concept of disease. *Bull. Hist. Med.* 1974;48:234–248.
15. Kant I. *Foundations of the Metaphysics of Morals.* New York: Bobbs-Merrill, 1959.
16. Mill JS. *On Liberty.* New York: Bobbs-Merrill, 1956.
17. Broome J. Discounting the future. *Philos. Public Aff.* 1994;23:128–156.
18. Parfit D. Energy policy and the further future: the social discount rate. In: MacLean D, Brown PG, editors *Energy and the Future.* Totowa, NJ: Rowman & Littlefield, 1983. pp. 31–37.
19. DeGrazia D. *Taking Animals Seriously: Mental Life and Moral Status.* New York: Cambridge University Press, 1996.
20. Singer P. *In Defense of Animals.* New York: Blackwell, 1985.
21. Beauchamp TL. Opposing views on animal experimentation: do animals have rights? *Ethics Behav.* 1997;7:113–121.
22. Merchant C. *The Death of Nature: Women, Ecology, and the Scientific Revolution.* San Francisco, CA: Harper & Row, 1979.
23. Weston A. Forms of Gaian ethics. *Environ. Ethics* 1987;9:121–134.
24. Carson R. *Silent Spring.* Boston, MA: Houghton Mifflin, 2002.
25. Independent Television Service. A Healthy Baby Girl: DES Timeline, 1997. http://www.itvs.org/external/babyg/timeline.html (accessed January 2010).
26. Food and Water Watch and Beyond Pesticides. What's Lurking in Your Soap? The Trouble with Triclosan, 2008. http://www.foodandwaterwatch.org/water/chemical-contaminants/what-is-lurking-in-your-soap (accessed December 2009).
27. FDA. Lipstick and Lead: Questions and Answers, 2010. http://www.fda.gov/Cosmetics/ProductandIngredientSafety/ProductInformation/ucm137224.htm#q6 (accessed January 2010).
28. Card RF. Conscientious objection and emergency contraception. *Am. J. Bioeth.* 2007;7:8–14.
29. Beauchamp DE. Community: the neglected tradition of public health. *Hastings Cent. Rep.* 1985;15:28–36.
30. Lever Brothers. Lifebuoy advertisement. *Graphic* 1916, 707.
31. Pulver CR. Animals do not have rights. In: Chathran H, editor *Animal Experimentation: Opposing Viewpoints.* San Diego, CA: Greenhaven Press, 2002. pp. 25–43.

CHAPTER 3

ROLE OF STRATUM CORNEUM IN PERMEABILITY BARRIER FUNCTION AND ANTIMICROBIAL DEFENSE

Peter M. Elias[1,2]

[1]Department of Dermatology, University of California San Francisco Medical Center, San Francisco, CA
[2]Dermatology Service, VA Medical Center, San Francisco, CA

3.1 INTRODUCTION

Since life in a terrestrial environment threatens mammals continuously with desiccation, the research thrust of biologists has focused on epidermal, structural, cellular, biochemical, and regulatory mechanisms that sustain permeability barrier homeostasis. Yet, the epidermis mediates a broad set of additional defensive ("barrier") functions that include antimicrobial defense at the level of the stratum corneum (SC) (Table 3.1). While these various functions are mediated largely by either the corneocytes ("bricks") or the extracellular matrix ("mortar"), recent studies suggest that these functions may not be discrete. For example, the permeability and antimicrobial functions of the stratum corneum are both coregulated and interdependent, overlapping through multiple features of the SC that limit pathogen colonization, including its low water content, acidic pH, resident (normal) microflora, and surface-deposited antimicrobial lipids (primarily free fatty acids, monoglycerides, and sphingols). In addition, both the localization and the organization of secreted hydrophobic lipids into characteristic lamellar bilayers are critical for permeability barrier function, while also providing a formidable physical and biochemical barrier to pathogen invasion. Though some antimicrobial peptides are cosecreted into the SC interstices along with lipids, their low constitutive levels of expression under basal conditions emphasize the key role of SC structural integrity in regulating cutaneous antimicrobial defense.

Innate Immune System of Skin and Oral Mucosa: Properties and Impact in Pharmaceutics, Cosmetics, and Personal Care Products, First Edition. Nava Dayan and Philip W. Wertz.
© 2011 John Wiley & Sons, Inc. Published 2011 by John Wiley & Sons, Inc.

TABLE 3.1 Multiple Protective Functions of Mammalian Stratum Corneum

Function	Principal compartment	Structural basis	Chemical basis within SC	How regulated?
Permeability[a]	Extracellular matrix	Lamellar bilayers	Ceramides, cholesterol, nonessential FA in proper ratio ≈1:1:1 molar	IL-1α, Ca^{++}, PPAR/LXR, SP (klk) activation (PAR2)
Antimicrobial[a]	Extracellular matrix	Lamellar bilayers	Antimicrobial peptides, FFA, Sph, monoglycerides	1,25 $(OH)_2D_3$; IL-1α, TNFα, IFNγ
Antioxidant+	Extracellular matrix	Lamellar bilayers	Secreted vit. E; redox gradient; ?chol., FFA	Not known
Cohesion (integrity) → desquamation[a]	Extracellular matrix	Corneodesmosomes; lamellar bilayers	Intercellular DSG1/DSC1 homodimers	pH → SP activation
Mechanical/rheological	Corneocyte	Cornified envelope; keratin filaments	γ-Glutamyl isopeptide bonds	Ca^{++}, $CholSO_4$, PPARs, LXR
Chemical (antigen exclusion)[a]	Extracellular matrix	Lamellar bilayers	Hydrolytic products of CD (lacunar pathway)	Not known
Neurosensory interface	Outer epidermis	Keratinocyte membrane receptors		pH, thermal, osmotic Δ's (TPRV1–4)
Hydration	Corneocyte cytosol; extracellular lacunae	Aguaporin channels; CD hydrolytic products	Filaggrin proteolytic products; glycerol	Δ's in relative humidity (TPRV1)
Electromagnetic radiation	Corneocyte cytosol	UV filtration	Structural proteins; trans-urocanic acid	Δ's in relative humidity → histidase activity
Initiation of inflammation (1° cytokine activation)[a]	Corneocyte	Cytosol	Proteolytic activation of pro-IL-1α/β	↑pH → SP activation

[a]Regulated by stratum corneum pH.

3.2 EPIDERMIS MEDIATES MULTIPLE PROTECTIVE FUNCTIONS

Life in a xeric terrestrial environment threatens mammals continuously with desiccation. Hence, the structural, cellular, biochemical, and regulatory mechanisms that sustain permeability barrier homeostasis have justifiably occupied much attention from epidermal biologists in recent years [1,2]. Yet, the outer layers of the epidermis mediate a broad set of not-yet-fully-appreciated protective ("barrier") functions against microbial pathogen challenges, oxidant stress, incident ultraviolet light, mechanical insults, and shear resistance. Moreover, these layers serve as a distal outpost of the immune system (Table 3.1).

It is now generally accepted that most of the defensive (barrier) functions of the epidermis localize to the stratum corneum [2]. These various barrier functions are largely mediated by either the corneocyte or the extracellular matrix, and they further localize to specific subcompartments in each (e.g., corneocyte envelope versus cytosol) (Table 3.1). However, it is not only the localization but also the organization of secreted hydrophobic lipids into characteristic lamellar bilayers that is critical both for permeability barrier function and for antimicrobial defense and the maintenance of SC integrity [3].

A key concept to emerge in recent years emphasizes the SC not as a dead tissue, but rather as possessing multiple types of metabolic (primarily catabolic) activity in both the cytosolic and the membrane/extracellular compartments [4]. Much of this activity (1) generates the various "barriers" described above; (2) regulates desquamation; (3) results in the generation of endogenous UV filters and osmotically active ingredients; and/or (4) activates primary cytokines (Table 3.1).

3.3 BRIEF REVIEW OF PERMEABILITY BARRIER FUNCTION

The major function of the epidermis is to provide a protective barrier between the external environment and the organism [1,2,5,6]. To fulfill this function, keratinocytes undergo a vectorial path of outward differentiation, which culminates in corneocyte formation [7,8]. The parallel generation of the extracellular matrix, organized into multilayers of lamellar membranes, forms the intact stratum corneum [6]. While the SC provides several defensive functions, we have focused on two of these (the hydrophobic *permeability barrier*, which not only prevents the outward movement of water and electrolytes but also simultaneously blocks the ingress of xenobiotes and chemicals, and the *cutaneous antimicrobial barrier*, which prevents cutaneous infections).

The extracellular lamellar membranes in the SC, which contain predominantly cholesterol, free fatty acids (FFAs), and ceramides, in an approximate 1:1:1 molar ratio, derive from the secretion of lamellar body contents at the stratum granulosum–SC interface [9,10]. To generate lamellar bodies, epidermis synthesizes three families of lipids: free sterols (primarily cholesterol), phospholipids (including sphingomyelin), and glucosylceramides [10]. Once secreted, the polar lipid precursors are rapidly metabolized to FFA and ceramides by cosecreted sPLA2,

TABLE 3.2 Shared Structural and Biochemical Features of Permeability and Antimicrobial Barriers

Feature	Permeability barrier	Antimicrobial defense
Cohesive stratum corneum	+	+
Replete lamellar matrix	+	+
Low H_2O content of SC	+	+
Acidic pH of SC	+	+
SC extracellular lipids (e.g., FFA)	+	+
Secreted epidermal AMP (e.g., LL-37)	+	+
Secreted protease inhibitors	+	+
Normal microbial flora	?	+

β-glucocerebrosidase, and acidic sphingomyelinase [11]. Together, the resultant FFA, ceramides, and cholesterol form the mature lamellar membranes that mediate permeability barrier function [9]. Yet, the phospholipid-derived FFAs are important as structural constituents of the lamellar bilayers and also account for ≈1 pH unit toward the acidification of the SC [12], with multiple, positive downstream consequences [13]. Furthermore, FFAs are a potent antimicrobial species [14–17]. Finally, FFAs also derive from partial hydrolysis of preformed ceramides by two isoforms of ceramidase that are present in SC [18,19]. Hydrolysis of ceramides generates not only more FFA but also sphingosine [20], another potent cutaneous antimicrobial lipid [21]. These observations demonstrate the dualistic nature of SC lipid constituents as multifunctional ingredients of importance for both permeability barrier homeostasis and antimicrobial defense (Table 3.2).

3.4 CLINICAL RELEVANCE OF BARRIER FUNCTION

As a general mechanism, acute insults to the permeability barrier stimulate cytokine production, which if repeated can lead to inflammation ("outside–inside" provocation) [22,23]. Although a variety of immune mechanisms sustain cutaneous inflammatory dermatoses, evidence is accumulating that primary barrier abnormalities may initiate their pathogenesis [24–26]. A pertinent example is the recent discovery that atopic dermatitis (AD), which occurs in up to 30% of Caucasians, is associated frequently with loss-of-function mutations in the *FILAGGRIN* (*FLG*) gene (reviewed in Refs 24–26). Using flaky-tail (flg-deficient) mice, we and others recently showed that flg deficiency produces a barrier abnormality, which allows sustained irritant and hapten ingress, including a th2 immune response, characteristic of human AD [27,28]. Pertinently, AD is also frequently complicated by *Staphyloccoccus aureus* and viral infections, attributable in part to Th2-cytokine-mediated downregulation of LL-37 and hBD2 in AD [29–31]. But abnormalities in extracellular lamellar bilayers [32] should not be overlooked in explaining *S. aureus* persistence and penetration in AD. Regardless of cause, *S. aureus*, once established, further exacerbates AD by a variety of other mechanisms [24,25] (Figure 3.2). Our recent studies show that both psychological stress (PS) and systemic or topical glucocorticoids (GC) not only compromise epidermal permeability barrier function [33,34] but also decrease levels of the murine homologues of at least two AMPs [35]. Therefore, PS and GC likely also contribute to an increased risk of infections in AD.

3.5 INTEGRATIVE ASPECTS OF VARIOUS EPIDERMAL BARRIERS

While each protective function of the skin can be considered as a discrete activity, these activities are often linked and even coregulated [3]. For example, one type of external stressor, an increase in SC pH, can impact several defensive functions of the SC [13,24,25,36,37]. For example, while an acidic pH is hostile to bacterial, yeast, and dermatophytic pathogens, elevations in pH support the growth of *S. aureus*, *S. pyogenes*, and other pathogenic species [38]. In contrast, the negative impact of an increased pH on permeability barrier homeostasis, SC integrity/cohesion, and the initiation of inflammation results from activation of serine proteases (kallikreins), followed by signaling of diverse downstream mechanisms [13,39].

As noted above, PS displays negative consequences for several epidermal functions, through an increase in endogenous GCs, which compromise permeability barrier homeostasis, SC integrity/cohesion [33,40], and antimicrobial defense [35]. A mechanism that largely accounts for these alterations comprises GC-mediated inhibition of epidermal lipid synthesis, resulting in a decline in lamellar body (LB) production [40,41]. Ultimately, less LB content gets delivered to the SC interstices, resulting in fewer extracellular lamellar membrane bilayers [34,40]. Since assembly of protein into LB requires prior or concurrent lipid sequestration [42], antimicrobial peptide (AMP) cargoes are not delivered to nascent LB [35]. For example, human β-defensin2 (hBD2) and its murine homologue, mBD3, as well as the carboxyterminal product of human cathelicidin, LL-37, and its murine homologue, CAMP, are first packaged within and then secreted from LB [35,43,44]. Furthermore, the negative effects of PS on SC integrity/cohesion are also linked to the GC-induced lipid synthesis/secretory abnormality, although the responsible pathophysiologic mechanisms have not yet been elucidated. Proof of the link between decreased lipid generation and these three functional abnormalities was demonstrated by the ability of topical physiologic lipid replenishment to largely or completely override these functional abnormalities in the face of ongoing PS/GC [34,35,40].

Another type of functional interaction that demonstrates how permeability barrier homeostasis and antimicrobial defense are intertwined relates to changes accompanying shifts in SC hydration. Prolonged exposure to extremes of external humidity produces parallel alterations in permeability barrier function and antimicrobial defense (Figure 3.1). Another example pertinent to this chapter would be that

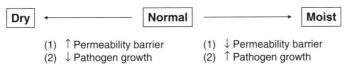

Figure 3.1   Changes in external humidity alter permeability and antimicrobial barriers in parallel.

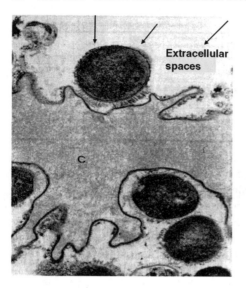

Figure 3.2 *S. aureus* penetrates via paracellular pathway. Biopsy specimen from culture-positive *S. aureus* skin infection. Gram-positive cocci may be seen intercalating between corneocytes (C) within stratum corneum; that is, via extracellular spaces, which are normally occupied by stratum corneum lipids. Note that corneocytes do not appear damaged and are not traversed by bacteria.

barrier perturbations, sufficient to accelerate transcutaneous water loss, simultaneously allow ingress of xenobiotics [45] and pathogenic microorganisms (Figure 3.2). Moreover, while external insults to the permeability barrier provoke inflammation by initiating a "cytokine cascade," some of these signaling molecules also signal certain physiologic responses that restore permeability barrier homeostasis [1,2,46–48], and activate hBD2 and hBD3 production by epidermal keratinocytes (see below).

Initiation of IL-1α and IL-1β activation at the level of the SC appears to occur through a pH-induced increase in the activity of at least one serine protease that is resident primarily within the SC (kallikrein 7 or SC chymotryptic enzyme) [49]. A further example of how permeability barrier function and antimicrobial defense are linked are the permeability barrier abnormalities that result from inherited defects of corneocyte proteins, for example, K1/K10 (epidermolytic hyperkeratosis), which result in an inadequate scaffold for the lamellar bilayers [50,51]. As noted above, an intact lamellar membrane system, which completely engorges the SC extracellular domains, is critical not only for permeability barrier homeostasis but also for antimicrobial defense (Table 3.2). In these disorders, the bilayer system is depleted or disorganized, and secondary infections frequently complicate these disorders.

3.6 COREGULATION AND INTERDEPENDENCE OF PERMEABILITY AND ANTIMICROBIAL BARRIERS

Certain characteristics of normal SC, including its low water content, acidic pH, cohesive geometric structure, resident normal flora, content of barrier lipids with antimicrobial activity, and the constitutive delivery of AMP to the SC interstices, render the SC resistant to pathogen colonization/invasion [52] (Table 3.2). With the notable exception of dermatophytes and *Candida albicans*, with elaborate proteases that allow these pathogens to enter corneocytes [53–55], ultrastructural studies

TABLE 3.3 Basis for Antimicrobial Defense at the Level of Stratum Corneum Under Basal Conditions

A. From normal microbial flora
   Niche occupancy
   Competition for nutrients
   Secrete inhibitory metabolic products: for example, acetic and propionic acids
   Produce specific antimicrobial compounds; for example, penicillin, azelaic acid
   Upregulate LL-37 production
B. Surface-deposited antimicrobials
   Sweat: for example, dermcidin, LL-37
   Sebum (lysozyme, FFA, RNase 7)
C. Intrinsic to stratum corneum
   Geometry of intact SC layer
   Replete lamellar bilayers
   SC lipids; for example, FFA, sphingosine
   Acidic pH, low water content
   Low, constitutive levels of hBD2 and LL-37 within extracellular matrix

suggest that the extracellular matrix is the pathway through which bacterial pathogens such as *S. aureus* breach the SC [14] (Figure 3.2). Therefore, the lamellar bilayers serve both as an important physical and as a chemical barrier. As noted above, epidermal LB deliver a family of lipids that form the permeability barrier, and some of these lipids, most notably free fatty acids and sphingosine, themselves exhibit potent activity against a variety of bacterial, yeast, and viral pathogens [14,16,21,56]. In addition, LB deliver several nonlipid proteins that display AMP activity (Tables 3.3 and 3.4; Figure 3.3), including LL-37 [44] and hBD2 [43], and their murine homologues [35], to the SC interstices. Thus, the colocalization of both dual-function lipids and peptides by LB to the SC supports the view that these two functions are intimately related.

The close relationship between permeability and antimicrobial function is most convincingly corroborated perhaps by the demonstration that expression of certain AMP (e.g., mBD3, CAMP, and catestatin) increases after acute disruption of the permeability barrier [3,35,57]. Although this relationship is readily explained by the fact that barrier disruption removes both the extracellular AMP and the lipids required for permeability barrier maintenance [3], the relationship between these two functions is more complex than simply a response to coremoval of extracellular lipids and peptides. In fact, AMP appears to be important not only for antimicrobial function but also, conversely, for permeability barrier homeostasis. Transgenic mice that fail to express CAMP, the murine homologue of LL-37, exhibit not only increased cutaneous streptococcal infections [58], but also a significant permeability barrier abnormality [35]. Ultrastructural studies suggest further that LL-37 (and perhaps other AMP) contribute to the supramolecular organization of the extracellular matrix into lamellar domains (op. cit.), perhaps through the requirement for relatively hydrophilic molecules for lamellar membrane organization. Thus, AMPs exercise a third set of functions in epidermis that extend beyond their well-established dual roles as

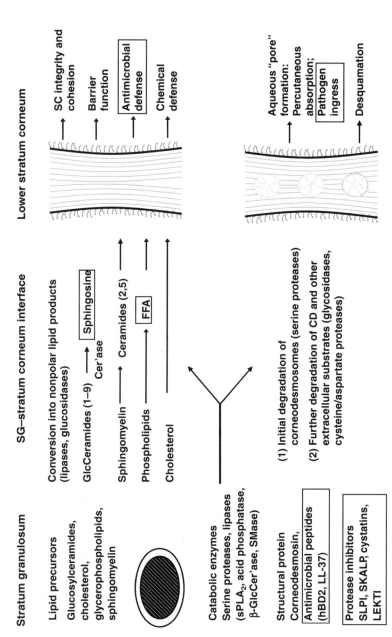

Figure 3.3 Lamellar body secretory system generates key components of the permeability and antimicrobial barriers.

antimicrobial and signaling molecules; that is, they are structural constituents of the epidermal permeability barrier.

3.7 DISTAL CONTRIBUTORS TO CUTANEOUS ANTIMICROBIAL DEFENSE

3.7.1 Physical–Chemical Characteristics of SC and Resident Normal Flora

The normal barrier to pathogenic microbes is diverse and multilayered, initially comprising certain amphiphilic lipids of epidermal and sebaceous gland origins, particularly sphingosine and FFA [17,59], AMP [59], a structurally cohesive SC replete with extracellular lamellar bilayers, and the normal microflora of the skin (Tables 3.2 and 3.3). These features, coupled with the acidic pH and low water content of the SC, provide a formidable physical–chemical barrier against the entry of pathogens [52]. The acidic pH of normal SC encourages the growth of normal flora, such as *S. epidermidis*, which inhibit the growth of pathogens by multiple mechanisms, including competition for niche occupancy and nutrients, elaboration of antimicrobial metabolites, and even stimulation of production of certain AMP, such as LL-37 [60]. Conversely, an absent or markedly abnormal SC, as occurs in burn patients, cutaneous ulcers, or in very premature infants' skin (≤ 33 weeks), can greatly increase the risk of infection.

3.7.2 Epidermal Antimicrobial Peptides

The SC is laced with AMP, an evolutionarily conserved component of the innate immune system that defends against invading bacteria, viruses, and fungi through membrane or metabolic disruption [59,61,62]. Their efficacy derives from their ability to quickly eradicate foreign pathogens through precise biochemical mechanisms. Human epidermal AMPs comprise several members of the β-defensin family (hBD1–4), the N-terminal and carboxyterminal products (LL-37 and cathelin moieties) of human cathelicidin (hCAP), calcium binding S100 proteins, particularly RNase 7, the S100A7 protein, psoriasin, and several other multifunctional proteins with antimicrobial activity, such as the neuroendocrine peptide, catestatin, secretory leukocyte protease inhibitor, elafin, and parotid secretory protein (PSP) [59,62]. Because their antimicrobial spectrum only partially overlaps (Table 3.4), these AMP are required collectively to repel a diversity of invading pathogens. Several protease inhibitors also exhibit antimicrobial activity, but most are substrates for transglutaminase 1, and therefore they may not be available for antimicrobial defense once they become cross-linked into the cornified envelope. We and others have shown that the expression of several of these AMP rapidly upregulates after the barrier is abrogated in mice (e.g., CAMP, mBD3, mBD14, psoriasin, and catestatin) and/or in response to external microbial challenges [35,57,63].

TABLE 3.4 Spectrum and Activities of Major Epidermal Antimicrobial Peptides

Chemicals	Lamellar body product	Killing mechanism	Organism class			
			Gram +	Gram −	Yeast	Viruses
Lipids						
(FFA, Sph)	+	?Detergent activity	+	Minimal	+	+
Proteins						
LL-37	+	Pore formation	+	+	+	+
hBD2	+	Pore formation	−	+	−	?
hBD3	?	Pore formation	+	−	−	?
Psoriasin	?	Trace element (Zn++, Cu++) sequestration	Minimal	+ (*E. coli*)	?	?
RNase7	?	Unknown	+	+ (*S. fecalis*)	+	?
Catestatin	?	Pore formation	+	?	?	?
Paratid secretory protein	?	?		− (Except *Pseudomonas*)	+	−

3.7.3 Cutaneous Antimicrobial Lipids

Several naturally occurring lipids (i.e., fatty alcohols, FFAs, monoglycerides, and sphingosine) exhibit antimicrobial activity against enveloped viruses, Gram-positive bacteria, *Candida*, and fungi [15,17], but little activity against Gram-negative organisms [14,15,17]. Since FFAs of both epidermal and sebaceous gland origin are present in large quantities on the skin surface and within the SC interstices, and since they exhibit antimicrobial activity in the micromolar range (as do AMP), they likely play an important role in host defense in the outer epidermis [15,16]. As noted above, FFAs are also key structural ingredients of the lamellar bilayers [64], as well as important contributors to the acidic pH of normal SC [12]. Thus, FFA influence cutaneous antimicrobial defense by multiple mechanisms. Moreover, FFA and sphingolipid levels decline significantly and selectively in humans with AD [65,66], accounting for increased susceptibility of AD skin to pathogen colonization. Thus, strategies that restore normal permeability barrier function in AD will likely improve antimicrobial defense.

The close relationship between permeability barrier function and antimicrobial defense is also shown under experimental conditions, such as psychological stress, where permeability barrier function and antimicrobial defense decline in parallel. We and others showed that various types of PS, such as psychological interviews, sleep deprivation, and marital separation/distress, compromise permeability barrier function in humans [67–70]. Moreover, in our cohort of students preparing for final exams [68], there was a clear dose effect, with the greatest deterioration in barrier function occurring in subjects who demonstrated the largest increases in PS, as measured by the perceived stress scale and the profile of mood states [68]. Then, in four different mouse models of PS (crowding; movement to an unfamiliar environment; immobilization [frustration]; and sleep deprivation), we showed that permeability barrier recovery is delayed following acute barrier disruption, as in PS humans [33,34], and importantly, that treatment with a sedative, chlorpromazine, blocks the adverse effects of PS [33]. In these models, we further identified four mechanisms by which PS impairs permeability barrier homeostasis: (1) decreased epidermal proliferation; (2) decreased expression of epidermal structural proteins (e.g., involucrin, loricrin, and filaggrin [34]); (3) reduced epidermal cholesterol, FFAs, and ceramide synthesis, leading to decreased production of epidermal lamellar bodies, and a paucity of secreted lipids [34]; and (4) PS compromises SC integrity, defined as the resistance to detachment of adjacent corneocytes and quantified as the rate of increase in TEWL levels with sequential tape strippings (SC cohesion = the amount of protein removed per stripping [12]). Normal SC integrity/cohesion allows the invisible, distal shedding of corneocytes (= desquamation), which is accomplished by the progressive, proteolytic degradation of corneodesmosomes (CDs), and its constituent proteins, desmoglein 1 (DSG1), desmocollin 1, and corneodesmosin [71–76]. The PS-induced decline in SC integrity is associated with reduced CD and its constituent proteins (e.g., desmoglein 1, DSG1) [34].

Accordingly, topical applications of the three physiologic lipids, which have no net effect on barrier recovery in normal skin [64,77], restore normal barrier recovery kinetics and SC integrity/cohesion in PS animals [34]. Thus, provision of extracellular lipids appears to leave adjacent CD less vulnerable to premature, PS/GC-induced proteolysis [78–80].

REFERENCES

1. Feingold KR, Schmuth M, Elias PM. The regulation of permeability barrier homeostasis. *J. Invest. Dermatol.* 2007;127(7):1574–1576.
2. Elias PM. Stratum corneum defensive functions: an integrated view. *J. Invest. Dermatol.* 2005; 125(2):183–200.
3. Elias PM, Choi EH. Interactions among stratum corneum defensive functions. *Exp. Dermatol.* 2005; 14(10):719–726.
4. Elias PM. Stratum corneum architecture, metabolic activity and interactivity with subjacent cell layers. *Exp. Dermatol.* 1996;5(4):191–201.
5. Madison KC. Barrier function of the skin: "la raison d'etre" of the epidermis. *J. Invest. Dermatol.* 2003;121(2):231–241.
6. Nemes Z, Steinert PM. Bricks and mortar of the epidermal barrier. *Exp. Mol. Med.* 1999;31(1):5–19.
7. Fuchs E. Epidermal differentiation. *Curr. Opin. Cell Biol.* 1990;2(6):1028–1035.
8. Eckert RL, Crish JF, Robinson NA. The epidermal keratinocyte as a model for the study of gene regulation and cell differentiation. *Physiol. Rev.* 1997;77(2):397–424.
9. Elias PM, Menon GK. Structural and lipid biochemical correlates of the epidermal permeability barrier. *Adv. Lipid Res.* 1991;24:1–26.
10. Feingold KR. Thematic review series: skin lipids. The role of epidermal lipids in cutaneous permeability barrier homeostasis. *J. Lipid Res.* 2007;48(12):2531–2546.
11. Holleran WM, Takagi Y, Menon GK, et al. Processing of epidermal glucosylceramides is required for optimal mammalian cutaneous permeability barrier function. *J. Clin. Invest.* 1993;91(4):1656–1664.
12. Fluhr JW, Kao J, Jain M, et al. Generation of free fatty acids from phospholipids regulates stratum corneum acidification and integrity. *J. Invest. Dermatol.* 2001;117(1):44–51.

13. Hachem JP, Man MQ, Crumrine D, et al. Sustained serine proteases activity by prolonged increase in pH leads to degradation of lipid processing enzymes and profound alterations of barrier function and stratum corneum integrity. *J. Invest. Dermatol.* 2005;125(3):510–520.

14. Miller SJ, Aly R, Shinefeld HR, Elias PM. *In vitro* and *in vivo* antistaphylococcal activity of human stratum corneum lipids. *Arch. Dermatol.* 1988;124(2):209–215.

15. Thormar H, Hilmarsson H. The role of microbicidal lipids in host defense against pathogens and their potential as therapeutic agents. *Chem. Phys. Lipids* 2007;150(1):1–11.

16. Georgel P, Crozat K, Lauth X, et al. A toll-like receptor 2-responsive lipid effector pathway protects mammals against skin infections with gram-positive bacteria. *Infect. Immun.* 2005; 73(8):4512–4521.

17. Drake DR, Brogden KA, Dawson DV, Wertz PW. Thematic review series: skin lipids. Antimicrobial lipids at the skin surface. *J. Lipid Res.* 2008;49(1):4–11.

18. Wertz PW, Downing DT. Ceramidase activity in porcine epidermis. *FEBS Lett.* 1990;268(1): 110–112.

19. Houben E, Holleran WM, Yaginuma T, et al. Differentiation-associated expression of ceramidase isoforms in cultured keratinocytes and epidermis. *J. Lipid Res.* 2006;47(5):1063–1070.

20. Wertz PW, Downing DT. Free sphingosine in human epidermis. *J. Invest. Dermatol.* 1990;94 (2):159–161.

21. Bibel DJ, Aly R, Shinefield HR. Antimicrobial activity of sphingosines. *J. Invest. Dermatol.* 1992;98 (3):269–273.

22. Nickoloff BJ, Naidu Y. Perturbation of epidermal barrier function correlates with initiation of cytokine cascade in human skin. *J. Am. Acad. Dermatol.* 1994;30(4):535–546.

23. Wood LC, Jackson SM, Elias PM, Grunfeld C, Feingold KR. Cutaneous barrier perturbation stimulates cytokine production in the epidermis of mice. *J. Clin. Invest.* 1992;90(2):482–487.

24. Elias PM, Hatano Y, Williams ML. Basis for the barrier abnormality in atopic dermatitis: outside–inside–outside pathogenic mechanisms. *J. Allergy Clin. Immunol.* 2008;121(6): 1337–1343.

25. Elias PM, Steinhoff M. "Outside-to-inside" (and now back to "outside") pathogenic mechanisms in atopic dermatitis. *J. Invest. Dermatol.* 2008;128(5):1067–1070.

26. Jung T, Stingl G. Atopic dermatitis: therapeutic concepts evolving from new pathophysiologic insights. *J. Allergy Clin. Immunol.* 2008;122(6):1074–1081.

27. Fallon PG, Sasaki T, Sandilands A, et al. A homozygous frameshift mutation in the mouse Flg gene facilitates enhanced percutaneous allergen priming. *Nat. Genet.* 2009;41(5):602–608.

28. Scharschmidt T, Man M, Hatano Y, et al. Filaggrin deficiency confers a paracellular barrier abnormality that reduces inflammatory thresholds to irritants and haptens. *J. Allergy Clin. Immunol.* 2009;124 (3):496–506.

29. Ong PY, Ohtake T, Brandt C, et al. Endogenous antimicrobial peptides and skin infections in atopic dermatitis. *N. Engl. J. Med.* 2002;347(15):1151–1160.

30. Howell MD, Novak N, Bieber T, et al. Interleukin-10 downregulates anti-microbial peptide expression in atopic dermatitis. *J. Invest. Dermatol.* 2005;125(4):738–745.

31. Nomura I, Goleva E, Howell MD, et al. Cytokine milieu of atopic dermatitis, as compared to psoriasis, skin prevents induction of innate immune response genes. *J. Immunol.* 2003;171 (6):3262–3269.

32. Chamlin SL, Kao J, Frieden IJ, et al. Ceramide-dominant barrier repair lipids alleviate childhood atopic dermatitis: changes in barrier function provide a sensitive indicator of disease activity. *J. Am. Acad. Dermatol.* 2002;47(2):198–208.

33. Denda M, Tsuchiya T, Elias PM, Feingold KR. Stress alters cutaneous permeability barrier homeostasis. *Am. J. Physiol. Regul. Integr. Comp. Physiol.* 2000;278(2):R367–R372.

34. Choi EH, Brown BE, Crumrine D, et al. Mechanisms by which psychologic stress alters cutaneous permeability barrier homeostasis and stratum corneum integrity. *J. Invest. Dermatol.* 2005;124 (3):587–595.

35. Aberg KM, Radek KA, Choi EH, et al. Psychological stress downregulates epidermal antimicrobial peptide expression and increases severity of cutaneous infections in mice. *J. Clin. Invest.* 2007; 117(11):3339–3349.

36. Cork MJ, Robinson DA, Vasilopoulos Y, et al. New perspectives on epidermal barrier dysfunction in atopic dermatitis: gene–environment interactions. *J. Allergy Clin. Immunol.* 2006;118(1):3–21;quiz 22–23.

37. Hachem JP, Fowler A, Behne M, et al. Increased stratum corneum pH promotes activation and release of primary cytokines from the stratum corneum attributable to activation of serine proteases. *J. Invest. Dermatol.* 2002;119(1):258.

38. Korting HC, Hubner K, Greiner K, Hamm G, Braun-Falco O. Differences in the skin surface pH and bacterial microflora due to the long-term application of synthetic detergent preparations of pH 5.5 and pH 7.0. Results of a crossover trial in healthy volunteers. *Acta Derm. Venereol.* 1990;70(5):429–431.

39. Hachem JP, Crumrine D, Fluhr J, et al. pH directly regulates epidermal permeability barrier homeostasis, and stratum corneum integrity/cohesion. *J. Invest. Dermatol.* 2003;121(2):345–353.

40. Kao JS, Fluhr JW, Man MQ, et al. Short-term glucocorticoid treatment compromises both permeability barrier homeostasis and stratum corneum integrity: inhibition of epidermal lipid synthesis accounts for functional abnormalities. *J. Invest. Dermatol.* 2003;120(3):456–464.

41. Choi EH, Demerjian M, Crumrine D, et al. Glucocorticoid blockade reverses psychological stress-induced abnormalities in epidermal structure and function. *Am. J. Physiol. Regul. Integr. Comp. Physiol.* 2006;291(6):R1657–R1662.

42. Rassner U, Feingold KR, Crumrine DA, Elias PM. Coordinate assembly of lipids and enzyme proteins into epidermal lamellar bodies. *Tissue Cell* 1999;31(5):489–498.

43. Oren A, Ganz T, Liu L, Meerloo T. In human epidermis, beta-defensin 2 is packaged in lamellar bodies. *Exp. Mol. Pathol.* 2003;74(2):180–182.

44. Braff MH, Di Nardo A, Gallo RL. Keratinocytes store the antimicrobial peptide cathelicidin in lamellar bodies. *J. Invest. Dermatol.* 2005;124(2):394–400.

45. Tsai JC, Guy RH, Thornfeldt CR, et al. Metabolic approaches to enhance transdermal drug delivery: 1. Effect of lipid synthesis inhibitors. *J. Pharm. Sci.* 1996;85(6):643–648.

46. Ye J, Garg A, Calhoun C, et al. Alterations in cytokine regulation in aged epidermis: implications for permeability barrier homeostasis and inflammation. I. IL-1 gene family. *Exp. Dermatol.* 2002; 11(3):209–216.

47. Barland CO, Elias PM, Ghadially R. *The aged epidermal barrier: basis for functional abnormalities.* In: Elias PM, Feingold KR. editors. *Skin Barrier.* New York: Marcel Dekker; 2005. pp. 535–552.

48. Jensen JM, Schutze S, Forl M, Kronke M, Proksch E. Roles for tumor necrosis factor receptor p55 and sphingomyelinase in repairing the cutaneous permeability barrier. *J. Clin. Invest.* 1999; 104(12):1761–1770.

49. Nylander-Lundqvist E, Egelrud T. Formation of active IL-1 beta from pro-IL-1 beta catalyzed by stratum corneum chymotryptic enzyme *in vitro*. *Acta Derm. Venereol.* 1997;77(3):203–206.

50. Schmuth M, Fluhr JW, Crumrine DC, et al. Structural and functional consequences of loricrin mutations in human loricrin keratoderma (Vohwinkel syndrome with ichthyosis). *J. Invest. Dermatol.* 2004;122(4):909–922.

51. Elias PM, Feingold KR. Coordinate regulation of epidermal differentiation and barrier homeostasis. *Skin Pharmacol. Appl. Skin Physiol.* 2001;14(Suppl. 1):28–34.

52. Elias PM. The skin barrier as an innate immune element. *Sem. Immunopath.* 2007;29(1):3–14.

53. Schaller M, Schackert C, Korting HC, Januschke E, Hube B. Invasion of *Candida albicans* correlates with expression of secreted aspartic proteinases during experimental infection of human epidermis. *J. Invest. Dermatol.* 2000;114(4):712–717.

54. Viani FC, Dos Santos JI, Paula CR, Larson CE, Gambale W. Production of extracellular enzymes by *Microsporum canis* and their role in its virulence. *Med. Mycol.* 2001;39(5):463–468.

55. Monod M, Capoccia S, Lechenne B, et al. Secreted proteases from pathogenic fungi. *Int. J. Med. Microbiol.* 2002;292(5–6):405–419.

56. Wille JJ, Kydonieus A. Palmitoleic acid isomer (C16:1delta6) in human skin sebum is effective against gram-positive bacteria. *Skin Pharmacol. Appl. Skin Physiol.* 2003;16(3):176–187.

57. Radek KA, Lopez-Garcia B, Hupe M, et al. The neuroendocrine peptide catestatin is a cutaneous antimicrobial and induced in the skin after injury. *J. Invest. Dermatol.* 2008;128(6):1525–1534.

58. Nizet V, Ohtake T, Lauth X, et al. Innate antimicrobial peptide protects the skin from invasive bacterial infection. *Nature* 2001;414(6862):454–457.

59. Radek K, Gallo R. Antimicrobial peptides: natural effectors of the innate immune system. *Semin. Immunopathol.* 2007;29(1):27–43.
60. Cogen A, Lai Y, Yamasaki K, et al. *Staphylococcus* epidermidis antimicrobial peptide functions as a surface antibiotic and induces keratinocyte TLR2-mediated expression of defensins and cathelicidin. *J. Invest. Dermatol.* 2009;129 (S1):S118.
61. Lehrer RI, Lichtenstein AK, Ganz T. Defensins: antimicrobial and cytotoxic peptides of mammalian cells. *Annu. Rev. Immunol.* 1993;11:105–128.
62. Barak O, Treat JR, James WD. Antimicrobial peptides: effectors of innate immunity in the skin. *Adv. Dermatol.* 2005;21:357–374.
63. Glaser R, Meyer-Hoffert U, Harder J, et al. The antimicrobial protein psoriasin (S100A7) is upregulated in atopic dermatitis and after experimental skin barrier disruption. *J. Invest. Dermatol.* 2009; 129(3):641–649.
64. Man MQ, Feingold KR, Thornfeldt CR, Elias PM. Optimization of physiological lipid mixtures for barrier repair. *J. Invest. Dermatol.* 1996;106(5):1096–1101.
65. Imokawa G, Abe A, Jin K, et al. Decreased level of ceramides in stratum corneum of atopic dermatitis: an etiologic factor in atopic dry skin? *J. Invest. Dermatol.* 1991;96(4):523–526.
66. Di Nardo A, Wertz P, Giannetti A, Seidenari S. Ceramide and cholesterol composition of the skin of patients with atopic dermatitis. *Acta. Derm. Venereol.* 1998;78(1):27–30.
67. Muizzuddin N, Matsui MS, Marenus KD, Maes DH. Impact of stress of marital dissolution on skin barrier recovery: tape stripping and measurement of trans-epidermal water loss (TEWL). *Skin Res. Technol.* 2003;9(1):34–38.
68. Garg A, Chren MM, Sands LP, et al. Psychological stress perturbs epidermal permeability barrier homeostasis: implications for the pathogenesis of stress-associated skin disorders. *Arch. Dermatol.* 2001;137(1):53–59.
69. Altemus M, Rao B, Dhabhar FS, Ding W, Granstein RD. Stress-induced changes in skin barrier function in healthy women. *J. Invest. Dermatol.* 2001;117(2):309–317.
70. Robles TF. Stress, social support, and delayed skin barrier recovery. *Psychosom. Med.* 2007; 69(8):807–815.
71. Serre G, Mils V, Haftek M, et al. Identification of late differentiation antigens of human cornified epithelia, expressed in re-organized desmosomes and bound to cross-linked envelope. *J. Invest. Dermatol.* 1991;97(6):1061–1072.
72. Haftek M, Simon M, Kanitakis J, et al. Expression of corneodesmosin in the granular layer and stratum corneum of normal and diseased epidermis. *Br. J. Dermatol.* 1997;137(6):864–873.
73. Fartasch M, Bassukas ID, Diepgen TL. Structural relationship between epidermal lipid lamellae, lamellar bodies and desmosomes in human epidermis: an ultrastructural study. *Br. J. Dermatol.* 1993;128(1):1–9.
74. Chapman SJ, Walsh A, Jackson SM, Friedmann PS. Lipids, proteins and corneocyte adhesion. *Arch. Dermatol. Res.* 1991;283(3):167–173.
75. Brysk MM, Rajaraman S. Cohesion and desquamation of epidermal stratum corneum. *Prog. Histochem. Cytochem.* 1992;25(1):1–53.
76. Caubet C, Jonca N, Brattsand M, et al. Degradation of corneodesmosome proteins by two serine proteases of the kallikrein family, SCTE/KLK5/hK5 and SCCE/KLK7/hK7. *J. Invest. Dermatol.* 2004;122(5):1235–1244.
77. Mao-Qiang M, Elias PM, Feingold KR. Fatty acids are required for epidermal permeability barrier function. *J. Clin. Invest.* 1993;92(2):791–798.
78. Komuves LG, Hanley K, Man MQ, et al. Keratinocyte differentiation in hyperproliferative epidermis: topical application of PPARalpha activators restores tissue homeostasis. *J. Invest. Dermatol.* 2000;115 (3):361–367.
79. Burdick AD, Bility MT, Girroir EE, et al. Ligand activation of peroxisome proliferator-activated receptor-beta/delta(PPARbeta/delta) inhibits cell growth of human N/TERT-1 keratinocytes. *Cell. Signal.* 2007;19(6):1163–1171.
80. Muga SJ, Thuillier P, Pavone A, et al. 8S-lipoxygenase products activate peroxisome proliferator-activated receptor alpha and induce differentiation in murine keratinocytes. *Cell Growth Differ.* 2000;11(8):447–454.

PART II

ANTIMICROBIAL LIPIDS AND PEPTIDES

CHAPTER 4

ANTIMICROBIAL LIPIDS OF THE SKIN AND ORAL MUCOSA

Kim A. Brogden, David R. Drake, Deborah V. Dawson,
Jennifer R. Hill, Carol L. Bratt, and Philip W. Wertz

Dows Institute, University of Iowa, Iowa City, IA

4.1 SKIN SURFACE LIPIDS

The surface of the skin is a major interface between the organism and its environment. Numerous factors contribute to the innate defense mechanisms of the skin including the impermeability of the stratum corneum, desquamation, relatively low moisture availability, and low pH [1]. In recent years, much attention has been focused on the roles of antimicrobial peptides in defense of the skin [2–4]. Although a role for lipids in immunity of the skin was recognized in the 1940s [5,6], this area has been largely neglected until recently [7,8]. The antimicrobial lipids at the human skin surface arise from two sources: epidermal (sphingosine, dihydrosphingosine, and 6-hydroxysphingosine) and sebaceous (lauric acid and sapienic acid). Structures of the antimicrobial lipids found at the skin surface are shown in Figure 4.1.

Lipids synthesized in the viable portion of the epidermis pass into the outer, cornified layer, or stratum corneum, and provide a hydrophobic permeability barrier [9,10]. This barrier primarily prevents water loss through the skin and also prevents the penetration of potentially harmful substances from the environment. The main lipids of the stratum corneum are ceramides, cholesterol, and long-chain fatty acids. There is ceramidase activity in the stratum corneum that acts on some of the ceramides to liberate free sphingosine in significant amounts [11–13]. The free sphingosine is a broad acting and potent antimicrobial agent [8,14–16]. Its production close to the skin surface is thought to be part of the innate immune system of the skin [8]. In addition to being a potent antimicrobial agent, sphingosine is a potent inhibitor of protein kinase c [17]. In this capacity, the sphingosine gradient generated by ceramidase action on stratum corneum ceramides may be important in regulating cell proliferation and differentiation.

In addition to the stratum corneum lipids, the skin surface is coated with a film of liquid-phase lipids synthesized in the sebaceous glands [6,18,19]. In human sebaceous glands, a mixture of triglycerides, wax monoesters, and squalene is synthesized.

Innate Immune System of Skin and Oral Mucosa: Properties and Impact in Pharmaceutics, Cosmetics, and Personal Care Products, First Edition. Nava Dayan and Philip W. Wertz.

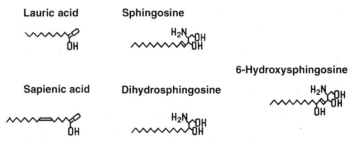

Figure 4.1   Chemical structures of antimicrobial lipids found on the surfaces of skin and oral mucosa.

Small amounts of cholesterol and cholesterol esters are derived from the initial membrane components of the sebocyte. This liquid-phase lipid mixture flows out through the follicle and over the skin surface. As sebum flows outward, some of the triglycerides are hydrolyzed to liberate free fatty acids. This process continues on the skin surface. The major free fatty acid derived from human sebum is a 16-carbon monoene called sapienic acid (C16:1Δ6). Among the sebaceous fatty acids, sapienic acid and lauric acid (C12:0) are uniquely bactericidal. Other fatty acids from the skin surface are bacteriostatic or inactive. Sapienic acid and lauric acid are both active against a range of Gram-positive bacteria, most notably *Staphylococcus aureus*, including antibiotic-resistant isolates [8]. Lauric acid is a minor sebaceous fatty acid in terms of abundance, but it is a potent antimicrobial.

4.2   ORAL MUCOSAL SURFACE LIPIDS

Factors contributing to protection of the oral mucosa include desquamation, antimicrobial peptides, IgA, and various enzymes, such as lysozyme [20,21].

The regions of the hard palate and the gingiva, like the skin, are covered by a stratum corneum [22]. The main lipids also consist of ceramides, cholesterol, and fatty acids, and significant levels of free long-chain bases have been found [23,24]. The buccal region and the floor of the mouth are covered by nonkeratinizing epithelia and so do not have a stratum corneum. The superficial layers in these epithelia do provide a permeability barrier, although it is not as effective as that in the keratinized oral regions [25]. The main lipids found in the superficial barriers are glucosylceramides, phospholipids, cholesterol, and fatty acids. Only small proportions of one ceramide are found, but free sphingoid bases are present [23]. The dorsum of the tongue is covered by a specialized epithelium, but it is well approximated as a mosaic of keratinized and nonkeratinized epithelia.

The vermilion border of the lip and all regions of the oral mucosa contain sebaceous follicles [26–29]. These are sebaceous glands without associated hairs. Although some sebaceous follicles are found in all regions of skin excluding the palmar and plantar regions, these secretory units uniquely surround all orifices of the body, including the vermilion border of the lip.

They are also present in the oral mucosa and the lining of the ear canals. This anatomic distribution suggests a protective function. The sebaceous follicles produce sebaceous lipids with the same composition as the pilosebaceous units of the skin [30]. In addition, sebaceous glands are found associated with the major salivary glands. As a result, sebaceous lipids, including sapienic acid, are found at the oral mucosal surfaces and in the saliva. The same antimicrobial lipids found at the skin surface are found in the oral cavity on mucosal surfaces and in saliva (Figure 4.1).

4.3 HISTORICAL PERSPECTIVES ON ANTIMICROBIAL LIPIDS

In 1942, Burtenshaw demonstrated that the lipids from ethyl ether extracts of the human skin surface killed a strain of *S. aureus* [5]. It was speculated that free fatty acids might be the active component, and it was subsequently shown that some fatty acids were antibacterial. It became an accepted dogma that sebaceous fatty acids were antimicrobial and contributed to the self-disinfecting properties of the skin surface. In a series of papers published between 1945 and 1947 (reviewed in Ref. 1), Rothman and coworkers noted that the onset of immunity to tinea capitis, ringworm of the scalp, caused by *Microsporon audouinii*, corresponded to the increase in sebum production at the onset of puberty. They found that the growth of this fungus was inhibited by sebum and that a free fatty acid fraction was responsible for this inhibition. In a remarkable study, the fatty acid fraction extracted from human hair clippings was converted to fatty acid methyl esters and analyzed by fractional distillation at reduced pressure [6]. The primary fractionation was by chain length. Fractions containing even and odd numbers of carbons from 7- to 22-carbons were collected. Unsaturated fatty acid methyl esters were obtained by removal of the saturated species by crystallization. The unsaturated species were then subjected to oxidation. Analysis of the products demonstrated that most of the unsaturated species were monounsaturated, and the position of the double bond was identified. The most abundant sebaceous fatty acid was 5,6-hexadecenoic acid ($C16:1\Delta6$, sapienic acid), and an 18-carbon monoene was identified as $C18:1\Delta8$. Lauric acid ($C12:0$) represented about 3.5% of the total. When each of the sebaceous fatty acids was tested for activity against *M. audouinii*, the shorter, odd carbon chain fatty acids ($C7:0$, $C9:0$, $C11:0$, $C13:0$) were responsible for the antifungal activity.

Short-chain fatty acids are also active against *Trichophyton mentagrophytes*, a fungus that causes athlete's foot [1]. The most active compound is undecylenic acid ($C11:1\Delta10$), a fatty acid found in sweat. Undecylenic acid is an active ingredient found in many over-the-counter preparations for treatment of foot fungus.

Rothman and Lorincz did not consider the possibility that some or all the shorter fatty acids might have originated from sweat rather than sebum [1]. They did point out that in addition to development of immunity to ringworm of the scalp coinciding with increased sebum output, fungal infections of the human skin in adults most frequently occur on the feet where there are relatively few sebaceous glands. With the advent of gas chromatography [31,32], the presence of the fatty acids at the skin surface with essentially the same chain-length distribution reported by Weitkamp *et al.* [6] was confirmed. Furthermore, the short C-7–C-12 entities were found in the skin surface triglycerides. Therefore, these short-chain fatty acids are of sebaceous origin.

Unfortunately, most subsequent work on sebaceous fatty acids either did not find or did not report fatty acids shorter than 12- or 14-carbons. This was either because these volatile constituents were lost during preparation of methyl esters for analysis or because they are minor in amount. Gas chromatography revealed that sebaceous fatty acids include iso, anteiso, and other methyl branched species [18].

4.4   LAURIC ACID AND SAPIENIC ACID

The epidermal fatty acids that reach the skin surface are principally straight chain, saturated species ranging from 20- to 28-carbons in length. These entities have not demonstrated antimicrobial activity. The sebaceous fatty acids, as noted above, range from 7- to 22-carbons in length. The major sebaceous fatty acids include 12- through 18-carbon straight-chained, saturated species, sapienic acid (C16:1Δ6) and the C18:1Δ8 produced by extending sapienic acid by two carbons. There are variable amounts of assorted methyl branched chain species as well. The structure–activity relationship for the straight chain, saturated sebaceous fatty acids versus *S. aureus* is shown in Figure 4.2. As shown, maximum activity is found at C12:0, lauric acid. Activity decreases sharply with either shorter or longer chain lengths. One methyl-branched fatty acid, 15-methylpalmitic acid, was found to have essentially the same activity as the parent palmitic acid. No other branched fatty acid was tested. Under similar conditions, C16:1Δ6 was similar to C12:0 in activity, and C18:1Δ8 was inactive. The minimum inhibitory concentration for C16:1Δ6 versus *S. aureus* was 30 µg/mL, and this fatty acid was capable of rapidly killing methicillin-resistant *S. aureus* [8].

Over 40 fatty acids and derivatives have been tested for antimicrobial activity against a range of microorganisms [33,34]. Lauric acid proved to be the most potent of the fatty acids. The relationship between chain length of the saturated fatty acids and activity was essentially as shown in Figure 4.2. Lauric acid was

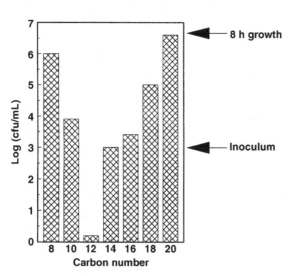

Figure 4.2   Antibacterial activity versus *S. aureus* of straight chain saturated fatty acids (1 mg/mL) as a function of chain length. Arrows to the right indicate the log(CFU)/mL in the initial inoculum and after 8 h growth in the absence of added fatty acid (Wertz PW, Drake DR, Dawson DV, Brogden KA, unpublished observation).

effective against a range of Gram-positive bacteria but not against Gram-negative bacteria or *Candida albicans*. MICs generally ranged from 16 to 62 µg/mL, depending upon the organism.

In support of the assertion that the endogenous sapienic acid is part of innate immunity, an inverse relationship between *S. aureus* colony forming units per unit area of skin and C16:1Δ6 content has been demonstrated for normal control subjects and subjects with atopic dermatitis [35]. The atopic subjects produced significantly less C16:1Δ6 than controls, which was thought to relate to their increased susceptibility to colonization by *S. aureus*. A similar relationship has not been sought for lauric acid. Since lauric acid represents only about 3.5% of the total sebaceous fatty acid, it might be argued that it is biologically unimportant. However, it is very potent as indicated by the range of MICs cited above. It should also be noted that the shorter chain sebaceous fatty acids that confer immunity to ringworm of the scalp represent only 0.1–0.3% of the total.

4.5 LONG-CHAIN BASES

Sphingosine, dihydrosphingosine, and 6-hydroxysphingosine have been reported to be present in significant amounts at the surfaces of the skin and oral mucosa [11,12,36]. These long-chain bases are thought to be liberated from ceramides through the action of one or more ceramidases [13].

Sphingoid bases have been shown to have broad antibacterial and antifungal activities [14–16]. Sensitive organisms include Gram-positive bacteria, Gram-negative bacteria, and yeast.

Ceramide concentrations in the stratum corneum are diminished in atopic dermatitis due to an error in sphingomyelin metabolism [37]. Individuals with atopic dermatitis generally have more bacterial colony forming units per unit area of skin. In this regard, *S. aureus* is prominent [38]. Recently, it has been shown that this increased carriage of *S. aureus* correlated with a reduction in free sphingosine [39]. In addition to an apparent contribution to the antimicrobial defenses of the skin surface, sphingosine is a potent inhibitor of protein kinase c [17]. As such, the sphingosine gradient could play a significant role in regulation of the rate at which cell division and differentiation occur in the viable epidermis. The sphingosine gradient may provide a means for the stratum corneum to communicate with the viable portion of the epidermis. MICs for the long-chain bases range from 2 to 40 µg/mL, depending upon the organism. The long-chain bases have been found to act synergistically with the antimicrobial peptide, LL37 [8]. Organisms sensitive to the long-chain bases include periodontal pathogens.

4.6 CONCLUSIONS

Short-chain, odd carbon saturated fatty acids (C7:0, C9:0, C11:0), lauric acid, sapienic acid, sphingosine, dihydrosphingosine, and 6-hydroxysphingosine are present at the surfaces of the human skin and oral mucosa. These fatty acids and long-chain bases have a range of antibacterial and antifungal activities. The short, odd carbon fatty acids from sebum are active against *M. audouinii* and confer immunity to scalp ringworm. Sapienic acid is active against Gram-positive bacteria, and the amount of sapienic acid per unit area of skin correlates inversely with the number of *S. aureus* colony forming units per unit area. Lauric acid, also derived from human sebum, is active against a range of Gram-positive bacteria. The long-chain bases are active against Gram-positive bacteria, Gram-negative bacteria, and yeast. In atopic dermatitis where colonization by *S. aureus* is higher than normal, the free sphingosine level is lower than normal. These observations all support the argument that endogenous lipids are part of the innate immune system of skin and mucosa.

REFERENCES

1. Rothman S, Lorincz AL. Defense mechanisms of the skin. *Ann. Rev. Med.* 1963;14:215–242.
2. Dorschner RA, Pestonjamasp VK, Tamakuwala S, Ohtake T, Rudisill J, Nizet V, Agerberth B, Gudmunder GH, Gallo RL. Cutaneous injury induces release of cathelicidin antimicrobial peptides active against group A *Strep. J. Invest. Dermatol.* 2001;117:91–97.
3. Schauber J, Gallo RL. Antimicrobial peptides and the skin immune defense system. *J. Allergy Clin. Immunol.* 2008;122:261–266.
4. Rivas-Santiago B, Serrano CJ, Enciso-Moreno A. Susceptibility to infectious diseases based on antimicrobial peptide production. *Infect. Immun.* 2009;77:4690–4695.
5. Burtenshaw JM. The mechanisms of self disinfection of the human skin and its appendages. *J. Hyg.* 1942;42:184–209.
6. Weitkamp AW, Smiljanic AM, Rothman S. The free fatty acids of human hair fat. *J. Am. Chem. Soc.* 1947;69:1936–1939.
7. Thormar H, Hilmarsson H. The role of microbiocidal lipids in host defense against pathogens and their potential as therapeutic agents. *Chem. Phys. Lipids* 2007;150:1–11.
8. Drake DR, Brogden KA, Dawson DV, Wertz PW. Antimicrobial lipids at the skin surface. *J. Lipid Res.* 2008;49:4–11.
9. Wertz PW. Biochemistry of human stratum corneum lipids. In: Feingold K, Elias PM, (editors) *Skin Barrier*. New York: Marcel Dekker, Inc., 2006. pp. 33–42.
10. Elias PM. The skin barrier as an innate immune element. *Semin. Immunopathol.* 2007;29:3–14.
11. Wertz PW, Downing DT. Free sphingosine in porcine epidermis. *Biochim. Biophys. Acta.* 1989;1002:213–217.
12. Wertz PW, Downing DT. Free sphingosine in human epidermis. *J. Invest. Dermatol.* 1990;94:159–161.
13. Wertz PW, Downing DT. Ceramidase activity in porcine epidermis. *FEBS Lett.* 1990;268:110–112.
14. Bibel DJ, Aly R, Shinefield HR. Antimicrobial activity of sphingosines. *J. Invest. Dermatol.* 1992;98:269–273.
15. Bibel DJ, Aly R, Shah S, Shinefield HR. Sphingosines: antimicrobial barriers of the skin. *Acta. Derm. Venereol.* 1993;73:407–411.
16. Payne CD, Ray TL, Downing DT. Cholesterol sulfate protects *Candida albicans* from inhibition by sphingosine *in vitro*. *J. Invest. Dermatol.* 1996;106:549–552.
17. Strum JC, Ghosh S, Bell RM. Lipid second messengers: a role in cell growth and cell cycle progression. *Adv. Exp. Med. Biol.* 1997;407:421–431.
18. Downing DT, Strauss JS. Synthesis and composition of surface lipids of human skin. *J. Invest. Dermatol.* 1974;62:228–244.
19. Wertz PW. Sebum secretion and acne. In: Rawlings AV, Webster T, (editors) *Acne and Its Therapy*. New York: Marcel Dekker, Inc., 2007. pp. 37–44.
20. Dale BA, Fredericks LP. Antimicrobial peptides in the oral environment: expression and function in health and disease. *Curr. Issues Mol. Biol.* 2005;7:119–134.

21. Puy CL. The role of saliva in maintaining oral health and as an aid to diagnosis. *Med. Oral Path. Oral Cir. Bucal.* 2006;11:E449–E455.
22. Wertz PW, Squier CA. Biochemical basis of the permeability barrier in skin and oral mucosa. In: Rathbone MJ, (editor) *Oral Mucosal Drug Delivery.* Wilmington: AAI Inc., 1996. pp. 1–26.
23. Steen Law SL, Squier CA, Wertz PW. Free sphingosine in oral epithelium. *Comp. Biochem. Physiol.* 1994;110B:511–513.
24. Law S, Wertz PW, Swartzendruber DC, Squier CA. Regional variation in content, composition and organization of porcine epithelial barrier lipids revealed by thin-layer chromatography and transmission EM. *Arch. Oral. Biol.* 1995;40:1085–1091.
25. Squier CA, Wertz PW. Structure and function of the oral mucosa and implications for drug delivery. In: Rathbone MJ, (editor) *Oral Mucosal Drug Delivery.* Wilmington: AAI Inc., 1996. pp. 1–26.
26. Gorski M, Buchner A, Fundoianu-Dayan D, Cohewn C. Fordyce's granules in the oral mucosa of adult Israeli Jews. *Comm. Dent. Oral. Epidemiol.* 1986;14:231–232.
27. Batsakis JG, el-Naggar AK. Sebaceous lesions of salivary glands and oral cavity. *Ann. Otol. Rhinol. Laryngol.* 1990;99:416–418.
28. Daley T. Pathology of intraoral sebaceous glands. *J. Oral. Pathol. Med.* 1993;22:241–245.
29. Olivier JH. Fordyce granules on the prolabial and oral mucous membranes of a selected population. *SADJ* 2006;61:72–74.
30. Nordstrom KM, McGinley KJ, Lessin SR, Leyden JJ. Neutral lipid composition of Fordyce's granules. *Brit. J. Dermatol.* 1989;121:669–670.
31. James AT, Wheatley VR. Studies of sebum. 6. The determination of component fatty acids of human forearm sebum by gas–liquid chromatography. *Biochem. J.* 1956;63:269–273.
32. Haahti E. Major lipid constituents of human skin surface with special reference to gas chromatographic methods. *Scand. J. Clin. Lab. Invest.* 1961;13(Suppl. 59):1–108.
33. Kabara JJ, Swieczkowski DM, Conley AJ, Truant JP. Fatty acid derivatives as antimicrobial agents. *Antimicrob. Agents Chemother.* 1972;2:23–28.
34. Kabara JJ, Vrable R. Antimicrobial lipids: natural and synthetic fatty acids and monoglycerides. *Lipids* 1977;12:753–759.
35. Takigawa H, Nakagawa H, Kuzukawa M, Mori H, Imokawa G. Deficient production of hexadecenoic acid is associated in part with the vulnerability of atopic patients to colonization by *Staphylococcus aureus. Dermatology* 2005;211:240–248.
36. Stewart ME, Downing DT. Free sphingosines of human skin include 6-hydroxysphingosine and unusually long-chain dihydrosphingosines. *J. Invest. Dermatol.* 1995;105:613–618.
37. Imokawa G. Lipid abnormalities in atopic dermatitis. *J. Am. Acad. Dermatol.* 2001;45(Suppl. 1): S29–S32.
38. Abeck D, Mempel M. *Staphylococcus aureus* colonization in atopic dermatitis and its therapeutic implications. *Brit. J. Dermatol.* 1998;139:13–16.
39. Arikawa J, Ishibashi M, Kawashima M, Takagi Y, Ichikawa Y, Imokawa G. Decreased levels of sphingosine, a natural antimicrobial agent, may be associated with vulnerability of the stratum corneum from patients with atopic dermatitis to colonization with *Staphylococcus aureus. J. Invest. Dermatol.* 2002;119:433–439.

CHAPTER 5

RESIDENT MICROFLORA AND ANTIMICROBIAL PEPTIDES OF SKIN

Shamim A. Ansari

Colgate-Palmolive Co., Technology Center, Piscataway, NJ

5.1   INTRODUCTION

Skin is the most exposed organ of human body and acts as the body's first line of defense against infection and illness. Skin is also the largest organ of the body with a surface area of about $2\,m^2$ in an average human adult. This vast organ is originally microbe free, but soon after birth microbes start to colonize on the stratum corneum and eventually establish a complex microbial ecosystem [1,2]. The health of skin depends upon the delicate balance between skin and millions of bacteria and other organisms such as fungi, viruses, and mites on the skin [3]. A variety of physico-chemical factors in skin such as acidic pH, moisture, and sebum content influence the growth of skin microflora.

In recent years, a comprehensive research expedition on skin microbiomes has been launched essentially to uncover and analyze all the skin microbes at the DNA and genome levels. Studies published so far have uncovered new findings [3–5]. Analysis of 16s ribosomal RNA gene sequence obtained from 20 distinct skin sites reveals the presence of a much wider array of bacteria than previously thought [3]. The study also found that body location greatly influences bacterial diversity. For example, the bacteria in the underarm are more similar among different individuals than the bacteria on the forearm.

Human skin is also equipped with a complex network of innate immune system to defend itself from microbial attacks and invasion. The skin's antimicrobial defense apparatus includes various physical and chemical factors. For example, the mechanical rigidity of the stratum corneum, increased phospholipase A_2 activity, low moisture content, lipids, lysozyme, and the continuous exfoliation process by which the outer layer of skin completely renewed every 15–28 days [6–8] are all part of the innate immune system. At cellular level, Langerhans' cells (also termed as dendritic cells) that reside in the epidermis play an important role as immune cells [9].

Innate Immune System of Skin and Oral Mucosa: Properties and Impact in Pharmaceutics, Cosmetics, and Personal Care Products, First Edition. Nava Dayan and Philip W. Wertz.
© 2011 John Wiley & Sons, Inc. Published 2011 by John Wiley & Sons, Inc.

Langerhans' cells alert the immune system about in-coming threats. They produce cytokines, signal molecules that influence the immune system to take action against various external stimuli such as sun, smoke, and other environmental assaults. Langerhans' cells also modulate biochemical imbalances that lead to inflammatory skin conditions. They are involved in boosting collagen synthesis and enhance wound repair process. Recent experimental evidences are emerging that propose different role for these important cells [9,10]. The role of these cells is discussed in detail elsewhere in this book.

Functionally, skin's innate immune system is also involved in the release of various immune mediators, such as cytokines and chemokines, recruitment and activation of phagocytes, and the production of defensins or antimicrobial proteins/peptides [11–14]. Antimicrobial peptides (AMPs) act as innate chemical shield, which provides a frontline defense against microbial invasion. Apart from exhibiting a broad spectrum microbicidal properties, AMPs are also involved in activation and modulation of the immune system. Thus, improving the skin's innate immune defenses is the best way to achieve a healthier skin and may also benefit overall health of the body. The aim of this chapter is to discuss the resident microflora and how this diverse population of bacteria reacts or parts with the skin under normal health or disease conditions. We will also discuss the antimicrobial peptides of skin and highlight their respective roles in health and disease, and provide a brief overview on skin cleansers and their impact on skin health and immunity.

5.2 RESIDENT MICROFLORA OF THE SKIN

Bacterial colonization of human skin begins during birth and the process continues in next several months and years to stabilize the microflora growth on the skin. Being the most exposed organ of human body, skin constantly encounters a variety of micro-organisms. Billions of bacteria reside on the skin. Bacteria–skin relationship can be commensal (i.e., the type of relationship between two organisms in which one organism benefits but the other is unaffected), symbiotic (i.e., close, often long-term relationship between different biological species), or parasitic (i.e., the relationship in which one organism, parasite, lives off another organism or host) relative to the host's overall physical and immune status. The status of microbes on skin can be temporary or transient and permanent or resident biota. Transient bacteria are those that come in contact with the skin and live temporarily due to unfavorable skin environment. On the other hand, permanent or resident microbiota are members of the normal flora that live in or on the body permanently without causing any harm to healthy individuals under normal conditions. Permanent colonization of a bacterial species depends on the adaptability of the organism to adhere to the skin epithelium, grow in a relatively dry and acidic environment, and establish relationships that are more mutualistic than commensalistic [15–17]. Bacterial adhesion or detachment from the skin could be mediated by (a) specific interactions via lectin or sugar binding, (b) hydrophobic interactions, and (c) electrostatic interactions [18,19].

The colonization of specific bacterial species and their population density on various location of the skin depend on physicochemical characteristics of the skin and environmental factors of that particular niche, for example, the anatomical location, amount of sebum and sweat production, pH, moisture content, temperature, and light exposure [20,21]. Skin's microbial composition and density are also influenced by the age, personal habits, and immune and hormonal status of the host [22,23]. Not all bacteria are able to reside on skin; only those bacteria that protect the host from pathogenic bacteria both directly and indirectly are allowed to take the resident status on skin. These resident bacteria provide protection to the host by producing antibiotics (e.g., bacteriocin) and toxic metabolites, inducing a low reduction–oxidation potential, depleting essential nutrients, preventing attachment of competing bacteria, inhibiting translocation by degrading toxins, and so on [15,22]. Minor racial and gender differences as factors in skin microflora have been suggested [4,24]. Interestingly, in a recent study, in which the taxonomic diversity, evenness, and richness of each sites' microbiome were examined using the ecological diversity statistics [3], revealed that the richest site with diverse microbiome was the volar forearm. The most even site was the politeal fossa; the least even sites were back, retroauricular crease, and toe web space. In general, the sebaceous sites were less diverse, less even, and less rich than moist and dry sites [3].

Common resident bacterial species on normal skin belong to Gram-positive bacteria that include *Staphylococcus, Micrococcus, Corynebacterium, Brevibacteria, Propionibacteria,* and *Acinetobacter* [20,22,25,26]. These bacterial species have specific affinity for different skin sites, some are more populated in underarm and groin area and others are more prominent in drier areas (Table 5.1).

The Gram-negative bacteria make up the minor constituents of the normal skin flora. Acinetobacter is one of the few Gram-negative bacteria commonly found on skin. Generally, *Staphylococcus aureus, Streptococcus pyogenes, Escherichia*

TABLE 5.1 Resident Skin Bacteria and Their Dominant Sites

Bacteria	Skin site
S. epidermidis	Upper trunk
S. hominis	Glabrous skin
S. aureus	Nostrils, sebaceous sites
S. capitis	Head
S. saccharoliticus	Forehead/antecubital
S. saprophyticus	Perineum
M. luteus	Forearm
Corynebacterium xerosis	Perineum, axilla, conjuctiva
C. minutissimum	Toe webs, axilla, intertriginous area
C. jeikeium	Intertriginous (e.g., axilla) area
P. acnes	Sebaceous gland, forehead
P. granulosum	Sebaceous gland, forehead, axilla
P. avidum	Axilla
Brevibacterium spp.	Axilla, toe webs
Dermabacter spp.	Forearm
Acinetobacter spp.	Forearm, forehead, toe webs

coli, and *Pseudomonas aeruginosa* can be isolated from skin as transient colonizers [25,27]. The presence of *E. coli* on the skin surface is indicative of fecal contamination. Yeasts and fungi are uncommon on the skin surface, but the lipophilic yeast *Pityrosporum ovalis* is occasionally found on the scalp.

In recent years, the advances in sophisticated molecular techniques have led to new discoveries in the microbiome of the human body including skin [28–33]. Using molecular tools some unknown species that had never before been identified on skin or described in the literature were identified [4,34]. A total of 182 species of bacteria were identified on human forearm skin, of which 8% were unknown species [35]. Roughly, half the bacteria identified in the samples were normal resident bacteria such as *Propionibacteria, Corynebacteria, Staphylococcus*, and *Streptococcus*. Interestingly, the study also noticed subtle individual and gender differences in the type of bacterial species isolated.

A recent study in which the palmar surfaces of the dominant and nondominant hands of 51 healthy young adults were examined using a novel pyrosequencing-based method for bacterial diversity and variability within and between individuals [36]. The study found highly diverse bacterial communities, >150 unique species-level bacterial phylotypes, and identified a total of 4742 unique phylotypes across all the hands examined [36]. The study also found a higher bacterial diversity in women than men, and bacterial community composition was greatly affected by handedness, time since the last hand washing, and gender.

5.3   PROTECTIVE ROLE OF RESIDENT MICROFLORA

The permanent residency of the skin flora is the direct result of a mutually beneficial relationship between the bacteria and the host. One of the attributes of skin's innate immune system is that it allows commensal bacteria to establish residency so that it prevents invasion by potential pathogenic organisms. Normal flora thrives on the host-generated nutrients and in turn the microflora acts as protective barrier and directly or indirectly prevents invasion and growth of pathogenic bacteria [37,38]. A healthy population of the resident bacteria effectively denies the colonization by transient bacteria including *E. coli*, coagulase positive *S. aureus*, group A *Streptococci* (GAS), *Pseudomonas* spp., and *Candida albicans*. Some resident bacteria produce antibiotics, for example, bacteriocins, toxic metabolites, create low reduction–oxidation potential, deplete essential nutrients, prevent attachment, and degrade toxins produced by the invading microbes. For example, *S. epidermidis* binds to keratinocyte receptors and prevents attachment of pathogenic *S. aureus* [39,40]. *S. aureus* strain 502A releases bacteriocin that inhibits other virulent staphylococci [40]. *Propionibacterium acnes* releases fatty acids from sebum breakdown, thus acidifying the milieu and inhibiting the growth of *S. pyogenes* [41].

It has also been suggested that skin pathogenic and commensal bacteria such as group A *Streptococci* and *S. epidermidis*, respectively, upregulate keratinocyte human β-defensin 2 (HBD2) utilizing different signaling pathways [42]. The signal transduction leads to the expression of antimicrobial peptides, proinflammatory cytokines, chemokines, and inducible enzymes. Indirectly, resident bacteria can induce host immune system; for example, they stimulate phagocytosis and augment interferon and other cytokines' production. This protective role of normal flora suggests that an excessive use of antimicrobial skin cleansers because of not exhibiting a selective mode of action may make the skin vulnerable to infection by more hostile Gram-negative bacteria rather than protecting it [43–45].

5.4 ROLE OF SKIN MICROFLORA IN SKIN DISEASES

One of the important benefits of the normal resident flora is preventing transient pathogenic organisms from colonizing the skin. Therefore, cutaneous invasion and infection depends on the health status of the skin, its local microenvironment, immune status, and pathogenic potential of invading microbes. Resident microbes can also cause skin infections and in some cases can lead to life-threatening conditions in the host, particularly immunocompromised people [46]. Among the transient Gram-negative organisms, *Pseudomonas aeruginosa*, *Pasteurella multocida*, *Klebsiella rhinoscleromatis*, and *Vibrio* spp. are known to cause skin infection. Pathogenicity of bacteria depends on their ability to attach to, grow on, and invade the host tissues [20]. Bacteria possess virulence genes that facilitate the invasion and subsequent disease process. For example, *S. aureus* and *S. pyogenes* produce toxins that may elicit superantigen response triggering a massive release of cytokines. These superantigens cause Staphylococcal scalded skin syndrome, toxic shock syndrome, and scarlet fever [47]. The normal flora also carries the opportunistic character. Resident organisms have been shown to play a role in noninfectious skin diseases such as atopic dermatitis [48], rosacea, psoriasis [49], and acne [50]. Bacteria otherwise nonpathogenic in normal skin condition can become pathogenic when the skin is compromised [23].

There is a selective shift in microbial community linked to some skin diseases. In atopic dermatitis, recurrent bacterial infection and heavy recolonization of *S. aureus* was linked to the antibiotic resistance, nasal carriage, and treatment contamination [51–53]. In psoriasis, the microbial population was higher than for other normal skin samples [5] and a substantial alteration in microbial flora was observed. Bacteria isolated from patients with rosacea have shown to function very differently from the same type of bacteria isolated from normal rosacea-free skin. Bacteria isolated from patients with rosacea also produced different types of proteins in different amounts at 37°C versus at 30°C temperature. These observations indicate that increase in facial skin temperature in rosacea patients is likely to play a role in altered bacterial protein synthesis [54]. A great deal of research is required to understand the shift in specific microbiota under disease condition, which would lead to novel approaches to control numbers of overrepresented organisms and help repopulate normal resident flora that diminish in disease.

5.5 INNATE ANTIMICROBIAL SKIN DEFENSES

The physical properties of skin, for example, dryness, acidic pH, and temperature lower than 37°C, act as defensive barriers are mostly unfavorable conditions for bacterial growth. The dead keratinized cells that are constantly being sloughed off in a way that removes the colonized organisms from skin acts as a "cleansing mechanism" that adds to the overall protective attributes. Chemical components of the antimicrobial defense include lysozymes, RNases, and antimicrobial lipids secreted via hair follicles and produced by sweat glands [55,56]. One of the key components of this natural immune defense system is a group of antimicrobial peptides such as cathelicidins and defensins produced by the epithelial cells. Evidence for the important role of antimicrobial peptides in innate immunity is well documented [57,58]. These antimicrobial proteins are gene-encoded endogenous proteins. Several *in vivo* studies have demonstrated that AMPs have a broad spectrum of activity and the capacity to protect the host against a wide range of bacteria, viruses, fungi, and parasites [59–62]. AMPs are capable of killing bacteria, fungi, viruses, and parasites at micro- and nanomolar concentrations. The minimal inhibitory concentration (MIC) of these peptides ranges from 0.1 to 100 µg/mL [63]. Production of these peptides is very limited under normal conditions; however, some of these AMPs are upregulated at sites of infection, inflammation, and tissue injury, such as human β-defensins 2 and 3 (HBD-2, HBD-3) and cathelicidin LL-37 [64–68].

Recent studies have revealed that some of these AMPs, especially cathelicidins, protect the skin through two distinct pathways: (1) by direct antimicrobial activity and (2) by inducing various immune apparatuses such as cytokine release, angiogenesis, and reepithelialization [69,70]. Most of these peptides are small 12–50 amino acids, positively charged with an amphipathic structure. Structurally, these AMPs can be divided into several categories such as peptides with an α-helix structure, peptides with a β-sheet structure stabilized by disulfide bridges, or peptides with an extended or loop structure. Beneath the epidermis of the skin are Langerhans' cells, the immature dendritic cells that phagocytose and kill microbes.

In human skin, major antimicrobial peptides include human β-defensins, cathelicidins or LL-37, dermacidin (DCD), and psoriasin [71]. In addition to these peptides, there are a number of other components (Table 5.2) such as BPI [72,73], sphingosins [74], lactic acid [75], lysozyme [63,76], RNase 7 [77] that play a role in host immune defense. These defense molecules are at work even before birth since

TABLE 5.2 Examples of Selected Defense Components of Human Skin

Defense component	Function	References
LL-37	Antimicrobial and immune modulatory activity	[14,86]
Beta-defensins	Antimicrobial, antienveloped viruses Activation of dendritic cells	[44,87–89,117]
Dermacidin	Antibacterial and antifungal	[90,127]
Psoriasin	Antibacterial and chemokine activity	[92,128]
BPI	Active against G (−) bacteria	[73]
Fatty acids	Prevent microbial growth	[53,56,75,134]
Sphingosine	Natural antibacterial agent	[74,129,130]
Lysozyme	Hydrolyzes bacterial cell wall peptidoglycan	[63,76]
RNase 7	Antimicrobial, ribonuclease activity	[77,93]

many of these molecules are present in the vernix caseosa (lipid-rich film) that attaches to fetal and neonatal skin [78].

The mode of action of most AMPs is not clearly understood; however, it is largely believed that most AMPs kill microbes by causing membrane leakage or disruption [79–81]. A number of models such as "barrel-stave" and "carpet-like" for membrane permeation by amphipathic α-helical peptides have been proposed, but these models may not properly reflect the complex processes involved in the killing of microorganism [80,82,83]. In the barrel-stave model, channel-forming peptides position in a ring, which is barrel-like, around an aqueous pore. Peptides or peptide complexes may constitute individual transmembrane spokes in the barrel, hence the term "stave" in the model. In the carpet mechanism, a high density of peptide acts upon the microbe and causes phospholipid displacement, changes in membrane fluidity, and/or reductions in membrane barrier properties, which lead to membrane disruption. The peptides initially bind to the membrane by electrostatic interactions, yet no quaternary structures are formed. Rather, the membrane integrity is lost after a sufficient concentration of peptides is reached, causing unfavorable membrane energetics. Peptides operating under this model do not form channel-like structures and may not integrate in the hydrophobic membrane core.

Cathelicidins and β-defensins are well characterized of the AMPs found in the skin. Methicillin-resistant *S. aureus* (MRSA) is an important public health problem. Skin AMPs are one of the key host factors that determine whether MRSA colonization/exposure results in infection of skin or soft tissue [84]. A better understanding of the biology of these compounds would clarify the pathophysiology of inflammatory and infectious diseases [85].

With the rise in antibiotic resistance in managing infectious diseases, these immune defense peptides may provide useful alternatives to conventional antibiotics. A brief description of key AMPs is given in the following sections.

5.5.1 Human Cathelicidin LL-37

Cathelicidins are effectors of innate immune defense in mammals. Humans and mice have only one cathelicidin gene, whereas domesticated animals such as cows, pigs, and horses have multiple cathelicidin genes. The human cathelicidin LL-37 is an α-helical, cationic antimicrobial peptide, and cathelicidin expression *in vivo* is highly resistant to proteolytic degradation. LL-37 is induced in normal keratinocytes in response to injury or inflammation or vitamin D [94,95]. However, in sebocytes, cathelicidin expression is both constitutive and inducible [96]. Cathelicidin LL-37 produced by sebocytes has been shown to kill microflora such as *S. aureus* and *P. acnes in vitro* [96]. It is now recognized that several cell types in the skin produce cathelicidin, including keratinocytes, mast cells, neutrophils, and ecrine glands [94,97–100].

Under normal conditions, LL-37 level is very minimal, but in wounded skin the LL-37 level can reach up to 2000 ng/mg of total protein [101,102]. In sweats and seminal fluids, the concentration of LL-37 can be as high as 360 ng/mL and 140 ng/mL, respectively [98]. Interestingly, some of the cathelicidins found in sweats and seminal fluids are suggested to be the novel processed cathelicidin with enhanced antimicrobial activity [103]. LL-37 shows activity against *C. albicans in vitro*, even in physiological saline. This indicates that LL-37 can function in salty environment such as the skin surface that is salty due to the presence of sweat and its subsequent evaporation. LL-37 acts as a potent antisepsis agent by inhibiting macrophage stimulation by bacterial LPS, lipoteichoic acid, and noncapped liporabinomannan [104]. A recent study suggests that LL-37 inhibits replication of vaccinia (pox) virus [86]. It was also demonstrated that LL-37 protects mice against endotoxemia.

Advances in cathelicidin research have revealed that LL-37 is a multifunctional peptide with receptor-mediated effects on eukaryotic cells and its involvement in chemotaxis, angiogenesis, and wound healing [67,105–110]. On the other hand, cathlicidin disfunction has been linked to many skin disorders such as atopic dermatitis and psoriasis [52,86,111]. In atopic dermatitis, cathelicidin production is suppressed [52], whereas in psoriasis, cathelicidin expression is increased that has been suggested to control excessive inflammation. Downregulation of LL-37 in atopic dermatitis predisposes patients to skin infection with *S. aureus* [52].

The role of sunlight in increased expression of LL-37 has been investigated. A number of recent studies indicated that there is a link between sunlight exposure to the function of the innate immune system [112]. Individuals exposed to UVB have shown increased synthesis of vitamin D and increased expression of LL-37 in epidermis [112,113]. Vitamin D was found to induce keratinocyte LL-37 and HBD expression and antimicrobial activity against *P. aeruginosa* through consensus vitamin D response elements [112]. These observations suggest that any local deficit of immunity can be compensated by stimulating skin's antimicrobial peptide expression mediated by UVB or sunlight. Therefore, the concept that sunlight exposure to a "certain degree" may be good for the immunity is gaining some ground.

5.5.2   Human β-Defensins

Like cathelicidins, defensins are small cationic peptides (about 3–5 kDa) with a broad-spectrum antimicrobial activity against bacteria, fungi, and enveloped viruses [114–117]. Different disulfide linkage patterns separate defensin peptides into α-, β-, and θ-defensins, although humans do not produce θ-defensins [116]. Resident skin cells have not been shown to produce α-defensins. Although genes of at least 30 different human β-defensins exist, only three of them (HBD-1, -2, and -3) are expressed by keratinocytes and have been widely studied [44,118,119]. The HBDs are a group of small (4.5–5 kDa) cationic peptides with six conserved cysteine residues and three intramolecular disulfide bonds [120]. HDB-1 is constitutively produced by keratinocytes and its broad spectrum of antimicrobial activity includes Gram-negative bacteria and *C. albicans*. HBD-2 is not expressed by normal skin, but in psoriasis and in inflammatory skin conditions. It is highly expressed by keratinocytes [44,121–124]. On the other hand, HBD-3 is produced by keratinocytes only in response to infectious or inflammatory stimuli. In psoriasis, the genomic copy number of beta defensin is reported to be increased [125]. The downregulation of HBD-2 and -3 along with LL-37 is found to be relevant for the pathogenesis of atopic dermatitis [126].

5.5.3 Dermacidin

Dermacidin (DCD) is a 47 amino acid peptide produced in ecrine sweat glands and is delivered to the skin surface via sweat. Dermacidin expression is constitutive and undergoes postsecretory proteolytic processing in sweat-yielding anionic and cationic DCD peptides. DCD has a broad spectrum of antibacterial activity against *E. coli, Enterococcus faecalis, S. aureus*, and *C. albicans* [90]. It is likely that DCD in sweat may play a role in regulating the density and composition of human skin flora. The mode of action of DCD peptides is reported to be different from that of the cathelicidin LL-37. DCD causes membrane depolarization and the provocation on the integrity of bacterial cell envelope plays a role in the antimicrobial activity of DCD [127].

5.5.4 Psoriasin

Psoriasin, also referred to as S100A7, is a small, cell-secreted, calcium binding protein that is overexpressed in psoriasis, other inflammatory skin diseases, and in cancer tissues [92]. Psoriasin is highly active against the Gram-negative *E. coli* [92]. Psoriasin acts by creating pores in microbial membrane that is pH dependent. At neutral pH, *E. coli* is killed without compromising its membrane, whereas at acidic pH *Bacillus megaterium* (Gram positive) is killed by permeabilization of its cytoplasmic membrane [128]. The antimicrobial activity of psoriasin and related protein is inhibited by zinc.

5.5.5 Antimicrobial Lipids

In human skin, sebum lipids play important role as a dynamic aspect of skin innate immunity [56,129–131]. The sources of these lipids can be varied. During epidermal differentiation, for example, sphingoid bases are synthesized locally in the epidermis and carried to the outer surface of skin where other lipids are secreted by sebaceous glands. Free sphingoid bases are known to have a broad antibacterial activity [130]. Like antimicrobial peptides, fatty acids are induced in skin upon injury or microbial stimuli through Toll-like receptor-dependent pathways [132,133]. Reduced levels of sebum fatty acids and antimicrobial peptides are found in atopic dermatitis [52,53]. Skin fatty acids prevent the production of virulence determinants and the induction of antibiotic resistance in *S. aureus* and other Gram-positive organisms. A purified human skin fatty acid was shown to be effective in treating topical and systemic infections caused by *S. aureus* [134].

5.5.6 RNase 7

Another antimicrobial protein expressed in human skin is RNase 7, a member of the RNase A superfamily. RNase 7 is characterized by homology with bovine ribonuclease A [55]. To date, 13 human RNase members (RNase 1–13) of the RNase superfamily have been identified [55]. However, the physiological role of these ribonucleases is not clear. A recent study suggests that RNase 7 may play a major role in skin defense and contributes to the high resistance of human skin against colonization with the Gram-positive enteric bacteria *E. faecium* [93].

5.6 EFFECTS OF SKIN-CLEANSING PRODUCTS ON SKIN MICROFLORA AND SKIN IMMUNITY

Historically, the use of soap as skin cleanser dates back to some 5000 years; however, industrial production of soaps started in 19th century. It is now a universal fact that the routine use of skin cleansers has multidimensional benefits to the user in terms of reducing/eliminating the transient organisms and maintaining the resident microflora at a healthy level. Soap is still the most commonly used form of skin cleanser. Commercially available skin cleansers come mainly in two forms: (1) solid as bar soaps and (2) liquid as liquid hand and body wash and facial cleansers and lotions. The major constituents in skin cleansers are surfactants (i.e., detergents and emulsifiers/soaps), which lower the surface tension on the skin due to the emulsification of fat, thus helping to remove dirt, oil, sweat, sebum, microbes, and dead corneocytes. In addition, surfactants aid in the normal exfoliation process of the skin. Water alone removes about 65% of oil and dirt from the skin. In some cases, skin cleansers remove not only dirt but also some beneficial lipids; especially the harsh surfactants may disrupt epidermal barrier function [135] resulting in accelerated transepidermal water loss (TEWL). The use of skin-cleansing products can also have effect on the skin flora [136].

An ideal skin cleanser should effectively remove dirt and oils, including the oil from cosmetic products used, environmental pollutants, and transient microbes from the skin without damaging the barrier properties or irritating the skin. One of the most important benefits of using skin-cleansing products, especially the hand wash products, is that these products prevent the spread of infectious diseases. Laboratory and community-based studies have shown the antimicrobial and degerming effects of these products [137,138]. It is now widely recognized that proper washing of hands with soap and water is regarded as one of the most important steps in preventing the spread of infectious diseases. A recent community-based study has shown that the use of skin-cleansing soap coupled with hand washing promotion resulted in 50% decrease in pneumonia, 53% reduction in diarrhea, and 34% reduction in impetigo (skin infection) in children under 5 years of age [139].

Depending on the type, surfactants can have harmful effects on the outermost layer of the skin, that is, stratum corneum, such as postwash skin tightness, dryness, barrier damage, redness, irritation, and itching. Surfactants in the cleansers can bind to the corneocyte proteins making them overhydrated and swell. This swelling may facilitate cleanser ingredients to penetrate into the skin where they interact with nerve endings and immune system inducing inflammatory response and itching. Once the water evaporates, it leaves the skin dryer than before. Skin cleansers can also remove the natural moisturizing factor (NMF) from the skin and damage the lipid structures causing a reduction in the amounts of lipids in the skin. NMF is a collection of free amino acids, along with other physiological chemicals such as lactic acid, urea, and salts; together these elements are known as "natural moisturizing factors." The interactions of surfactants with the skin have been extensively studied in the past [140]. In general, skin-cleansing surfactants are broadly divided into soap-based surfactants and synthetic detergent-based (syndet) surfactants. Soaps are chemically the alkali salt of fatty acids with a pH between 9 and 10. On the other hand, chemically, a synthetic detergent can be anionic, cationic, nonionic, or amphoteric depending on its chemistry and surfactant type [141]. Examples of various skin-cleansing products are listed in Table 5.3.

5.6.1 Plain Alkaline Bar Soap

The effects of skin-cleansing products on the pH, moisture, and fat content of the skin are well documented [142]. The alkaline bar soaps significantly increase the skin pH. In general, all skin cleansers remove fats and oil from skin, but alkaline bar soap has been shown to cause the highest reduction in fat content [142]. Increase in pH irritates the skin and long-term usage of these products has been shown to alter the skin surface pH and affect the skin microflora [143–145]. The use of an alkaline soap results in higher skin surface pH and significantly increases the number of *Propionibacteria* [142,146]. Compared to acidic syndet bar soap, washing of facial skin with alkaline soap in acne-prone young adults was reported to cause more inflammatory reaction [147]. On the other hand, although washing with an acidic skin cleanser (pH of 5.5) in adults was shown to increase the skin surface pH, this increase was significantly less than the increase caused by the alkaline soap [142,148,149]. On the forehead, there was a clear correlation between bacterial counts and skin pH both with *Propionibacteria* and with *Staphylococci*, but on the forearm only *Propionibacteria* count was higher with higher pH. The number of *Propionibacteria* was significantly linked to the skin pH [146]. In a crossover clinical study, Korting et al. [150] have shown that when soap was used, compared to syndet, the skin pH increased and the number of *Propionibacteria* was increased significantly, but no change in the coagulase-negative staphylococci counts was observed.

The soaps commonly recommended and used by the population at large have a pH, which is neutral to alkaline in most cases, ranging between 7 and 9. Those skin cleansers that exhibit a pH value closer to the pH of the normal skin (pH 4.5–6) are less drying and mild to skin. It is evident from the available studies that the pH of the skin changes depending on the pH of the cleanser used. This has a multifold impact on the skin in terms of the barrier damage, moisture content, the irritability, and the bacterial flora. Thus, before recommending a cleanser to a patient especially in case of atopic dermatitis, sensitive and acne-prone skin, one should carefully consider the pH of the cleanser in use.

5.6.2 Antibacterial Soap

Unlike plain soap, antibacterial soaps contain an antibacterial active that is bacteriostatic or bactericidal in nature. In addition to cleansing the skin off dirt, bacteria, body sweat, oil, and other odorous by-products, antibacterial soaps reduce/inhibit the bacterial growth on skin. The bacteriostatic or bactericidal efficacy depends on the nature of the antibacterial active and the delivery of the active on the skin surface. The

TABLE 5.3 Examples of Skin-Cleansing Products

Type of cleanser	Chemistry/additives	Usage and attributes	References
Alkaline bar soap	Saponification of fats and oils with strong alkali	Hand and body wash; drying, irritating, raises skin pH, hard water creates soap scum	[141,145,151–153]
Syndet bar	Synthetic surfactants	Hand, body, and facial wash; cleansing, high lather, mildness, skin-feel	[145,150,154]
Combar (soap + synthetic surfactants)	Combination of superfatted soap and synthetic surfactants	Hand and body wash; less irritating than soap; less mild than syndet bars	[142,147,154]
Beauty bar soap	Synthetic anionic surfactants, also contain emollients	Hand and body wash; less drying and irritating, causes follicular plugging, keeps the skin pH near neutral to alkaline	[154,156]
Antibacterial bar soap	Saponification of fats and oils with strong alkali	Hand, body, and facial wash; kills/inhibits skin bacteria; eliminates transient bacteria; long-lasting residual efficacy	[153,155,156]
Dermatologic bars/cakes	Amphoteric, anionic, and nonionic surfactants	Hand and body wash; may raise skin pH, emollients added to reduce dryness and irritation; antiacne	[150,157,158]
Cosmetic liquid cleansers	Nonionic, aninonic, amphoteric surfactants; other additives may include silicone, moisturizers, emollients, bioactive molecules	Hand, body, and facial wash; mild, skin protectant, moisturizing, and less irritating, pH around acidic similar to skin, high rinsibility factor. Antiacne	[159,160]
Antiseptic, antibacterial liquid cleansers	Amphoteric, anionic, and nonionic surfactants. Examples of antibacterial actives: triclosan, TCC, PCMX, CHG, Quats	Hand, body, and facial wash; potentially less drying and irritating than topical bactericide, may raise skin pH, adjunct to acne treatment, may help control bacteria	[161–165]

commercialization of antibacterial soap started around mid-twentieth century. During the past five decades, the use of antibacterial soap in homes, hospitals, and other institutional settings has increased significantly. A recent survey indicates that 45% of the commercially available soaps contain antibacterial agents [165]. Initially, the bar soaps with antibacterial actives were developed and marketed as deodorant soaps, but were later marketed for their antibacterial benefits as well. The most commonly used antibacterial actives in soap products includes triclosan (TCS), chlorohexidine gluconate, triclocarban (TCC), benzalkonium chloride (BKC), benzethonium chloride (BTC), and parachlorometaxylenol (PCMX).

It is widely believed that the overuse of antibiotics in human illnesses and in livestock has contributed to the emergence of antibiotic-resistant bacteria in the community. Does the regular use of antibacterial soap by general population could lead to the emergence of resistant pathogens? This issue has been widely debated in the scientific community [166–169]. Although there may be some similarities in the mechanism of action of antibacterial actives used in skin-cleansing products and antibiotics, there has been no evidence of the development of cross-resistance to antibiotics due to the use of antibacterial wash products in the community [170,171]. Multiple community-based studies have demonstrated significant reductions in infections, specifically in enteric diseases as a result of hand hygiene interventions [172–178]. A laboratory-based clinical hand wash study demonstrated significantly less transfer of *Shigella felxineri* from artificially contaminated hands to melon balls following hand washing with an antibacterial soap compared to a plain soap, suggesting potential infection reduction benefits of antibacterial soap [138].

Few laboratory-based studies [169,179,180] have reported that bacteria may develop resistance to triclosan when exposed to sublethal doses of triclosan over time. However, to date no organism originally known to be sensitive to triclosan has been found on human skin that became resistant due to the use of triclosan-containing products. A recent retrospective study (personal communication) found no increased antibiotic resistance in *Staphylococcus* isolates from groups regularly using antibacterial wash products containing TCC or triclosan, compared to the groups using wash products containing no TCC or TCS. In addition, none of the 317 study isolates was resistant to vancomycin, and the rate of MRSA detected was appreciably less than that reported in the literature for both inpatient and outpatient isolates of MRSA.

There are also some misconceptions that regular use of antibacterial soap would lead to sterile condition and increase the risk of invasion by pathogenic organisms. Interestingly, several studies have actually reported higher postwash count than prewash [181–183]. This might be due to increased shedding of the skin during the washing and increased dispersion of bacterial microcolonies. Moreover, Larson et al. found that those using the plain soap were significantly more likely to have larger proportion of higher postwash counts compared to prewash count after 1 year of use [184]. These observations may indicate that mere washing of skin with plain or antibacterial soap does not disturb or alter the bacterial population in any significant way. Antimicrobials may cause reduction in the density of the skin flora for a short duration, and the skin flora tend to regrow to the previous level within 24–48 h. While the use of antimicrobials may induce irritant and allergic contact dermatitis in some users, no evidence exists that the use of antimicrobial products may alter the ecology of resident skin bacteria that would lead to the overgrowth of pathogenic bacteria [185]. Clearly, more work would be needed to clearly understand the effect of long-term usage of antimicrobial-containing skin cleansers on skin microflora.

Pathogenic bacteria and viruses are known to survive very well on human hands [186,187]. Pathogens are also known to be transferred from person to person via hand contact [161,188]. Proper hand washing is one of the most important intervention steps in disease transmission and control because it reduces and/or inactivates the microbial load on the hands and decreases the chance of self-inoculation or spread of microorganisms from the contaminated hands to other hands or inanimate objects and food products [138,186,189–191]. Studies conducted on human hands have shown that the use of antibacterial soaps provides greater reduction in the number of bacteria on the hands compared to the use of regular soaps [138]. Furthermore, antibacterial soap may substantially reduce the transmission of bacteria from the hands to inanimate objects and food items [138,190].

A comparative study on the effects of antibacterial deodorant soap containing triclocarban versus a plain soap on the skin flora found no significant difference in total colony counts [192]. However, more *S. epidermidis* was observed with plain soap, while washing with deodorant soap resulted in higher colonization of *Acinetobacter calcoaceticus* and *Micrococcus luteus*. A new antibacterial soap preparation containing TCC was compared in laboratory tests with commercially available hexachlorophene soap and a control, nongermicidal soap. Both antibacterial soaps showed significant reductions in the skin flora; however, there was no difference between the two preparations. More recently, an 18-month-long study conducted in a ward showed that the use of TCC soap significantly reduced the transmission of staphylococci [193]. In a clinical study involving patients with atopic dermatitis, those who bathed with soap containing 1.5% TCC had greater reductions in *S. aureus* colonization and in the severity and extent of skin lesions than those who used plain soap [194].

Chlorhexidine gluconate (CHG)-containing skin cleansers have also been shown to be effective against bacteria, fungi, and viruses [162]. CHG is an FDA-approved antimicrobial agent for topical application in products for use as surgical scrub, healthcare personnel hand wash, and patient preoperative scrub [195]. CHG-containing skin cleansers are commercially available in various liquid and foam bases at 2% and 4% concentrations. CHG-containing hand wash products have been shown to reduce skin microflora in a single wash and further reductions in subsequent multiple washes. The concentration of CHG may also impact the level of bacterial reduction; for example, in one study [196], although not significantly different, the reductions in flora among those using the 2% CHG product were less than among those using the products with 4% CHG. CHG-containing skin cleansers are mostly used in healthcare settings as surgical scrub and preoperative skin preparation and are not used as daily hand wash regimen due to its adverse effect on skin.

Alcohol or ethanol is widely used in many topical products with direct exposure to the human skin. One of the growing trends is the use of alcohol-based hand sanitizer for hand disinfection [197]. The antimicrobial effect of alcohol-based hand sanitizers is of a fast-acting nature, but due to evaporation it does not provide a lasting residual efficacy. Ethanol also dries the skin, extracts secreted lipids, and may serve as penetration enhancer that leads to irritation. Opposing arguments on the safety of topical applications of alcohol can be found in the scientific literature and warrant further studies on this topic [198]. On the other hand, cationic chlorohexidine strongly binds with the skin resulting in persistent antimicrobial effect. Antiseptic hand wash products intended for use by healthcare workers are regulated by the US Food and Drug Administration as over-the-counter or OTC drug products. The requirements for *in vitro* and *in vivo* testing of these products as well as surgical hand scrubs are described in the FDA Tentative Final Monograph for Health-care Topical Antiseptic Drug Products issued in 1994 [199].

The antimicrobial wash products do not exhibit moisturizing properties to skin. Lotions have been developed to provide antimicrobial activity to inactivate/ destroy microorganisms on the surface of the skin while also providing a moisturizing benefit. Moisturizing lotions usually contain emollients such as glycerin that has been shown to improve the hydration of the horny layer of skin [200,201]. Skin cleansing particularly in institutional settings such as hospital, nurseries, day care centers, and food establishments requires potent antimicrobial agents to kill and/or eliminate germs from hands of care-givers and also provide, in conjunction with antimicrobial properties, skin moisturizing benefit. Excessive hand washing with soaps is not totally harmless. In particular, harsh soaps can alter the acidic mantle of the skin that can hinder some of the protective fatty acid secretions. Excessive washing can also remove protective microflora leaving the newly exposed skin susceptible to colonization by other potentially pathogenic microorganisms. People working in healthcare settings who scrub their hands frequently are prone to sustain barrier damage and skin infections. Dry and barrier-damaged skin also suffers from irritation and inflammation.

Although a number of studies have been published on the role of surfactants in affecting the skin pH, depletion of proteins, and lipids, there has been very little work done to understand the effects of skin cleansers on skin's innate immunity. In recent years, there has been a growing interest in developing skin care products that boost skin immunity and its defense mechanisms. Enhancing the skin's natural antimicrobial defenses would help to prevent infection and maintain skin health and can possibly improve the over-all health. Patients with atopic dermatitis are susceptible to bacterial skin infections because patients with atopic dermatitis fail to produce effective amounts of the antimicrobial peptides LL-37 and β-defensin 2 and 3. These findings suggest that boosting the synthesis of antimicrobial peptides may ameliorate the skin conditions. Skin's immunity provides skin with power to repair and regenerate and maintain a healthy balance between the host and microbe and the environment. As skin gets older, its natural immune system starts to slow down. As a result, skin loses its power to effectively protect, prevent, and repair damages due to biological, chemical, or physical factors.

5.7   CONCLUDING REMARKS

Skin is a vital organ of the human body responsible for protecting the body from various physical, chemical, biological, and environmental stressors. In that role, skin possesses a network of defensive apparatuses. The resident microflora, antimicrobial peptides, antimicrobial lipids, and other immune components play respective roles in defending the skin. The resident microflora protects the skin from invasion by pathogenic microbes by producing antibiotics and enzymes, making the local environment hostile for the invading microbes, and preventing unwanted inflammation. The acidic pH of the skin also plays a role in controlling the microbial colonization of skin. Under normal conditions, skin microflora is in a mutualistic relationship with the host; however, in altered circumstances, the same resident bacteria can get involved in skin conditions such as atopic dermatitis, rosacea, psoriasis, and acne. Recent advances in human microbiome project have uncovered interesting variations within and between individuals in microbial ecology. Such observations in a way will help in defining what constitutes a healthy bacterial community of the skin.

Among the various immune components that constitute skin's innate immunity, antimicrobial peptides, especially cathelicidin LL-37 and human β-defensins 1 and 2, are the key players involved in the protective mechanisms. Normally, production of these peptides is minimal; however, their synthesis is upregulated at the site of infection, inflammation, and tissue injury. These antimicrobial peptides are very important in maintaining a healthy skin as evident from some of the instances where downregulation of HBD-2 and -3 and LL-37 has been linked to the pathogenesis of atopic dermatitis. Recent advances in this area indicate that some of these antimicrobial peptides not only kill microorganisms but are also involved in immune regulation and other functions. Antibacterial lipids present in the epidermis are also a factor in skin's protective mechanism. Further work is required to fully understand how antibacterial lipids are synthesized and what is their mode of action. Based on *in vitro* and *in vivo* studies [202,203] on the antimicrobial activities of lipids, the possibilities of using such lipids as active ingredients in skin-cleansing products should be considered. A better understanding of skin microflora and its innate immunity will advance the treatment of skin diseases, prevent skin infection, and improve the skin health.

The use of skin-cleansing products both removes dirt, sweat, and oil and reduces the microbial load on the skin. Skin-cleansing products with exfoliating agents also help skin cell differentiation and exfoliation. Skin cleansers with antibacterial actives further help to prevent the growth of skin flora including the odor-causing bacteria. Antibacterial hand wash products are known to be effective in eliminating transient and potentially pathogenic organisms from hands. In hospital and other institutional settings, the use of antibacterial wash products has led to the reduction in the outbreaks of infectious diseases. A clear evidence for infection reduction in homes due to the use of antibacterial wash products is yet to be demonstrated.

Skin-cleansing products, especially those formulated with harsh surfactants, may cause skin dryness due to loss of natural moisturizing factors and beneficial lipids. Resident bacteria otherwise nonpathogenic in normal skin condition can become pathogenic when skin becomes damaged [23]. Investigations in this area would lead to novel skin cleansers that would enhance local immunity and at the same time maintain healthy microflora. Generally, surfactant-based skin-cleansing products help to maintain skin's normal physiology; however, surfactant-induced barrier disruption triggers immune response resulting in irritation and inflammation. In order to minimize skin barrier damage, skin care products supplemented with emollients, humectants, and lipid analogues may protect skin from drying and irritation. The selection of a skin cleanser is very important to maintain a healthy skin. An ideal skin cleanser should remove unwanted waste materials and microbes from skin, leaving beneficial components behind to continue to nourish and protect the skin. Delivery of bioactive materials such as vitamins and antioxidants on skin via skin cleansers would also help the skin to neutralize environmental stresses.

REFERENCES

1. Aly R. Cutaneous microbiology. In: Orkin M, Maibach HI, Dahl MV, editors. *Dermatology*. Los Altos: Appleton & Lange, 1991. pp. 22–25.
2. Leyden J, McGinley K, Hoelzle E, Labows JN, Kligman AM. The microbiology of the human axilla and its relationship to axillary odor. *J. Invest. Dermatol.* 1981;77:413–416.
3. Grice EA, Kong HH, Conlan S, Deming CB, Davis J, et al. Topographical and temporal diversity of the human skin microbiome. *Science*, 2009;324:1190–1192.
4. Gao Z, Tseng CH, Pei Z, Blaser MJ. Molecular analysis of human forearm superficial skin bacterial biota. *Proc. Natl. Acad. Sci. USA* 2007;104:2927–2932.
5. Gao Z, Tseng C-H, Strober BE, Pie Z, Blaser MJ. Substantial alternations of the cutaneous bacterial biota in psoriatic lesions. *PLoS ONE* 2008;3(7):e2719.
6. Ansari SA. Skin pH and skin flora. In: Barel AO, Paye M, Maibach HI, editors. *Handbook of Cosmetic Science and Technology*, 3rd ed. New York: Informa Healthcare USA Inc., 2008. pp. 221–233.
7. Fluhr JW, Kao J, Jain M, Ahn SK, Feingold KR, Elias PM. Generation of free fatty acids from phospholipids regulates stratum corneum acidification and integrity. *J. Invest. Dermatol.* 2001;117:44–51.
8. Öhman H, Vahlquist A. The pH gradient over the stratum corneum differs in X-linked recessive and autosomal dominant ichthyosis: a clue to the molecular origin of the "acid skin mantle". *J. Invest. Dermatol.* 1998;111:674–677.
9. Mathers AR, Larregina AT. Professional antigen presenting cells of the skin. *Immunol. Res.* 2006;36:127–136.
10. Kaplan DH, Jenison MC, Saeland S, Shlomchik WD, Shlomchil MJ. Epidermal Langerhans cell-deficient mice develop enhanced contact hypersensitivity. *Immunity* 2005;23:611–620.
11. Lai Y, Gallo R. AMPed up immunity: how antimicrobial peptides have multiple role in immune defense. *Trends Immunol.* 2009;30:131–141.
12. Kai-Larsen Y, Agerberth B. The role of multi-functional peptide LL-37 in host defense. *Front. Biosci.* 2008;13:3760–3767.
13. Niyonsaba F, Someya A, Hirata M, Ogawa H, Nagaoka I. Evaluation of the effects of peptide antibiotics human beta-defensins-1/-2 and LL-37 on histamine release and prostaglandin D(2) production from mast cells. *Eur. J. Immunol.* 2001;31:1066–1075.
14. Yang D, Chertov O, Oppenheim JJ. Participation of mammalian defensins and cathelicidins in anti-microbial immunity: receptors and activities of human defensins and cathelicidin (LL-37). *J. Leukoc. Biol.* 2001;69:691–697.
15. Costerton JW, Geesey GG, Cheng KJ. How bacteria stick. *Sci. Am.* 1978;238:86–95.
16. Lambers H, Piessens S, Bloem A, Pronk H, Finkel P. Natural skin surface pH is on average below 5, which is beneficial for its resident flora. *Int. J. Cosmet. Sci.* 2006;28:359–370.
17. Rippke F, Schriener V, Schwantiz H-J. The acidic milieu of the horny layer: new findings on the physiology and pathophysiology of skin. *Am. J. Clin. Dermatol.* 2002;3:261–272.
18. Ansari SA, Scala D, Kaplan S, Jones K, Ghaim J, Polefka T. A novel skin cleansing technology that reduces bacterial attachment to the skin. Poster Abstract, 102nd General Meeting of the American Society for Microbiology, Salt Lake City, Utah, USA, 2002.
19. Ofek I, Beachy EH. General concepts and principles of bacteria adherence in animals and man. In: Beachy EH,editor. *Bacterial Adherence*. London: Chapman and Hall, 1980. pp. 3–29.

20. Feingold DS. Bacterial adherence, colonization, and pathogenicity. *Arch. Dermatol.* 1986;122:161–163.
21. Jacobi U, Gautier J, Sterry W, Lademann J. Gender-related differences in the physiology of the stratum corneum. *Dermatology* 2005;211:312–317.
22. Chiller K, Slekin BA, Murakawa GJ. Skin microflora and bacterial infections of the skin. *J. Invest. Dermatol. Symp. Proc.* 2001;6:170–174.
23. Roth RR, James WD. Microbial ecology of the skin. *Annu. Rev. Microbiol.* 1988;42:441–464.
24. Ogawa T, Katsuoka K, Kawano K, Nishiyama S. Comparative study of the staphylococcal flora on the skin surface of atopic dermatitis patients and healthy subjects. *J. Dermatol.* 1994;21:453–460.
25. Akiama H, Morizane S, Yamazaki O, Oono T, Iwatsuki K. Assessment of *Streptococcus pyogenes* microcolony formation in infected skin by confocal laser scanning microscopy. *J. Dermatol. Sci.* 2003;32:193–199.
26. Noble WC. Observations on the surface flora of the skin and on skin pH. *Brit. J. Dermatol.* 1968;80:279–281.
27. Wesley NO, Maibach HI. Racial (ethnic) differences in skin properties: the objective data. *Am. J. Clin. Dermatol.* 2003;4:843–860.
28. Bik EM, Eckburg PB, Gill SR, Nelson KE, Purdom EA, et al. Molecular analysis of the bacterial microbiota in the human stomach. *Proc. Natl. Acad. Sci. USA* 2006;103:732–737.
29. Dethlefsen L, McFall-Ngai M, Relman DA. An ecological and evolutionary perspective on human–microbe mutualism and disease. *Nature* 2007;449:811–818.
30. Eckburg PB, Bik EM, Bernstein CN, Purdom E, Dethlefsen L. Diversity of the human intestinal microbial flora. *Science* 2005;308:1635–1638.
31. Fredricks DN. Microbial ecology of human skin in health and disease. *J. Invest. Dermatol. Symp. Proc.* 2001;6:167–169.
32. Hayashi H, Takahashi R, Nishi T, Sakamoto M, Benno Y. Molecular analysis of jejunal, ileal, caecal and reco-sigmoidal human colonic microbiota using 16S rRNA gene libraries and terminal restriction fragment length polymorphisim. *J. Med. Microbiol.* 2003;54:1093–1101.
33. Turnbaugh PJ, Ley RE, Hamady M, Fraser-Liggett CM, Knight R, et al. The human microbiome project. *Nature* 2007;449:804–810.
34. Dekio I, Hayashi H, Sakamoto M, Kitahara M, Nishikawa T, et al. Detection of potentially novel bacterial components of the human skin microbiota using culture-independent molecular profiling. *J. Med. Microbiol.* 2005;54:1231–1238.
35. Behne MJ, Barry NP, Hanson KM, Aronchik I, Clegg RW, et al. Neonatal development of the stratum corneum pH gradient: localization and mechanisms leading to emergence of optimal barrier function. *J. Invest. Dermat.* 2003;120:998–1006.
36. Fierer N, Hamady M, Lauber CL, Knight R. The influence of sex, handedness, and washing on the diversity of surface bacteria. *Proc. Natl. Acad. Sci.* 2008;105:17994–17999.
37. Forfar JO, Gould JC, MacCabe AF. Effect of hexachlorophene on incidence of staphylococcal and Gram-negative infection in the newborn. *Lancet*, 1968;ii:177–180.
38. Puhvel SM, Reisner RM, Amirian DA. Quantification of bacteria in isolated pilosebaceous follicles in normal skin. *J. Invest. Dermatol.* 1975;65:525–531.
39. Bibel DJ, Aly R, Shinefield HR, Maibach HI. The *Staphylococcus aureus* receptor for fibronectin. *J. Invest. Dermatol.* 1983;80:494–496.
40. Peterson PK, Verhoef J, Sabath LD, Quie PG. Extracellular and bacterial factors influencing staphylococcal phagocytosis and killing by human polymorphonuclear leukocytes. *Infect. Immun.* 1976;14:496–501.
41. Hentges DJ. The anaerobic microflora of the human body. *Clin. Infect. Dis.* 1993;16:175–180.
42. Chung WO, Dale BA. Innate immune response of oral and foreskin keratinocytes: utilization of different signaling pathways by various bacterial species. *Infect. Immun.* 2004;72:352–358.
43. Elias PM, Menon GK. Structural and lipid biochemical correlates of the epidermal permeability barrier. *Adv. Lipid Res.* 1991;24:1–26.
44. Harder J, Bartels J, Christophers E, Schroder JM. A peptide antibiotic from human skin. *Nature* 1997;387:861.

45. Van der Hoeven E, Hinton, NA. An assessment of the prolonged effect of antiseptic scrubs on the bacterial flora of the hands. *Can. Med. Assoc. J.* 1968;99:402–407.

46. Cogen AL, Nizet V, Gallo RL. Skin microbiota: a source of disease or defence? *Brit. J. Dermatol.* 2008;158:442–455.

47. Hackett SP, Stevens DL. Super-antigens associated with staphylococcal and streptococcal toxic shock syndrome are potent inducers of tumor necrosis factor-beta synthesis. *J. Infect. Dis.* 1993;168:232–235.

48. Baker BS. The role of microorganisms in atopic dermatitis. *Clin. Exp. Immunol.* 2006;144:1–9.

49. Paulino LC, Tseng CH, Strober BE, Blaser MJ. Molecular analysis of fungal microbiota in samples from healthy human skin and psoriatic lesions. *J. Clin. Microbiol.* 2006;44:2933–2941.

50. Holland KT, Cunliffe WJ, Roberts CD. Acne vulgaris: an investigation into the number of anaerobic diphtheroids and members of the Micrococcaceae in normal and acne skin. *Brit. J. Dermatol.* 1977;96:623–626.

51. Gilani SJK, Gonzalez M, Hussain I, Finlay AY, Patel GK. Staphylococcus re-colonization in atopic dermatitis: beyond the skin. *Clin. Exp. Dermatol.* 2005;30:10–13.

52. Ong PY, Ohtake T, Brandt C, Strickland L, Boguniewics M, Ganz T, Gallo RL, Leung DY. Endogenous antimicrobial peptides and skin infections in atopic dermatitis. *N. Engl. J. Med.* 2002;347:1151–1160.

53. Takigawa H, Nakagawa H, Kuzukawa M, Mori H, Imokawa G. Deficient production of hexadecanoic acid in the skin is associated in part with vulnerability of atopic dermatitis patients to colonization by *Staphylococcus aureus. Dermatology* 2005;211:240–248.

54. Dahl MV, Ross AJ, and Schlievert PM. Temperature regulated bacterial protein production: possible role in rosacea. *J. Am. Acad. Dermatol.* 2004;50:266–272.

55. Dyer KD, Rosenberg HF. The RNase a superfamily: generation of diversity and innate host defense. *Mol. Divers.* 2006;10:585–597.

56. Wertz PW. The nature of the epidermal barrier: biochemical aspects. *Adv. Drug Deliv. Rev.* 1996;18:283–294.

57. Lemaitre B, Nicolas E, Michaut L, Reichhart JM, Hoffmann JA. The dorsoventral regulatory gene cassette spatzle/Toll/cactus controls the potent antifungal response in *Drosophila* adults. *Cell* 1996;86:973–980.

58. Wilson CL, Ouellette AJ, Satchell DP, Ayabe T, Lopez-Boado YS, et al. Regulation of intestinal beta-defensin activation by the metalloproteinase matrilysin in innate host defense. *Science* 1999;286:113–119.

59. Andreu D, Rivas L. Animal antimicrobial peptides: an overview. *Biopolymers* 1998;47:415–420.

60. Chromek M, Slamova Z, Bergman P, Kovacs L, Podracka L, et al. The antimicrobial peptide cathelicidin protects the urinary tract against invasive bacterial infection. *Nat. Med.* 2006;12:636–641.

61. Hancock REW, Scott MG. The role of antimicrobial peptides in animal defenses. *Proc. Natl. Acad. Sci. USA* 2000;97:8856–8861.

62. Nizet V, Ohtake T, Lauth X, Trowbridge J, Rudisill J, et al. Innate antimicrobial peptides protect the skin from invasive bacterial infection. *Nature* 2001;414:454–457.

63. Bals R. Epithelial antimicrobial peptides in host defense against infection. *Respir. Res.* 2000;1:141–150.

64. DeSmet K, Contreras R. Human antimicrobial peptides: defensins, cathelicidins and histatins. *Biotechnol. Lett.* 2005;27:1337–1347.

65. Dorschner RA, Pestonjamasp VK, Tamakuwala S, Ohtake T, Rudisill J, et al. Cutaneous injury induces release of cathelicidin antimicrobial peptides active against group A *Streptococcus. J. Invest. Dermatol.* 2001;117:91–97.

66. Schröder JM, Harder J. Antimicrobial skin peptides and proteins. *Cell Mol. Life Sci.* 2006;63:469–486.

67. Zanetti M. Cathelicidins, multifunctional peptides of the innate immunity. *J. Leukoc. Biol.* 2004;75:39–48.

68. Zasloff M. Antimicrobial peptides of multicellular organisms. *Nature* 2002;415:389–395.

69. Braff MH, Bardan A, Nizet V, Gallo RL. Cutaneous defense mechanisms by antimicrobial peptides. *J. Invest. Dermatol.* 2005;125:9–13.

70. Schauber J, Gallo RL. Expanding the roles of antimicrobial peptides in skin: alarming and arming keratinocytes. *J. Invest. Dermatol.* 2007;127:510–512.
71. Lehrere RI. In defense of skin. *J. Invest. Dermatol.* 2005;125:108–115.
72. Elsbach P, Weiss J. Bactericidal/permeability-increasing protein (BPI), a potent element in host-defense against Gram-negative bacteria and lipopolysaccharide. *Immunology* 1993;187:417–429.
73. Takahashi M, Horiuchi Y, Tezuka T. Presence of bactericidal/permeability-increasing protein in human and rat skin. *Exp. Dermatol.* 2004;13:55–60.
74. Arikawa J, Ishibashi M, Kawashima M, Takagi Y, Ichikawa Y, et al. Decreased levels of sphingosine, a natural antimicrobial agent, may be associated with vulnerability of the stratum corneum from patients with atopic dermatitis to colonization by *Staphylococcus aureus. J. Invest. Dermatol.* 2002;119:433–439.
75. Bibel DJ, Miller SJ, Brown BE, Pandey BB, Elias PM, et al. Antimicrobial activity of stratum corneum lipids from normal and essential fatty acid-deficient mice. *J. Invest. Dermatol.* 1989;92:632–638.
76. Niyonsaba F, Ogawa H. Protective roles of the skin against infection: implication of naturally occurring human antimicrobial agents β-defensins, cathelicidin LL-37 and lysozyme. *J. Dermatol. Sci.* 2005;40:157–168.
77. Harder J, Schröder JM. RNase 7, a novel innate immune defense antimicrobial protein of healthy human skin. *J. Biol. Chem.* 2002;277:46779–46784.
78. Marchini G, Lindow S, Brismar H, Stabi B, Berggren V, et al. The newborn infant is protected by an innate antimicrobial barrier: peptide antibiotics are present in the skin and vernix caseosa. *Brit. J. Dermatol.* 2002;147:1127–1134.
79. Brogden KA, Ackermann M, McCray PB, Jr., Tack BF. Antimicrobial peptides in animals and their role in host defenses. *Int. J. Antimicrob. Agents* 2003;22:465–478.
80. Henzler Wildman KA, Lee DK, Ramamoorthy A. Mechanism of lipid bilayer disruption by the human antimicrobial peptide, *LL-37. Biochemistry* 2003;42:6545–6558.
81. Shai Y. Mode of action of membrane active antimicrobial peptides. *Biopolymers* 2002;66:236–248.
82. Gutsmann T, Hagge SO, Larrick JW, Seydel U, Wiese A. Interaction of CAP18-derived peptides with membranes made from endotoxins or phospholipids. *Biophys. J.* 2001;80:2935–2945.
83. Yamasaki K, Gallo RL. Antimicrobial peptides in human skin disease. *Eur. J. Dermatol.* 2008;18:11–21.
84. Harrison CJ. Innate immunity as a key element in host defense against methicillin resistant *Staphylococcus aureus. Minerva Pediatr.* 2009;61:503–514.
85. Doss M, White MR, Tecle T, Hartshorn KL. Human defensins and LL-37 in mucosal immunity. *J. Leukoc. Biol.* 2010;87:79–92.
86. Howell MD, Jones JF, Kisich KO, Streib JE, Gallo RL, Leung DY. Selective killing of vaccinia virus by LL-37: implications for eczema vaccinatum. *J. Immunol.* 2004;172:1763–1767.
87. Liu L, Wang L, Jia HP, Zhao C, Heng HH, Schutte BC, et al. Structure and mapping of the human beta-defensin HBD-2 gene and its expression at sites of inflammation. *Gene* 1998;222:237–244.
88. Biragyn A, Ruffini PA, Leifer CA, Klyushnenkova, E, Shakhov A, et al. Toll-like receptor 4-dependent activation of dendritic cells by beta-defensin 2. *Science* 2002;298:1025–1029.
89. Ding J, Chou YY, Chang TL. Defensins in viral infections. *J. Innate Immun.* 2009;1:413–420.
90. Schittek B, Hipfel R, Sauer B, Bauer J, Kalbacher H, Stevanovic S, et al. Dermcidin: a novel human antibiotic peptide secreted by sweat glands. *Nat. Immunol.* 2001;12:1133–1137.
91. Murakami M, Ohtake T, Dorschner RA, Schittek B, Garbe C, et al. Cathelicidin antimicrobial peptide expression in sweat, an innate defense system for the skin. *J. Invest. Dermatol.* 2002;119:1090–1095.
92. Glaser R, Harder J, Lange H, Bartels J, Christophers E, et al. Antimicrobial psoriasin (S100A7) protects human skin from *Escherichia coli* infection. *Nat. Immunol.* 2005;6(1):57–64.
93. Köten B, Simanski M, Gläser R, Podschun R, Schröder J-M, et al. RNase 7 contributes to the cutaneous defense against *Enterococcus faecium. PLoS One* 2009;4:e6424.
94. Frohem M, Agerberth B, Ahangari G, Stahle-Backdahl M, Linden S, et al. The expression of the gene coding for the antimicrobial peptide LL-37 is induced in human keratinocytes during inflammatory disorders. *J. Biol. Chem.* 1997;272:15258–15263.

95. Weber G, Heilborn JD, Chamorro Jimenez CI, Hammarsojo A, et al. Vitamin D induces the antimicrobial protein hCAP18 in human skin. *J. Invest. Dermatol.* 2005;124:1080–1082.

96. Lee DY, Yamasaki K, Rudsil J, Zouboulis CC, Park GT, et al. Sebocytes express functional cathelicidin antimicrobial peptides and can act to kill *Propionibacterium acnes. J. Invest. Dermatol.* 2008;128:1863–1866.

97. Di Nardo A, Vitiello A, Gallo RL. Cutting edge: mast cell antimicrobial activity is mediated by expression of cathelicidin antimicrobial peptide. *J. Immunol.* 2003;170:2274–2278.

98. Murakami M, Dorschner RA, Stren LJ, Lin KH, Gallo RL. Expression and secretion of cathelicidin antimicrobial peptides in murine mammary glands and human milk. *Pediatr. Res.* 2005;57:10–15.

99. Sorensen OE, Cowland JB, Theilgaard-Monch K, Liu I, et al. Wound healing and expression of antimicrobial peptides/polypeptides in human keratinocytes, a consequence of common growth factors. *J. Immunol.* 2003;170:5583–5589.

100. Turner I, Cho Y, Dinh NN, Waring AI, Lehrer RI. Activities of LL-37, a cathelicidin-associated antimicrobial peptide of human neutrophils. *Antimicrob. Agents Chemother.* 1998;42:2206–2214.

101. Dorschner RA, Pestonjamasp VK, Tamakuwala S, Ohtake T, Rudisill J, et al. Cutaneous injury induces the release of cathelicidin antimicrobial peptides active against group A *Streptococcus. J. Invest. Dermatol.* 2001;117:91–97.

102. Zaiou M, Gallo RL. Cathelicidins, essential gene-encoded mammalian antibiotics. *J. Mol. Med.* 2002;80:549–561.

103. Murakami M, Lopez-Garcia B, Braff M, Dorschner RA, Gallo RL. Post-secretory processing generates multiple cathelicidins for enhanced topical antimicrobial defense. *J. Immunol.* 2004;172:3070–3077.

104. Scott MG, Davidson DJ, Gold MR, Bowdish D, Hancock RE. The human antimicrobial peptide LL-37 is a multifunctional modulator of innate immune responses. *J. Immunol.* 2002;169:3883–3891.

105. Bals R, Wilson JM. Cathelicidin: a family of multifunctional antimicrobial peptides. *Cell Mol. Life Sci.* 2003;60:711–720.

106. Barlow PG, Li Y, Wilkinson TS, Bowdish DME, Lau E, et al. The human cationic host defense peptide LL-37 mediates contrasting effects on apoptotic pathways in different primary cells of the innate immune system. *J. Leukoc. Biol.* 2006;80:509–520.

107. Gudmundsson GH, Agerbert B. Neutrophil antibacterial peptides, multifunctional effector molecule in the mammalian immune system. *J. Immunol. Methods* 1999;232:45–54.

108. Kamysz W, Okroj M. Novel properties of antimicrobial peptides. *Acta Biochim. (Polish)* 2003;50:461–469.

109. Risso A. Leukocyte antimicrobial peptides: multifunctional effector molecules of innate immunity. *J. Leukoc. Biol.* 2000;68:785–792.

110. Zaiou M, Nizet V, Gallo RL. Antimicrobial and protease inhibitory functions of the human cathelicidins (hCAP18/LL-37) prosequence. *J. Invest. Dermatol.* 2003;120:810–816.

111. Leung DY, Bieber T. Atopic dermatitis. *Lancet* 2003;361(9395):151–160.

112. Wang TT, Nestel FP, Bourdeau V, Nagai Y, et al. Cutting edge: 1,25-dihydroxyvitamin D3 is a direct inducer of antimicrobial peptide gene expression. *J. Immunol.* 2004;173:2909–2912.

113. Mallbris L, Edstrom DW, Sunblad L, Granath F, Stahle M. UVB up-regulates the antimicrobial protein hCAP18 mRNA in human skin. *J. Invest. Dermatol.* 2005;125:1072–1074.

114. Ganz T, Selsted ME, Szklarek D, Harwig SS, Daher K, et al. Defensins: natural peptide antibiotics of human neutrophils. *J. Invest. Dermatol.* 1985;76:1427–1435.

115. Hoover DM, Wu Z, Tucker K, Lu W, Lubkowski J. Antimicrobial characterization of human beta-defensin 3 derivatives. *Antimicrob. Agents Chemother.* 2003;47:280–289.

116. Lehrer RT, Ganz T. Antimicrobial peptides in mammalian and insect host defense. *Curr. Opin. Immunol.* 1999;11:23–27.

117. Lehrer RT, Daher K, Ganz T, Selsted ME. Direct inactivation of viruses by MCP-1 and MCP-2, natural peptide antibiotics from rabbit leukocytes. *J. Virol.* 1985;54:467–472.

118. Duits LA, Ravensbergen B, Rademaker M, Hemstra PS, Nibbering PH. Expression of beta-defensin 1 and 2 mRNA by human monocytes, macrophages and dendritic cells. *Immunology* 2002;106:517–525.

119. Fang XM, Shu Q, Chen QX, Book M, Sahl G, et al. Differential expression of alpha- and beta-defensins in human peripheral blood. *Eur. J. Clin. Invest.* 2003;33:82–87.
120. Lehrer RI. Primate defensins. *Nat. Rev. Microbiol.* 2004;2:727–738.
121. Ali RS, Falconer A, Ikram M, Bissett CE, Cerio R, Quinn AG. Expression of the peptides antibiotics human beta defensin-1 and human beta defensin-2 in normal human skin. *J. Invest. Dermatol.* 2001;117:106–111.
122. Bals R, Wang X, Wu Z, Freeman T, Bafna V, Zasloff M,et al Human beta-defensin 2 is a salt-sensitive peptide antibiotic expressed in human lung. *J. Clin. Invest.* 1998;102:874–880.
123. Chronnell CM, Ghali LR, Ali RS, Quinn AG, Holland DB, et al. Human beta defensin-1 and -2 expression in human pilosebaceous units: upregulation in acne vulgaris lesions. *J. Invest. Dermatol.* 2001;117:1120–1125.
124. Liu L, Roberts AA, Ganz T. By IL-1 signaling, monocyte-derived cells dramatically enhance the epidermal antimicrobial response to lipopolysaccharide. *J. Immunol.* 2003;170:575–580.
125. Hollox EJ, Huffmeier U, Zeeuwen PL, Palla R, Lascorz J, et al. Psoriasis is associated with increased beta-defensin genomic copy number. *Nat. Genet.* 2008;40:23–25.
126. Rupec R, Boneberger S, Ruzicka T. What is really in control of skin immunity: lymphocytes, dentritic cells, or keratinocytes? Facts and controversies. *Clin. Dermatol.* 2010;28:62–66.
127. Senyurek I, Paulmann M, Sinnberg T, Kalbacher H. et al. Dermicidin-derived peptides show a different mode of action than the cathelicidin LL-37 against *Staphylococcus aureus*. *Antimicrob. Agents Chemother.*, 2009;53:2499–2509.
128. Michalek M, Gelhaus C, Hecht O, Podschun R, Schröder JM, Leippe M, Grötzinger J. The human antimicrobial protein psoriasin acts by permeabilizing of bacterial membranes. *Dev. Comp. Immunol.* 2009;33:740–746.
129. Bibel DJ, Aly R, Shah S, Shinefield HR. Sphingosines: antimicrobial barriers of the skin. *Acta Derm. Venereol.* 1993;73:407–411.
130. Drake DR, Brogden KA, Dawson DV, Wertzi PW. Antimicrobial lipids at the skin surface. *J. Lipid Res.* 2008;49:4–11.
131. Thormar H, Hilmarsson H. The role of microbicidal lipids in host defense against pathogens and their potential as therapeutic agents. *Chem. Phys. Lipids* 2007;150:1–11.
132. Georgel P, Crozat K, Lauth X, Makrantonaki E, Seltmann H. A toll-like receptor 2-responsive lipid effector pathway protects mammals against skin infections with Gram-positive bacteria. *Infect. Immun.* 2005;73:4512–4521.
133. Schauber J, Dorschner RA, Coda AB, Buchau AS, Liu PT, et al. Injury enhances TLR2 function and antimicrobial peptide expression through a vitamin D-dependent mechanism. *J. Clin. Invest.* 2007;117:803–811.
134. Clarke SR, Mohamed R, Bian Li, Routh AF, Kokai-Kun JF, Mond JJ, Tarkowski A, Foster SJ. The *Staphylococcus aureus* surface protein IsdA mediates resistance to innate defenses of human skin. *Cell Host Microbe*, 2007;1:199–212.
135. Okuda M, Yoshiike T, Ogawa H. Detergent-induced epidermal barrier dysfunction and its prevention. *J. Dermatol. Sci.* 2002;30:173–179.
136. Holland KT, Bojar RA. Cosmetics: what is their influence on the skin microflora? *Am. J. Clin. Dermatol.* 2002;3:445–449.
137. Ansari SA, Sattar SA, Springthrope VS, Wells GA, Tostowaryk W. *In vivo* protocol for testing efficacy of hand-washing agents against viruses and bacteria: experiments with rotavirus and *Escherichia coli*. *Appl. Environ. Microbiol.* 1989;55:3113–3118.
138. Fischler GE, Fuls JL, Dail EW, Duran MH, Rodgers ND, et al. Effect of hand wash agents on controlling the transmission of pathogenic bacteria from hands to food. *J. Food Prot.* 2007;70:2873–2877.
139. Luby SP, Abogatwalla M, Felkin DR, Painter J, Billhimer W, et al. Effect of handwashing on child health: a randomized controlled trial. *Lancet* 2005;366:225–233.
140. Rhein L. *In vitro* interactions: biochemical and biophysical effects of surfactants on skin. In: Rieger MM, Rhein LD, editors. *Surfactants in Cosmetics*, 2nd ed., vol. 68 New York: Marcel Dekker, Inc., 1997. pp. 397–426.
141. Friedman M, Wolf R. Chemistry of soaps and detergents: various types of commercial products and their ingredients. *Clin. Dermatol.* 1996;14:7–13.

142. Gfatter R, Hackl P, Braun F. Effects of soap and detergents on skin surface pH, stratum corneum hydration and fat content in infants. *Dermatology* 1997;195:258–262.
143. de Almeida e Borges LF, Silva BL, Gontijo Filho P.P. Hand washing: changes in the skin flora. *Am. J. Infect. Control* 2007;35:417–420.
144. Korting HC, Megele M, Mehringer L, Vieluf D, Zienicke H, et al. Influence of skin cleansing preparation acidity on skin surface properties. *Int. J. Cosmet. Sci.* 1991;13:91–102.
145. Thune P, Nilsen T, Hansatad IK, Gustavsen T, Lovig Dahl H. The water barrier function of the skin in relation to the water content of stratum corneum, pH and skin lipids. The effect of alkaline soap and syndet on dry skin in elderly, non-atopic patients. *Acta Derm. Venereol.* 1988;68:277–283.
146. Aly R, Maibach HI, Rahman R, Shinefield HR, Mandel AD. Correlation of human *in vivo* and *in vitro* cutaneous antimicrobial factors. *J. Infect. Dis.* 1975;131:579–583.
147. Korting HC, Bruan-Falco O. The effect of detergents on skin pH and its consequences. *Clin. Dermatol.* 1996;14:23–27.
148. McGinley KJ, Labows JN, Zechman JM, Nordstrom KM, Webster GF, et al. Analysis of cellular components, biochemical reactions, and habitat of human cutaneous lipophilic diphtheroids. *J. Invest. Dermatol.* 1985;85:374–377.
149. Visscher M, Hoath SB, Conroy E, Wickett R. Effect of semipermeable membranes on skin barrier repair following tape stripping. *Arch. Dermatol. Res.* 2001;293:491–499.
150. Korting HC, Ponce-Poschi E, Klovekorn W, Schmotzer G, Arens-Corell M, et al. The influence of the regular use of a soap or an acidic syndet bar on pre-acne. *Infection* 1995;23:89–93.
151. Barel AO, Lambrecht R, Clarys P, Morrison BM, Jr., Paye M. A comparative study of the effects on the skin of a classical bar soap and a syndet cleansing bar in normal use conditions and in soap chamber test. *Skin Res. Technol.* 2001;7:98–104.
152. Corraza M, Lauriola MM, Zappaterra M, Bianchi A, Virgili A. Surfactants, skin cleansing protagonists. *J. Eur. Acad. Dermatol. Venereol.* 2010;24:1–6.
153. Lakshmi C, Srinivas CR, Anand CV, Mathew AC. Irritancy ranking of 31 cleansers in the Indian market in a 24-h patch test. *Int. J. Cosmet. Sci.* 2008;30:277–283.
154. Ananthapadmanabhan KP, Moore DJ, Subramanyan K, Misra M, Meyer, F. Cleansing without compromise: the impact of cleansers on the skin barrier and the technology of mild cleansing. *Dermatol. Ther.* 2004;17 S1:16–25.
155. Billhimer WL, Berge CA, Englehart JS, Rains GY, Keswick BH. A modified cup scrub method for assessing the antibacterial substantivity of personal cleansing products. *J. Cosmet. Sci.* 2001;52:369–375.
156. Ertel K. Modern skin cleansers. *Dermatol. Clin.* 2000;18:561–575.
157. Draelos ZD, Ertel K, Hartwig P, Rains G. The effect of two skin cleansing systems on moderate xerotic eczema. *J. Am. Acad. Dermatol.* 2004;50:883–888.
158. Draelos ZD. Concepts in skin care maintenance. *Cutis* 2005;76:19–25.
159. Draelos ZD. The effect of a daily facial cleanser for normal to oily skin on the skin barrier of subjects with acne. *Cutis* 2006;78(Suppl. 1):34–40.
160. Kuehl BL, Fyfe KS, Shear NH. Cutaneous cleansers. *Skin Therapy Lett.* 2003;8:1–4.
161. Ansari SA, Sattar SA, Springthorpe VS, Wells GA, Tostowaryk W. *In vivo* protocol for testing efficacy of hand-washing agents against viruses and bacteria: experiment with rotavirus and *Escherichia coli*. *Appl. Environ. Microbiol.* 1989;55:3113–3118.
162. Leyden JJ, McGinley KJ, Kaminer MS, et al. Computerized image analysis of full-hand touch plate: a modified method for quantification of surface bacteria on hands and the effect of antimicrobial agents. *J. Hosp. Infect.* 1991;18(Suppl. B):13–22.
163. Morrison BM, Jr., Scala D, Fischler GE. Topical antibacterial wash products. In: Rieger M, Rhein LD, editors. *Surfactants in Cosmetics*, 2nd ed. New York: Marcel Dekker, Inc., 1997. pp. 331–356.
164. Oughton MT, Loo VG, Dendukuri N, Fenn S, Libman MD. Hand hygiene with soap and water is superior to alcohol rub and antiseptic wipes for removal of *Clostridium defficile*. *Infect. Control Hosp. Epidemiol.* 2009;30:939–944.
165. Perencevich EN, Wong MT, Harris AD. National and regional assessment of the antibacterial soap market: a step toward determining the impact of prevalent antibacterial soaps. *Am. J. Infect. Control* 2001;29:281–283.

166. Aiello AE, Larson EL, Levy SB. Consumer antibacterial soaps: effective or just risky? *Clin. Infect. Dis.* 2007;45:S137–S147.
167. Gerba CP. Benefits of antibacterial products well documented. *Am. J. Infect. Control* 2002;30:257–258.
168. Russell AD. Antibiotic and biocide resistance in bacteria: comments and conclusions. *J. Appl. Microbiol.* 2002;92:171S–173S.
169. Russell AD. "Whither triclosan?" *J. Antimicrob. Agents Chemother.* 2004;53:693–695.
170. Cole EC, Addison RM, Rubino JR, Leese KE, Dulaney PD, et al. Investigation of antibiotic and antibacterial agents cross-resistance in target bacteria from homes of antibacterial product users and nonusers. *J. Appl. Microbiol.* 2003;95:664–676.
171. Aiello AE, Marshall B, Levy SB, et al. Relationship between triclosan and susceptibilities of bacteria isolated from hands in the community. *Antimicrob. Agents Chemother.* 2004;48: 2973–2979.
172. Aiello AE, Coulborn RM, Perez V, Larson EL. Effect of hand hygiene on infectious disease risk in the community setting: a meta-analysis. *Am. J. Public Health* 2008;98:1372–1381.
173. Black RE, Dykes AC, Anderson KE, Wells JG, Sinclair SP, et al. Handwashing to prevent diarrhea in day-care centers. *Am. J. Epidemiol.* 1981;113:445–451.
174. Carabin H, Gyorkos TW, Soto JC, Joseph L, Payment P, et al. Effectiveness of a training program in reducing infections in toddlers attending day care centers. *Epidemiology* 1999;10:219–227.
175. Falsey AR, Criddle MM, Kolassa JE, McCann RM, Brower CA, et al. Evaluation of a handwashing intervention to reduce respiratory illness rates in senior day-care centers. *Infect. Control Hosp. Epidemiol.* 1999;20:200–202.
176. Luby SP, Agboatwalla M, Painter J, Altaf A, Billhimer W, et al. Combining drinking water treatment and hand washing prevention, a cluster randomized controlled trial. *Trop. Med. Int. Health* 2006;11:479–489.
177. Peterson AF, Rosenberg A, Alatary SD. Comparative evaluation of surgical scrub preparations. *Surg. Gynecol. Obstet.* 1978;146:63–65.
178. Shahid NS, Greenough WB, 3rd, Samadi AR, Huq MI, Rahman N. Hand washing with soap reduces diarrhoea and spread of bacterial pathogens in a Bangladesh village. *J. Diarrhoeal Dis. Res.* 1996;14:85–89.
179. Heath RJ, Rubin JR, Holland DR, Zhang E, Snow ME, et al. Mechanism of triclosan inhibition of bacterial fatty acid synthesis. *J. Biol. Chem.* 1999;274:11110–11114.
180. McMurry LM, Oethinger M, Levy SB. Triclosan targets lipid synthesis. *Nature* 1998;394:531–532.
181. Larson EL, Hughes CA, Pyrek JD, Sparks SM, Cagatay EU, et al. Changes in bacterial flora associated with skin damage on hands of health care personnel. *Am. J. Infect. Control* 1998;26:513–521.
182. Larson EL, Aiello AE, Gomez-Duarte C, Lin SX, Lee L, et al. Bioluminescence ATP monitoring as a surrogate marker for microbial load on hands and surfaces in the home. *Food Microbiol.* 2003;20:735–739.
183. Meers PD, Yeo GA. Shedding of bacteria and skin squames after hand washing. *J. Hygiene (London)* 1978;81:99–105.
184. Larson EL, Aiello A, Lee LV, Della-Latta P, Gomez-Duarte C, Lin S. Short- and long-term effects of handwashing with antimicrobial or plain soap in the community. *J. Community Health* 2003;28:139–150.
185. Elsner P. Antimicrobials and skin physiological and pathological flora. *Curr. Probl. Dermatol.* 2006;33:3–41.
186. Ansari SA, Sattar SA, Springthorpe VS, Wells GA, Tostowaryk W. Rotavirus survival on human hands and transfer of infectious virus to animate and nonporous inanimate surfaces. *J. Clin. Microbiol.* 1988;26:1513–1518.
187. Ansari SA, Springthorpe VS, Sattar SA. Survival and vehicular spread of human rotaviruses: possible relation to seasonality of outbreaks. *Rev. Infect. Dis.* 1991;13:448–461.
188. Rusin P, Maxwell S, Gerba CP. Comparative surface-to-hand and fingertip-to-mouth transfer efficiency of Gram-positive bacteria, Gram-negative bacteria, and phage. *J. Appl. Microbiol.* 2002;93:585–592.

189. Bloomfield S, Exner M, Fara GM, Scott EA. Prevention of the spread of infection: the need for a family-centered approach to hygiene promotion. *Euro. Surveill.* 2008;3:18889.
190. Fuls JL, Rodgers ND, Fischler GE, Howard JM, Patel M, et al. Alternative hand contamination technique to compare the activities of antimicrobial and non-antimicrobial soaps under different test conditions. *Appl. Environ. Microbiol.* 2008;74:3739–3744.
191. Scott E, Duty S, Callahan M. A pilot study to isolate *Staphylococcus aureus* and methicillin-resistant *S. aureus* from environmental surfaces in home. *Am. J. Infect. Control* 2008;36:458–460.
192. Bibel DJ. Ecological effects of a deodorant and a plain soap upon human skin bacteria. *J. Hyg. (London)* 1977;78:1–10.
193. Wilson PE. A comparison of methods for assessing the value of antibacterial soaps. *J. Appl. Microbiol.* 2008;33:574–581.
194. Breneman DL, Hanifin JM, Berge CA, Keswick BH, Neuman PB. The effect of antibacterial soap with 1.5% triclocarban on *Staphylococcus aureus* in patients with atopic dermatitis. *Cutis* 2003;66:296–300.
195. Bruch, M. Newer germicides: what they offer. In: Maibach H, Aly R.editors. *Skin Microbiology: Relevance to Clinical Infection.* New York: Springer-Verlag, 1981. pp. 103–112.
196. Larson EL, Laughon BA. Comparison of four antiseptic products containing chlorhexidine gluconate. *Antimicrob. Agents Chemother.* 1987;31:1572–1574.
197. Bloomfield SF, Aiello AE, Cookson B, O'Boyle C, Larson EL. The effectiveness of hand hygiene procedures in reducing the risks of infection in home and in community settings including hand washing and alcohol-based hand sanitizers. *Am. J. Infect. Control* 2007;35:S27–S64.
198. Lachenmeier DW. Safety evaluation of topical applications of ethanol on the skin and inside the oral cavity. *J. Occup. Med. Toxicol.* 2008;3:26–31.
199. Food and Drug Administration. Tentative final monograph for healthcare antiseptic drug products: proposed rule. *Fed. Regist.* 1994;59(116):31402–31452.
200. Fluhr JW, Darlenski R, Surber C. Glycerol and the skin: holistic approach to its origin and functions. *Brit. J. Dermatol.* 2008;159:23–34.
201. Gloor M, Bettinger J, Gehring W. Modification of stratum corneum quality by glycerin-containing external ointments. *Hauarzt* 1998;49:6–9.
202. Bergsson, G, Arnfinnsson J, Steingrimsson O, Thormar, H. Killing of Gram-positive cocci by fatty acids and monoglycerides. *APMIS* 2001;09:670–678.
203. Thormar H, Hilmarsson H, Bergsson G. Stable concentrated emulsions of 1-monoglyceride of capric acid (monocaprin) with microbicidal activities against the foodborne bacteria *Campylobacter jejuni*, *Salmonella* spp. and *Escherichia coli*. *Appl. Environ. Microbiol.* 2006;72:522–526.

CHAPTER 6

DEFENSINS

Neelam Muizzuddin

Estee Lauder Companies and SUNY Stony Brook, Melville, NY

6.1 INTRODUCTION

Defensins and cathelicidins are the two major families of mammalian antimicrobial proteins. They contribute to innate, antimicrobial defense of the host both by disrupting the integrity of the bacterial cell membrane and by having chemotactic effects on host cells. These antimicrobial peptides have distinct, host-target cell spectra [1]. Mammalian defensins are a family of 2–6 kDa, cationic, cysteine-rich microbicidal peptides. They are active against many Gram-negative and Gram-positive bacteria, fungi, and enveloped viruses [2]. Cells of the immune system and almost all epithelial cells contain these peptides to assist in the elimination of phagocytized bacteria.

6.2 CLASSIFICATION

On the basis of their size and pattern of disulfide bonding, mammalian defensins are classified into alpha, beta, and theta categories [3,4].

α-*Defensins* are abundant both in neutrophils and in NK cells and certain T lymphocyte subsets. DEFA5 and DEFA6 are expressed in Paneth cells of the small intestine, where they may regulate and maintain microbial balance in the intestinal lumen [5].

β-*Defensins* consist of 36–42 residues [5] and are the most widely distributed. These are secreted by leukocytes and epithelial cells of many kinds. For example, they can be found on the tongue, skin, cornea, salivary glands, kidneys, esophagus, and respiratory tract. Human beta-defensins (hBD)-1, -2, and -3 have been detected in the stratified squamous epithelium. hBD-1 is constitutively expressed in epithelial cells whereas hBD-2 and -3 are expressed upon stimulation with proinflammatory cytokines such as IL-1β, TNFα IFNγ, and microorganisms [6–8].

Innate Immune System of Skin and Oral Mucosa: Properties and Impact in Pharmaceutics, Cosmetics, and Personal Care Products, First Edition. Nava Dayan and Philip W. Wertz.
© 2011 John Wiley & Sons, Inc. Published 2011 by John Wiley & Sons, Inc.

θ-*Defensins* are rare and thus far have been found only in the leukocytes of the rhesus macaque and the olive baboon, *Papio anubis*, as they are vestigial in humans and other primates [5].

6.3   HUMAN BETA-DEFENSINS

The human genome project indicates that the family of beta-defensins contains more than 20 potentially expressed genes, and about 6 human defensin peptides have been characterized to date. Three closely related defensins, human neutrophil peptides HNP-1, -2, and -3, are major components of the dense azurophil granules of neutrophils, and a fourth, HNP-4, is found in the same location but is much less abundant. The three most recently characterized defensins, HBD-1 [9,10], HBD-2 [11], and HBD-3 [8,12], differ slightly from the classical α-defensins in spacing and connectivity of their cysteines. Their mRNAs are expressed in epithelia, with HBD-1 being most abundant in the kidney and HBD-2 and -3 in inflamed skin [8,13]. The synthesis and secretion of HBD-2 (and presumably HBD-3) are regulated in a dual fashion, first by direct epithelial responses to LPS and other microbial stimuli and second by cytokines. The former, higher threshold effect is most likely mediated by epithelial CD14, Toll-like receptors, and the transcription factor NF-κB [14]. The lower threshold, cytokine-mediated response is triggered primarily by the encounter of microbes with local macrophages. These cells then produce IL-1α and IL-1β and other cytokines [15], which in turn act on epithelial cytokine receptors to increase epithelial defensin synthesis.

HBD-2 is a cysteine-rich cationic low molecular weight antimicrobial peptide present in psoriatic lesional skin. It is produced by epithelial cells and exhibits potent antimicrobial activity against Gram-negative bacteria and *Candida*, but not against Gram-positive *Staphylococcus aureus*. HBD-2 represents the first human defensin that is produced following stimulation of epithelial cells by contact with micro-organisms such as *Pseudomonas aeruginosa* or cytokines such as TNF-α and IL-1β. The HBD-2 gene and protein are locally expressed in keratinocytes associated with inflammatory skin lesions such as psoriasis and in the infected lung epithelia of patients with cystic fibrosis. It has been suggested that HBD-2 is a dynamic component of the local epithelial defense system of the skin and respiratory tract, playing a role in protecting surfaces from infection and providing a possible reason why skin and lung infections with Gram-negative bacteria are rather rare [7].

6.3.1   Distribution

Human beta-defensin-2 expression is variable and is readily detectable in facial skin. Human beta-defensin 1 and 2 are localized within interfollicular skin and Malpighian layer of the epidermis and stratum corneum. There are interindividual and site-specific differences in intensity of immunostaining and the pattern of peptide localization. The localization of human beta-defensins to the outer layer of the skin is consistent with the hypothesis that human beta-defensins play an essential part in cutaneous innate immunity [16,17].

HBD-2 is stored both in the lamellar bodies (LBs) of the keratinocytes of the spinous layer of the epidermis and in the intercellular space [18], suggesting that HBD-2 is released with the contents of the lamellar bodies. Thus, the lipid "permeability" barrier of the skin contains antimicrobial substances [19].

6.3.2 Activation of Defensins via Toll-like Receptors

The innate immune recognition of pathogens is mediated by specific receptors called pattern recognition receptors (PRRs) [20], also called Toll-like receptors (TLRs) [21–23]. TLRs comprise a family of type I transmembrane receptors, which are characterized by an extracellular leucine-rich repeat (LRR) domain and an intracellular Toll/IL-1 receptor (TIR) domain.

Recognition of microbial components by TLRs initiates signaling transduction pathways that induce gene expression [24]. Activation of signal transduction pathways by TLRs leads to the induction of various genes that function in host defense, including inflammatory cytokines, chemokines, major histocompatibility complex (MHC), and costimulatory molecules. Mammalian TLRs also induce multiple effector molecules such as inducible nitric oxide synthase and antimicrobial peptides, which can directly destroy microbial pathogens [25]. TLRs and IL-1Rs activate NF-κB and can induce some of the genes that transcribe into defensin (Figure 6.1) [26].

Ten different human TLRs with ligand specificity have been identified and characterized. TLR4 is associated with CD14 and primarily mediates cellular signaling induced by Gram-negative bacteria [27,28].

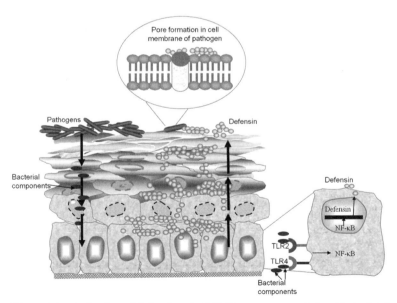

Figure 6.1   Activation of defensins via Toll-like receptors and the effect of defensin on bacterial destruction via pore formation.

Two members of the TLR family, TLR2 and TLR6, together coordinate macrophage activation by Gram-positive bacteria and the yeast cell wall particle, zymosan. TLR6 and TLR2 both are recruited to the macrophage phagosome, where they recognize peptidoglycan, a Gram-positive pathogen component. By contrast, TLR2 recognizes another component, bacterial lipopeptide, without TLR6. The requirement for TLR cooperation is supported by the finding that TLR2 needs a partner to activate tumor necrosis factor-alpha production in macrophages. TLRs sample the contents of the phagosome independent of the nature of the contents and can establish a combinatorial repertoire to discriminate among the large number of pathogen-associated molecular patterns found in nature [29].

Moreover, human alpha-defensins can enhance or suppress the activation of the classical pathway of complement *in vitro* by binding to solid-phase or fluid-phase complement C1q, respectively.

6.3.3 Activity

Defensins are produced constitutively and/or in response to microbial products or proinflammatory cytokines [30]. Human neutrophil alpha-defensins are chemotactic for resting, naïve CD45RA/CD4 T cells, CD8 T cells, and immature dendritic cells. Human beta-defensins are also chemotactic for immature dendritic cells, but induce the migration of memory T cells. In contrast, cathelicidin/LL-37 is chemotactic for neutrophils, monocytes, and T cells but not for dendritic cells. Thus, these antimicrobial peptides have distinct, host-target cell spectra. The chemotactic activities of human beta-defensins and cathelicidin/LL-37 are mediated by human CC chemokine receptor 6 and formyl peptide receptor-like 1, respectively. The capacity of defensins and cathelicidins to mobilize various types of phagocytic leukocytes, immature dendritic cells, and lymphocytes, together with their other effects such as stimulating IL-8 production and mast cell degranulation, provide evidence of their participation in alerting, mobilizing, and amplifying innate and adaptive antimicrobial immunity of the host [1]. Defensin-related peptide 1 (Defr1) displays chemoattractant activity for CD4(+) T cells and immature DC (iDC), but not for mature DC cells or neutrophils [31].

Some defensins are also called corticostatins (CS) because they inhibit corticotropin-stimulated corticosteroid production. The mechanism by which microorganisms are killed and/or inactivated by defensins is not understood completely. However, it is generally believed that killing is a consequence of disruption of integrity of the microbial membrane. The polar topology of defensins, with spatially separated charged and hydrophobic regions, allows them to intercalate themselves into the phospholipid membranes so that their hydrophobic regions are buried within the lipid membrane interior and their charged (mostly cationic) regions interact with anionic phospholipid head groups and water. Subsequently, some defensins can aggregate to form "channel-like" pores; others might bind to and cover the microbial membrane in a "carpet-like" manner [12]. The net outcome is the disruption of membrane integrity and function, which ultimately leads to the lysis of microorganisms [8]. Some defensins are synthesized as propeptides that may be relevant to this process.

Estimates of defensin concentrations in the phagocytic vacuoles of neutrophils are in the milligrams per milliliter range, a concentration that should be sufficient to overcome inhibition by extracellular ion concentrations [32]. The concentration of HBD-2 in desquamated inflamed skin is in the range of 10 μg/mL [11], again sufficient to inhibit or kill many microbes.

6.4   DEFENSINS AND INFLAMMATION

Neutrophils are recruited to sites of injury, but their timely removal is considered to be vital in preventing the exacerbation of inflammation. In addition, the recognition of apoptotic cells by the innate immune system provides potent anti-inflammatory and anti-immunogenic signals. Human neutrophils dying from apoptosis or necrosis release anti-inflammatory peptides, the alpha-defensins [33]. The alpha-defensins effectively inhibit the secretion of multiple proinflammatory cytokines and nitric oxide (NO) from macrophages, the main innate immune cell found at the sites of chronic inflammation. Hence, their effects may be far-reaching and serve to kill microbes while regulating a potentially tissue-destructive inflammatory response [34].

6.5   CONSEQUENCES OF DEFENSIN IMBALANCE

Acne may be characterized by an imbalance of defensins in the skin [35,36]. An upregulation of beta-defensin expression has been noticed in acne vulgaris lesions compared to controls suggesting that beta-defensins may be involved in the pathogenesis of acne vulgaris [35,37]. Sebocytes are capable of producing proinflammatory cytokines/chemokines and antimicrobial peptides, which may have a role in acne pathogenesis. On the other hand, overexpression of antimicrobial peptides can lead to increased protection against skin infections as seen in patients with psoriasis [7] and rosacea that are inflammatory skin diseases rarely resulting in superinfection [17].

Defensins may play a key role in the mechanism of host defense and might provide a new therapeutic approach to infectious diseases [38]. Patients with atopic dermatitis have problems with *S. aureus* skin infection due to increased levels of cytokines, which inhibit keratinocyte mobilization of human beta-defensin-3 [39]. *S. aureus* induces the upregulation of both proinflammatory cytokines and HBD-2, thereby resulting in induction of the persistent eczematous skin lesions in atopic dermatitis [40]. Ong et al. reported that induction of human beta-defensin-2 in the skin could be used in the prevention of atopic dermatitis [41].

6.6   SUMMARY

Defensins enhance phagocytosis, promote neutrophil recruitment, enhance the production of proinflammatory cytokines, suppress anti-inflammatory mediators, and regulate complement activation and thus upregulate innate host inflammatory defenses against microbial invasion.

Defensins and cathelicidins belong to antimicrobial peptides (AMPs), also called the natural antibiotics. These molecules have been described in bacteria, invertebrates, vertebrates, and mammals including humans. The amino acid sequence has been determined for about 880 antimicrobial peptides, and their classification is difficult and complex. These oligo- and polypeptides kill the microbes or inhibit their growth, act as bactericidal to Gram-negative and Gram-positive bacteria, neutralize toxins, and demonstrate antiviral activity. AMPs are multifunctional molecules, playing the first line of defense in humans as effectors of unspecific immunity, with a broad spectrum of activity against pathogens, are characterized by controlling the physiological bacterial flora, often acting synergistically, and are produced in different cells as defense against mechanisms of microbial resistance. They are chemotactic to neutrophils and T cells, and activate the dendritic cells. In humans, defensins are expressed in several cells and tissues; in neutrophils, platelets, and epithelial cells; and in liver, skin, and eye conjunctiva. Deficiency of defensins or cathelicidins causes pathological symptoms in atopic allergies or in Kostmann disease. Several synthetic peptides are at the final phase of clinical trials for the treatment of various bacterial infections. Defensins or cathelicidins could also be efficient as adjuvants or carriers for vaccines and could be used in dairy industry as preservatives. This chapter presents some problems concerning the occurrence of AMPs, especially defensins and cathelicidins of mammals, their classification, structure, various functions, and mechanisms of bactericidal activity, and also their use in treatment of some infectious diseases.

ACKNOWLEDGMENT

Paolo Giacomoni and Tom Mammone for helpful discussion.

REFERENCES

1. Yang D, Chertov O, Oppenheim JJ. Participation of mammalian defensins and cathelicidins in antimicrobial immunity: receptors and activities of human defensins and cathelicidin (LL-37). *J. Leukoc. Biol.* 2001;69(5):691–697.
2. Selsted ME, White SH, Wimley WC. Structure, function, and membrane integration of defensins. *Curr. Opin. Struct. Biol.* 1995;5(4):521–527.
3. Ganz T, Lehrer RI. Defensins. *Curr. Opin. Immunol.* 1994;6(4):584–589.
4. Lehrer RI, Ganz T. Antimicrobial peptides in mammalian and insect host defence. *Curr. Opin. Immunol.* 1999;11(1):23–27.
5. Bals, R. Epithelial antimicrobial peptides in host defense against infection. *Respir. Res.* 2000;1(3):141–150.
6. Diamond G, Bevins CL. Beta-defensins: endogenous antibiotics of the innate host defense response. *Clin. Immunol. Immunopathol.* 1998;88(3):221–225.
7. Schröder JM, Harder J. Human beta-defensin-2. *Int. J. Biochem. Cell, Biol.* 1999;31(6):645–651.
8. Harder J, Bartels J, Christophers E, Schroder JM. Isolation and characterization of human beta-defensin-3: a novel human inducible peptide antibiotic. *J. Biol. Chem.* 2001;276(8):5707–5713.
9. Bensch KW, Raida M, Magert HJ, Schulz-Knappe P, Forssmann WG. hBD-1: a novel beta-defensin from human plasma. *FEBS Lett.* 1995;368:331–335.

10. Valore EV, Park CH, Quayle AJ, Wiles KR, McCray PB, Jr., Ganz T. Human beta-defensin-1: an antimicrobial peptide of urogenital tissues. *J. Clin. Invest.* 1998;101:1633–1642.

11. Harder J, Bartels J, Christophers E, Schroeder J-M. A peptide antibiotic from human skin. *Nature* 1997;387:861–862.

12. Jia HP, Schutte BC, Schudy A, Linzmeier R, Guthmiller JM, Johnson GK, Tack BF, Mitros JP, Rosenthal A, Ganz T, McCray PB, Jr., Discovery of new human beta-defensins using a genomics-based approach. *Gene* 2001;263:211–218.

13. Zhao CQ, Wang I, Lehrer RI. Widespread expression of beta-defensin HBD-1 in human secretory glands and epithelial cells. *FEBS Lett.* 1996;396:319–322.

14. Becker MN, Diamond G, Verghese MW, Randell SH. CD14-dependent lipopolysaccharide-induced beta-defensin-2 expression in human tracheobronchial epithelium. *J. Biol. Chem.* 2000; 275:29731–29736.

15. Singh PK, Jia HP, Wiles K, Hesselberth J, Liu L, Conway BA, Greenberg EP, Valore EV, Welsh MJ, Ganz T, Tack BF, McCray PB, Jr., Production of β-defensins by human airway epithelia. *Proc. Natl. Acad. Sci. USA* 1998;95:14961–14966.

16. Ali RS, Falconer A, Ikram M, Bissett CE, Cerio R, Quinn AG. Expression of the peptide antibiotics human beta defensin-1 and human beta defensin-2 in normal human skin. *J. Invest. Dermatol.* 2001;117(1):106–111.

17. Schittek B, Paulmann M, Senyürek I, Steffen H. The role of antimicrobial peptides in human skin and in skin infectious diseases. *Infect. Disord. Drug Targets* 2008;(3):135–143.

18. Huh WK, Oono T, Shirafuji Y, Akiyama H, Arata J, Sakaguchi M, Huh NH, Iwatsuki K. Dynamic alteration of human beta-defensin 2 localization from cytoplasm to intercellular space in psoriatic skin. *J. Mol. Med.* 2002;80(10):678–684.

19. Oren A, Ganz T, Liu L, Meerloo T. In human epidermis, beta-defensin 2 is packaged in lamellar bodies. *Exp. Mol. Pathol.* 2003;74(2):180–182.

20. Kopp EB, Medzhitov R. The Toll-receptor family and control of innate immunity. *Curr. Opin. Immunol.* 1999;11(1):13–18.

21. Takeuchi O, Hoshino K, Akira S. Cutting edge: TLR2-deficient and MyD88-deficient mice are highly susceptible to *Staphylococcus aureus* infection. *J. Immunol.* 2000;165(10):5392–5396.

22. Zhang G, Ghosh S. Toll-like receptor-mediated NF-kappaB activation: a phylogenetically conserved paradigm in innate immunity. *J. Clin. Invest.* 2001;107(1):13–19.

23. Baroni A, Orlando M, Donnarumma G, Farro P, Iovene MR, Tufano MA, Buommino E. Toll-like receptor 2 (TLR2) mediates intracellular signalling in human keratinocytes in response to *Malassezia furfur*. *Arch. Dermatol. Res.* 2006;297(7):280–288.

24. Arancibia SA, Beltrán CJ, Aguirre IM, Silva P, Peralta AL, Malinarich F, Hermoso MA. Toll-like receptors are key participants in innate immune responses. *Biol. Res.* 2007;40(2):97–112.

25. Thoma-Uszynski S, Stenger S, Takeuchi O, Ochoa MT, Engele M, Sieling PA, Barnes PF, Rollinghoff M, Bolcskei PL, Wagner M, Akira S, Norgard MV, Belisle JT, Godowski PJ, Bloom BR, Modlin RL. Induction of direct antimicrobial activity through mammalian Toll-like receptors. *Science* 2001;291:1544–1547.

26. Medzhitov R. Toll-like receptors and innate immunity. *Nat. Rev. Immunol.* 2001;1(2):135–145.

27. Chow JC, Young DW, Golenbock DT, Christ WJ, Gusovsky F. Toll-like receptor-4 mediates lipopolysaccharide-induced signal transduction. *J. Biol. Chem.* 1999;274(16):10689–10692.

28. Hoshino K, Takeuchi O, Kawai T, Sanjo H, Ogawa T, Takeda Y, Takeda K, Akira S. Cutting edge: Toll-like receptor 4 (TLR4)-deficient mice are hyporesponsive to lipopolysaccharide: evidence for TLR4 as the Lps gene product. *J. Immunol.* 1999;162(7):3749–3752.

29. Ozinsky A, Underhill DM, Fontenot JD, Hajjar AM, Smith KD, Wilson CB, Schroeder L, Aderem A. The repertoire for pattern recognition of pathogens by the innate immune system is defined by cooperation between Toll-like receptors. *Proc. Natl. Acad. Sci. USA* 2000;97(25): 13766–13771.

30. Oppenheim JJ, Biragyn A, Kwak LW, Yang D. Roles of antimicrobial peptides such as defensins in innate and adaptive immunity. *Ann. Rheum. Dis.* 2003;62(Suppl. 2):ii17–ii21.

31. Taylor K, Rolfe M, Reynolds N, Kilanowski F, Pathania U, Clarke D, Yang D, Oppenheim J, Samuel K, Howie S, Barran P, Macmillan D, Campopiano D, Dorin R. Defensin-related peptide 1 (Defr1) is allelic

to Defb8 and chemoattracts immature DC and CD4 + T cells independently of CCR6. *Eur. J. Immunol.* 2009;39(5):1353–1360.

32. Knowles MR, Boucher RC. Mucus clearance as a primary innate defense mechanism for mammalian airways. *J. Clin. Invest.* 2002;109:571–577.

33. Rehaume LM, Hancock RE. Neutrophil-derived defensins as modulators of innate immune function. *Crit. Rev. Immunol.* 2008;28(3):185–200.

34. Miles K, Clarke DJ, Lu W, Sibinska Z, Beaumont PE, Davidson DJ, Barr TA, Campopiano DJ, Gray M. Dying and necrotic neutrophils are anti-inflammatory secondary to the release of alpha-defensins. *J. Immunol.* 2009;183(3):2122–2132.

35. Philpott M. Defensins and acne. *Mol. Immunol.* 2003;40(7):457–462.

36. Schlapbach C, Yawalkar N, Hunger RE. Human beta-defensin-2 and psoriasin are overexpressed in lesions of acne inversa. *J. Am. Acad. Dermatol.* 2009;61(1):58–65.

37. Chronnell CM, Ghali LR, Ali RS, Quinn AG, Holland DB, Bull JJ, Cunliffe WJ, McKay IA, Philpott MP, Muller-Rover S. Human beta defensin-1 and -2 expression in human pilosebaceous units: upregulation in acne vulgaris lesions. *J. Invest. Dermatol.* 2001;117(5):1120–1125.

38. Tomita T, Nagase T. Defensins as a mechanism of host defense and innate immunity. *Nippon Ronen Igakkai Zasshi* 2001;38(4):440–443.

39. Kisich KO, Carspecken CW, Fiéve S, Boguniewicz M, Leung DY. Defective killing of *Staphylococcus aureus* in atopic dermatitis is associated with reduced mobilization of human beta-defensin-3. *J. Allergy Clin. Immunol.* 2008;122(1):62–68.

40. Cho JW, Cho SY, Lee KS. Roles of SEA-expressing *Staphylococcus aureus*, isolated from an atopic dermatitis patient, on expressions of human beta-defensin-2 and inflammatory cytokines in HaCaT cells. *Int. J. Mol. Med.* 2009;23(3):331–335.

41. Ong PY, Ohtake T, Brandt C, Strickland I, Boguniewicz M, Ganz T, Gallo RL, Leung DY. Endogenous antimicrobial peptides and skin infections in atopic dermatitis. *N. Engl. J. Med.* 2002;347(15): 1151–1160.

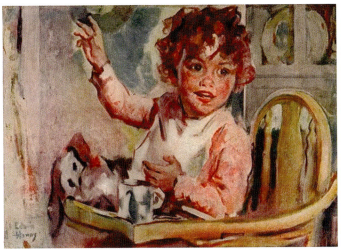

Figure 1.2   Listerine was not originally a mouthwash, instead it was used to wash hands in both the hospital and home. This 1930 advertisement for Listerine advocates mothers washing their hands in "undiluted" Listerine before bathing or feeding the baby in order to kill harmful germs [80]. Courtesy of Johnson and Johnson.

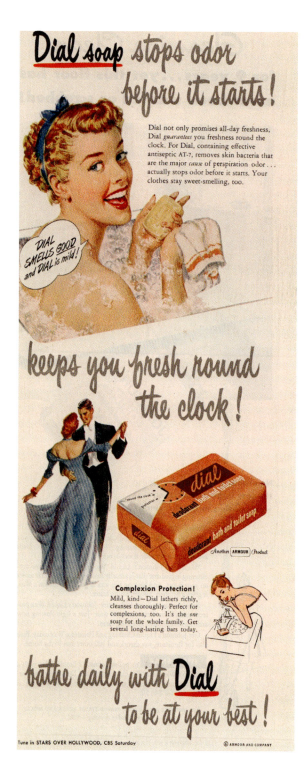

Figure 1.3 Dial soap was introduced in 1948. This 1955 magazine advertisement illustrates how its germ-killing ability was focused on the germs that caused body odor. Courtesy of Henkel of America, Inc.

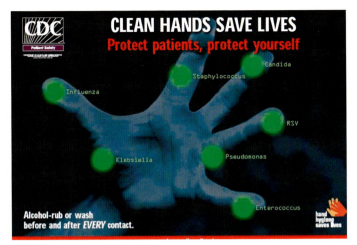

Figure 1.4   In 2005, the Centers for Disease Control first offered this poster on its web site to promote hand hygiene in health care facilities. (*See text for full caption.*)

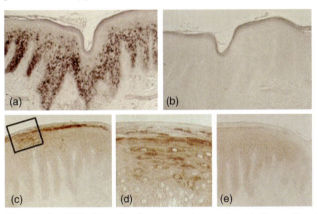

Figure 7.3   hBD-2 localization in gingival oral epithelium. (*See text for full caption.*)

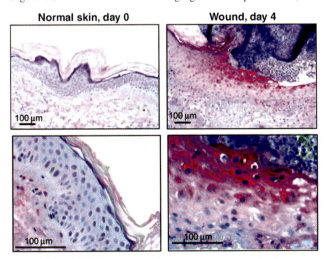

Figure 7.4   hBD-3 expression in a cutaneous wound. (*See text for full caption.*)

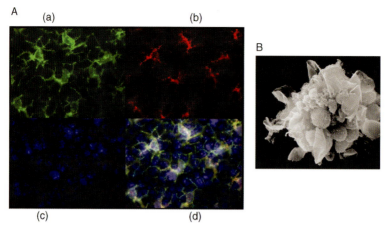

Figure 10.1 A. Appearance of murine dendritic cells. (*See text for full caption.*)

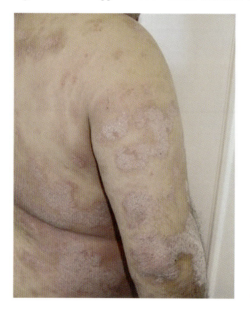

Figure 11.4 Psoriasis vulgaris involving the back and right arm of a man.

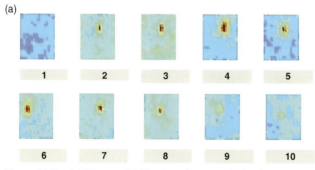

Figure 11.7 (a) Tissue viability imaging: a polarization spectroscopy technique has been used to produce serial images of the erythematous component of a minimal, full-thickness wound protocol [162] induced by a bleeding time lancet with dimensions 1 mm broad and 2 mm depth on ventral forearm skin. (*See text for full caption.*)

CHAPTER 7

ANTIMICROBIAL PEPTIDES OF SKIN AND ORAL MUCOSA

Whasun O. Chung[1] and Henrik Dommisch[1,2]

[1]*Department of Oral Biology, University of Washington, Seattle WA*
[2]*Department of Periodontology, Operative and Preventive Dentistry, University of Bonn, Bonn, Germany*

7.1 INTRODUCTION

Multiple microbial species harbor within the oral cavity, yet most individuals maintain healthy homeostasis. Maintenance of a healthy status can be achieved only when a sufficient interplay between microbial colonization and immune defense mechanisms is sustainable by the host. This interplay takes place on the oral epithelial surface. The oral cavity is lined with stratified squamous epithelium that functions as a barrier between the outside environment and the oral cavity in multiple ways. For one, the oral epithelium provides a rigid physical barrier that protects against mechanical impacts, for example, during mastication. In addition, the oral mucosa also produces a chemical barrier represented by a number of different antimicrobial peptides (AMPs) [1,2]. Similarly, epidermal surfaces are also colonized with multiple species of bacteria, but a healthy balance is maintained in most cases with host innate immune responses that include different AMPs. In fact, two of the AMPs, human beta-defensin-2 and human beta-defensin-3, were first discovered and isolated from psoriatic skin lesions [3–5].

AMPs are defined as proteins that are smaller than 100 amino acids with a molecular weight typically ranging between 3.5 and 6.5 kDa [2]. These small peptides provide a broad spectrum of antimicrobial activity both against Gram-negative and Gram-positive bacteria and against yeast and some viruses [6–8]. In humans, AMPs are represented by a number of different molecules, for example, human alpha-defensins, beta-defensins (hBDs), some C–C and C–X–C chemokines, and the cathelicidin LL-37 [6,9,10]. While alpha-defensins are synthesized in the intestines and as part of the nonoxidative defense mechanism in neutrophils, beta-defensins are mainly of epithelial origin [6,11]. Although both defensins and LL-37

Innate Immune System of Skin and Oral Mucosa: Properties and Impact in Pharmaceutics, Cosmetics, and Personal Care Products, First Edition. Nava Dayan and Philip W. Wertz.
© 2011 John Wiley & Sons, Inc. Published 2011 by John Wiley & Sons, Inc.

show a broad spectrum of antimicrobial activity, they are expressed in varying locations of the mucosa and may therefore play different and possibly synergistic roles in specific sites.

In this chapter, we will closely examine the properties of AMPs and how effective they are against various inflammatory diseases of skin and oral mucosa. We will also focus on the roles AMPs play in overall epidermal and oral health, and assess future therapeutic potential of these AMPs and AMPs from other origins.

7.2 NATURE OF PERIODONTAL DISEASES AND SKIN INFECTIONS

7.2.1 Nature of Periodontal Diseases

Despite the presence of physical and the chemical barriers in periodontium, various extents of periodontal diseases occur in more than 60% of the human population, where the prevalence is continually increasing with age. In the oral cavity, gingivitis and periodontitis are the most frequent inflammatory diseases, and periodontitis in particular may have an impact on systemic diseases such as cardiovascular disease. Therefore, better understanding of oral defense mechanisms against pathogenic bacteria is very important with respect to the increasing aging population.

The periodontal apparatus (periodontium) is represented by a complex of different tissues, including blood vessels, cementum, and periodontal ligaments that keep the teeth attached to the alveolar bone. Like the rest of the oral cavity, the periodontal apparatus is covered by stratified squamous epithelium [1,12]. The gingival epithelium not only possesses tight intercellular junctions between the differentiated epithelial cells toward the oral cavity but also forms an attachment and seal around the tooth surface via hemidesmosomes covering the periodontal ligament space. This sealing portion of gingival epithelium is called junctional epithelium. Since the intercellular space within the junctional epithelium is wider and allows the passage of crevicular fluid, this area is highly susceptible to potential invasion by pathogenic periodontal bacteria [13–15].

In general, periodontal disease can be of inflammatory, traumatic, metabolic, developmental, and/or genetic origin. In most cases, periodontal disease results in an inflammatory reaction of the periodontium to pathogenic microorganisms. Aerobic and anaerobic microorganisms make up bacterial biofilm that accumulates on the tooth surface adjacent to the gingiva [16]. Here, bacteria first form a supragingival biofilm attached to the tooth surface, and once they have passed the junctional epithelium, bacteria may enter the gingival crevice to form subgingival biofilm. Subgingival biofilm provides an optimal environment for anaerobic bacteria to colonize and reproduce [17]. The number of Gram-negative anaerobic bacteria increases during development and maturation of the dental biofilm. Certain clusters of bacterial species, including *Porphyromonas gingivalis*, *Tannerella forsythia*, and *Treponema denticola*, have been identified to be associated with periodontal disease [18]. Infection of the subgingival periodontal tissue is accompanied by the release of bacterial leukotoxins, collagenases, and other proteases that are secreted by these and a number of other microorganisms that are part of the dental plaque. Periodontal disease may be interpreted as the consequence of the imbalance between the pathogenic potential of the biofilm and the host immune defense properties. In addition, genetic and/or environmental factors, such as smoking, contribute to occurrence and progression of periodontal disease [19–22].

Periodontal inflammation undergoes different stages of severity accompanied by all the classical signs of inflammation (redness, welling, pain, and increased temperature, and in advanced instances, loss of function). The early stage of periodontal inflammation is called gingivitis, because it is limited to the gingival soft tissue, and is not associated with loss of attachment structures, such as the Sharpey's fibers. While gingivitis may be completely reversible, the more severe stage of periodontal inflammation, periodontitis, may not be. Periodontitis is characterized by inflamed gingival soft tissue plus clinical attachment loss accompanied by alveolar bone resorption leading to pronounced periodontal pockets (Figure 7.1). The progress of periodontitis can be of chronic (slow progress) or

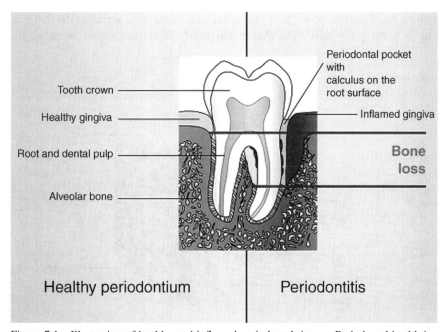

Figure 7.1 Illustration of healthy and inflamed periodontal tissues. Periodontal health is characterized by a sufficient epithelial seal around the tooth (junctional epithelium) and a stable attachment between teeth and alveolar bone (intact ligaments, Sharpey's fibers). In the course of periodontal disease (gingivitis and periodontitis), the epithelial seal around the tooth loosens so that pathogenic periodontal bacteria may penetrate the ligament space. Here, bacteria form the subgingival biofilm, which leads to inflammatory reactions in the surrounding tissues. This inflammatory host response subsequently leads to destruction of the ligament (Sharpey's fibers), while the periodontal pocket deepens and biofilm may calcify on the root surface. In general, calculus on teeth causes enhanced biofilm retention and is therefore critical during the development and progression of periodontal disease. Consequently, reduction of bone height occurs, leading to tooth loss.

aggressive (rapid progress) nature. Without proper treatment, inflammation ultimately leads to complete destruction of the periodontal ligament and alveolar bone, and subsequently to tooth loss [23].

7.2.2 Nature of Skin Infections

Healthy skin provides important barrier functions to protect the host from the outside environment. This protective barrier is disrupted during skin diseases, such as psoriasis, which may lead to severe infections entering deeper tissues (Figure 7.2). Psoriasis is an inflammatory skin disease characterized by morphological epidermal abnormalities and a cellular infiltrate of activated T cells [24]. Psoriatic skin is the site where AMPs hBD-2 and hBD-3 were first discovered [3–5]. In lesional skin of psoriasis patients, both mRNA and protein expression levels of cathelicidin and hBD-2 are increased, as are the levels of protease inhibitors SKALP/elafin and SLPI [3,5,25,26].

Atopic dermatitis is another inflammatory skin disease associated with severe epidermal barrier disruption. Since the epidermal barrier that serves as the first line of defense is compromised and also innate immunity is impaired in patients with

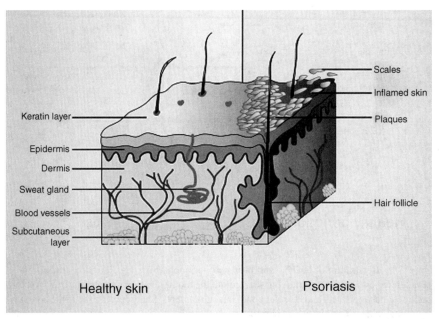

Figure 7.2   Illustration of healthy and inflamed skin. Healthy skin provides important barrier functions protecting the host from the microbial environment. This protective barrier is disrupted during skin diseases, such as psoriasis, which may lead to severe infections entering deeper tissues. Inflammatory skin diseases can be of multiple etiologies. The large number of various microorganisms can potentially cause a wide range of skin alterations, which eventually result in an inflammatory reaction of the skin and the underlying tissue. Ultimately, the loss of skin's protective barrier may cause severe generalized infections.

atopic dermatitis, these patients are at an increased risk of recurrent skin infections [27,28]. The inflammation in atopic dermatitis is mediated by T helper type 2 (Th2), and although genetic and environmental factors are suspected to play a role, the exact mechanisms leading to the onset of this chronic disease is still not well understood [27,29,30]. Gram-positive bacterium *Staphylococcus aureus* is the most commonly found microbe among atopic dermatitis patients, colonizing over 90% of the patients, compared to less than 5% of normal individuals [28]. AMPs LL-37 and hBD-3 have been shown to be effective against *S. aureus*, while hBD-2 needs to work synergistically with other AMPs to be effective [4,5,31].

7.3 PROPERTIES AND FUNCTIONS OF ANTIMICROBIAL PEPTIDES

Epithelial tissues function as the first line of defense between the host and the outside environment, which includes a variety of bacteria. Many studies have demonstrated that these tissues protect the host by not only providing a physical barrier but also stimulating innate immune responses in the form of antimicrobial peptides [1,2]. These antimicrobial peptides have a broad spectrum of activity against both Gram-negative and Gram-positive bacteria and against yeast and viruses [7,32]. In humans, these antimicrobial peptides include defensins and a cathelicidin family member LL-37 in skin and oral mucosa and other epithelia [9,10,32]. The human defensins include the alpha-defensins of intestinal and neutrophil origin and the beta-defensins of skin and oral mucosa and other epithelia.

7.3.1 Defensin Antimicrobial Peptides

Antimicrobial peptides are defined as proteins that are smaller than 100 amino acids with molecular weights typically ranging between 3.5 and 6.5 kDa [1]. Alpha-defensins are expressed in neutrophils as part of their nonoxidative antimicrobial mechanisms [33,34]. Alpha-defensins are also found in Paneth cells in the intestine [35,36]. They are synthesized as precursors that are proteolytically activated and released during inflammation [37,38]. The human beta-defensins (hBDs) are small, cationic antimicrobial peptides made primarily of epithelial cells and expressed in all human epithelia examined to date [1]. Both alpha- and beta-defensins have a compact structure that contain three disulfide bonds, consisting of six conserved cysteine residues, and the location of these disulfide bonds differs in alpha- and beta-defensins [39]. However, the genes encoding the alpha-defensins and the beta-defensins are clustered, suggesting a common origin [40]. The presence of arginine and lysine residues contributes to the cationic nature of beta-defensins. Their cationic charge and amphipathic structure with polar and hydrophobic surfaces allow the hBDs to bind to bacterial outer membranes and aggregate to form pores to disrupt membrane integrity. Others also suggest that these peptides have cytoplasmic targets [41]. Because of this mechanism and rapid action, bacterial resistance to hBDs is rare.

The defensins are secreted in biological fluids, including urine, bronchial fluids, nasal secretions, saliva, and gingival crevicular fluid [42–45]. hBDs were first

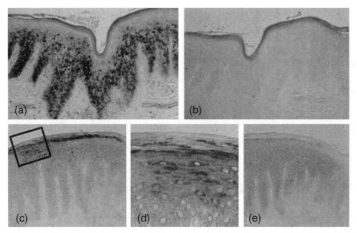

Figure 7.3   hBD-2 localization in gingival oral epithelium. *In situ* hybridization; antisense probe (a) and control sense probe (b). Localization of peptide by immunoreactivity with polyclonal hBD-2 antibody. (c) Low magnification and (d) high magnification views showing hBD-2 reactivity in cytoplasm in mid- and upper epithelial layers; (e) normal rabbit serum control showing nonspecific general epithelial reaction; (a–c, e) 610 original magnification and (d) 640 original magnification. Note that the mRNA (a) is most strongly expressed in the spinous layers, while the peptide is expressed mainly in the granular layer with some spinous layer staining. Serial sections are from a biopsy fixed in neutral buffered formalin and are representative results from multiple uninflamed and inflamed samples. (*See the color version of this figure in Color Plate section.*) (Permission to reprint granted by Wiley-Blackwell Publishing) [55].

identified in tracheal epithelial cells and subsequently found in many epithelia including kidney and urinary tract, oral mucosa, and skin [42,46–48]. hBD-1 is expressed constitutively in epithelial tissues, whereas hBD-2 and hBD-3 are expressed when epithelia are stimulated with bacteria, *Candida albicans*, IL-1, or TNF-α [49–54]. hBD-4 has not been well characterized, but its mRNA expression has been observed in skin [24]. Although hBD-2 is induced and expressed only in inflamed sites in most tissues, in the oral epithelium it is also expressed in normal uninflamed gingival tissue in the granular, spinous, and cornified layers, presumably because of the high level of exposure of this tissue to commensal organisms (Figure 7.3) [55–57]. The regulation of expression of multiple additional defensins is not yet known, although genes for 28 hBDs have been identified [58]. Surprisingly, nonpathogenic commensal organisms, such as *Fusobacterium nucleatum* and *Streptococcus gordonii* (oral), and *Staphylococcus epidermidis* (skin), are excellent stimulants for hBD-2 expression in cultured human gingival epithelial cells and foreskin keratinocytes [53].

hBDs are suspected to play a role in mucosal and skin defense not only by their direct antimicrobial action but also as signaling potential between the innate and the acquired immune responses [59,60]. Defensins may act as adjuvants in antibody production [61]. In addition, hBD-2 attracts immature dendritic cells (iDCs) via CCR6 receptor and stimulates maturation of iDC, eventually leading to activation and upregulation of IL-8 [62]. Thus, hBD-2 not only provides direct antimicrobial properties but also indirectly stimulates the long-term immune response. Other AMPs can also heighten immune functions indirectly by altering gene expression in epithelia. Human alpha-defensins, hBDs and LL-37 have all been shown to increase the expression and secretion of IL-8 and/or IL-18 in oral, skin, and respiratory epithelia [63–65]. In concert with the findings for hBD-2, it was shown that the C–C chemokine ligand 20 (CCL20) also attracts iDCs via CCR6 [66]. Like hBD-2, CCL20 is an antimicrobial peptide with a broad spectrum of antimicrobial activity, and the gene expression is also stimulated by the pathogenic periodontal bacterium *P. gingivalis* [54,66,67].

7.3.2 Signaling Pathways Involved in Defensin Regulation

In the oral cavity, the bacteria–host communication takes place via a number of signal transduction pathways, but different bacteria may induce different signals from the host. Conversely, various host immune responses may interfere with the way nonpathogens (commensals) and pathogens communicate to form biofilm, although this means of defense is poorly understood. Gingival epithelial cells utilize different membrane or cytoplasmic receptors in the induction of innate immune responses to various bacteria. How the host distinguishes pathogens from commensals is still not well understood, but several lines of evidence suggest that epithelial cells use different mechanisms of regulation for hBD-2 induction in response to commensals and pathogens and that hBD-2 regulation may differ in oral mucosa and the simple epithelium of trachea [53,68].

hBD-2 is induced by both pathogenic and commensal bacteria in cultured keratinocytes derived from the epidermis and oral gingiva [51,53,54]. In the oral epithelium, which is a stratified epithelium, hBD-2 is also induced by TNF-α, IL-1, and PMA, but not by bacterial LPS [49,51]. This is in contrast to tracheal epithelium, a pseudostratified epithelium, in which LPS stimulates hBD-2 mRNA expression [46,69]. Antibodies against CD14, a cell-surface receptor for LPS, inhibit this transcription [46,69]. CD14 interacts with TLRs, important receptors in innate immune response to microbial challenge, to activate NFκB [70]. Nevertheless, LPS from *P. gingivalis*, *F. nucleatum*, and *E. coli* was a poor stimulant of hBD-2 in cultured gingival epithelial cells even in the presence of human serum to provide CD14. The upregulation of hBD-2 by the commensal oral bacterium, *F. nucleatum*, was independent of other innate immune responses, such as the expression of IL-8, a neutrophil chemoattractant [51]. The mRNA expression of hBD-2 is associated with epithelial differentiation [55]. The promoter region of hBD-2 contains multiple binding sites for AP-1, which is a transcription factor involved in cell differentiation and proliferation [40]. Since MAP kinases activate AP-1, these kinases are expected to regulate the expression of hBD-2. MAP kinases p38 and JNK are involved in the upregulation of hBD-2 in response to commensal and pathogenic bacteria in both skin and oral keratinocytes [53,68,71]. However, NFκB is utilized in the induction of hBD-2 only in epithelial responses to pathogenic bacteria, illustrating the diversity of pathways utilized in hBD-2 induction in both skin and oral keratinocytes [53,68,71]. In addition to MAPK and NFκB, the pathogenic periodontal bacterium *P. gingivalis* utilizes protease-activated receptor-2 (PAR-2) leading to hBD-2 gene expression in oral epithelial cells [54,72]. Furthermore, endogenous hBDs stimulate epidermal keratinocyte production of proinflammatory cytokines and chemokines via G-protein and phospholipase C signaling pathway, suggesting a significant role hBDs play in innate immune responses [73].

7.3.3   Cathelicidins and Alpha-Defensins

LL-37 is an amphipathic cationic peptide and the only cathelicidin identified so far in humans. It is transcribed by CAMP (cathelicidin antimicrobial peptide) gene, which translates to an 18 kDa proprotein, which consists of the cathelin domain and C-terminal cationic domain [74,75]. The C-terminal domain is posttranscriptionally cleaved, giving rise to an active cathelicidin [75,76]. The nomenclature hCAP18 (human cationic antimicrobial protein 18 kDa) is commonly used along with LL-37, whose name is derived from its sequence that starts with Leucine–Leucine and includes 37 amino acids. LL-37 is expressed in various epithelial cell types, including inflamed epidermal keratinocytes and in human tongue, buccal mucosa and saliva following inflammatory stimulation [30,77–79]. Immunohistochemistry studies found that LL-37 is expressed in the junctional epithelium, where IL-8 is also expressed [55]. Since IL-8 expression upon bacterial stimulation follows a gradient that leads to directional migration of neutrophils into the gingival sulcus, it is suspected that the expression of LL-37 in gingival epithelium may be the result of neutrophil migration through the tissue [11,55,80,81]. Cathelicidin is a cationic peptide, much like hBDs, thus directly binds to cell wall of microbes, compromising the permeability of the cell wall [82]. It has a broad spectrum of activity against invading microorganisms, including Gram-negative and Gram-positive bacteria, vaccinia virus, and *C. albicans* [83–85]. In oral models, LL-37 has been shown to be effective against periodontal pathogen *Aggregatibacter actinomycetemcomitans*, while little effect is shown against cariogenic bacteria *Streptococcus mutans*, *Streptococcus sobrinus*, and *Actinomyces viscosus*, as well as another periodontal pathogen *P. gingivalis* [86].

LL-37 also induces cytokines and chemokines in human keratinocytes. In addition, it mobilizes calcium and triggers keratinocyte migration via activation of epidermal growth factor receptors STAT-1 and STAT-3 [73,87]. Similar to hBD-2, LL-37 also plays an additional role in modulating immune functions by recruiting neutrophils, monocytes, and T cells via binding to formyl peptide receptor-like 1 (FPRL1) [88,89]. LL-37 also stimulates secretion of IL-8 in human epidermal keratinocytes by activating epidermal growth factor receptor, while inducing IL-18 by LL-37 signals via p38 and ERK MAP kinases [65,87].

In humans, six different alpha-defensins have been identified so far. They include four neutrophil peptides (HNP1–4) and two human defensins 5 and 6 (HD-5, HD-6) [90–92]. HNP1–3 are expressed in saliva, Paneth cells both in the intestine and in the polymorphonuclear neutrophils in the undifferentiated junctional epithelium [33–36,55,93]. Increased levels of alpha-defensins have been observed in patients with oral inflammation [93,94]. HNP1 has antifungal activity against *C. albicans*, while HNP3 shows minimal activity against this microbe [95].

7.4   ROLE OF ANTIMICROBIAL PEPTIDES IN ORAL MUCOSA

Epithelial tissues function as the first line of defense between the outside environment and the host. In the oral cavity, gingival epithelial cells are one of the first host cell types that encounter colonizing bacteria. As a consequence, gingival epithelial cells respond to the presence of bacteria through an elaborate signaling network, producing AMPs and cytokines, leading to host innate immune responses [2,96,97]. The AMPs have a broad spectrum of activity both against Gram-negative and Gram-positive bacteria and against yeast and viruses [7,32]. In humans, these antimicrobial peptides include defensins and a cathelicidin family member LL-37 in skin and oral mucosa and other epithelia [9,10,32].

7.4.1   The Role of Cathelicidins and Defensins in Oral Health

Reduced HNP1–3 concentrations have been reported in patients with neutrophil disorders [98]. In particular, patients with Kostmann syndrome, an inherited bone marrow disorder and a congenital neutropenia, lack LL-37 in saliva and plasma, and have reduced concentrations of HNP1–3. On the other hand, patients with a bone marrow transplant show normal concentration of LL-37 in their saliva and plasma [99]. Interestingly, when patients with Kostmann syndrome have their levels of neutrophils restored by treatment with recombinant granulocyte colony-stimulating factor, they still experience recurring periodontal infections [99,100]. These studies suggest that the lack of salivary LL-37 is the likely reason for chronic periodontitis in patients with Kostmann prior to bone marrow transplant, highlighting the important role cathelicidins play in oral health.

Another important role AMPs play in oral health has been reported in a study that showed the level of HNP1–3 was significantly higher in children with no caries than in children with caries [101]. Although it is not clear how HNPs protect against caries, the presence of HNPs in saliva is thought to result in caries protection via direct antimicrobial properties or by binding to outer membranes of bacteria, thus preventing biofilm formation [101,102].

Another way AMPs participate in oral health has been documented in the studies on hBD gene polymorphisms and host susceptibility to oral pathogens. Multiple single nucleotide polymorphisms (SNPs) have been found in genes encoding hBD-1 and hBD-2 [103–105]. A study by Jurevic et al. found that the presence of an SNP in the gene encoding hBD-1 is associated with protection from oral *Candida* carriage [106]. Although type I diabetic patients generally have threefold more *Candida* carriage than nondiabetics in oral mucosa, those patients who carry the SNP have low level of *Candida* carriage [106]. How the presence of SNP protects individuals from oral *Candida* is still not well understood, but this finding underlines the significant role defensins play in innate immunity, especially in individuals who are more susceptible to opportunistic infections [80]. Other genes encoding defensins, hBD-2, hBD-3, hBD-4, HNP1, and HNP3, have also been found to have various copy numbers in different individuals [107,108], but more studies are needed to better understand the effects of copy number on defensin peptide expression and oral health.

7.4.2   Role of hBDs in Periodontal Disease and Oral Cancer

The expression of hBDs has been studied in gingival samples from different stages of periodontal disease (gingivitis and periodontitis). In all studies, high inter-individual variances were demonstrated when analyzing the expression of hBDs [56,57,109,110]. In some studies, analysis of mRNA expression by quantitative PCR showed the gene expression of hBD-1, -2, and -3 was less frequently detected in gingival samples with gingivitis and periodontitis compared to healthy samples [57,111]. In contrast, another study observed little difference in quantitative PCR analysis of gingival tissue samples from both gingivitis and periodontitis, where mRNA for hBD-1, -2, and -3 was detected, compared to samples from healthy gingiva [56]. Comparable results have also been demonstrated when analyzing the presence of mRNA and proteins for hBDs by *in situ* hybridization and immunohistochemistry, respectively [109,110,112]. In one study, the expression of hBD-1 and hBD-2 was investigated in gingival samples with gingivitis and with both chronic and aggressive periodontitis [113]. Here, the expression level for hBD-1 in samples from gingiva with chronic periodontitis was significantly higher compared to samples with gingivitis or aggressive periodontitis. On the other hand, the analysis of gingival samples with aggressive periodontitis showed significantly higher hBD-2 level than those with gingivitis and chronic periodontitis [113]. Immunohistological studies showed that hBD-1 and hBD-2 are mostly located in the granular and spinous cell layer of healthy and inflamed gingival tissue samples, whereas hBD-3 was found in the basal layer of healthy gingival samples, and in both the basal and the spinous layer in gingiva with periodontitis [109,110]. Taken together, it seems difficult to draw conclusions regarding the role of hBDs in periodontal disease. These differential expression patterns of hBDs in periodontal disease suggest complex regulatory mechanisms during local innate immune responses. In general, data from these studies suggest that hBDs play a crucial role in the maintenance of periodontal health and may exhibit preventive properties, but their role in the development and progression of established periodontal lesions remains to be identified.

Several recent studies suggested an important role AMPs play in various oral cancers. In one study, overexpression of hBD-3 at both mRNA and protein levels was observed in surgical biopsies from patients with oral squamous cell carcinoma (OSCC) compared to those from healthy subjects [114]. On the contrary, the mRNA expression of hBD-1 decreased 50-fold in biopsies from OSCC compared to those from healthy gingiva, while the expression decreased between 2.5- and 5-fold in benign and premalignant lesions [115]. This suggests that the loss of hBD-1 might contribute to the malignant progression of OSCC [115]. In another study from the same group, traceable expression of hBD-1, -2, and -3 was observed by immunohistochemistry both in healthy salivary gland tissue and in benign and malignant salivary gland tumors [116]. In particular, hBD-1 expression was detected in the cytoplasm of healthy salivary glands and benign salivary gland tumors, while its expression shifted and accumulated in the nucleus in malignant salivary gland tumors, suggesting a possible role hBD-1 may play in the oncogenesis of salivary gland tumors [116]. All these studies present a potential role AMPs play in the pathogenesis of oral cancer and a possibility of developing therapeutic alternatives to treat oral cancer based on natural AMPs or synthetic derivatives of AMPs.

7.4.3   Antimicrobial Activity of AMPs Toward Oral Microbes

Among different beta-defensins, hBD-1 has a weak antimicrobial activity against Gram-negative organisms and hBD-2 is more effective against Gram-negative bacteria, while hBD-3 is found to be effective against both Gram-positive and Gram-negative species [3,4,8,117]. Both hBD-2 and hBD-3 have been demonstrated to be effective against cariogenic bacteria *S. mutans* and *S. sanguis*, while LL-37 was found slightly less effective against Streptococcal species [117–120]. Interestingly, the minimum inhibitory concentrations (MICs) vary greatly for periodontal pathogens: the MIC for hBD-3 for *P. gingivalis* is 6 µg/mL for ATCC strain 33277, but greater than 250 µg/mL for strain W50. Similarly, the MIC for hBD-3 for *A. actinomycetemcomitans* ranges from 10 µg/mL for strain 1200 to more than 250 µg/mL for ATCC strain 29523 [118]. On the contrary, oral *Candida* species, *C. albicans*, *C. krusei*, and *C. parapsilosis*, are susceptible to hBD-2 and hBD-3 at low micromolar concentrations, while *C. glabrata* strains are resistant to hBD-2 and hBD-3 [118,121]. It is interesting to note that both hBD-2 and hBD-3 are able to inhibit the adherence of *C. glabrata* to epithelial cells, suggesting the physiological effectiveness of beta-defensins [121].

The apparent inability of HIV to transmit via oral mucosa may be partially due to the action of AMPs in saliva and in cells within the epithelia [11]. The effect of defensins has been documented against viruses, especially hBD-2 and hBD-3 against HIV [122–124]. In particular, the effect of hBD-3 against HIV has been reported to be due to its binding to the CXCR4 receptor without receptor signaling and its ability to compete for natural ligands and HIV for this receptor [125]. In addition to the oral mucosa, a number of different AMPs are also synthesized by oral salivary glands and thus are present in saliva [11]. The antimicrobial activity of LL-37, alpha-, and beta-defensins is salt sensitive, although hBD-3 is less affected by salt concentration [117,126]. The low salt environment of saliva may aid antimicrobial activity of AMPs, and their activity *in vivo* may also be aided by synergistic interactions between antimicrobials and other proteins in saliva.

7.5   ROLE OF ANTIMICROBIAL PEPTIDES IN SKIN INFECTIONS AND WOUND HEALING

Skin provides the outermost barrier against potentially harmful environmental factors, including pathogenic organisms. In addition to providing physical barrier, human skin is inhabited by multiple species of nonpathogenic commensal bacteria that aid in maintaining a healthy homeostasis of skin. Other major contributors in host skin defense include AMPs hBDs, cathelicidin LL-37, dermcidin, and S100A7/ psoriasin [127–129]. These AMPs are frequently found at the site of inflamed and injured epithelia and have a broad spectrum of activity against a wide range of pathogenic organisms, including bacteria, viruses, and fungi [8,83,85]. hBD-1 is constitutively expressed in epithelial tissues, while the expression of hBD-2, hBD-3, and LL-37 has been shown to be upregulated when epithelia are stimulated with bacteria *C. albicans*, IL-1, or TNF-α [50–53,104,130].

In epidermal lesion of psoriasis patients, the expression of hBD-2 and hBD-3 is significantly increased, while their expression decreases in atopic dermatitis, suggesting an important role these AMPs play in cutaneous innate immunity [5,128,131]. In particular, hBD-2 is highly expressed in psoriatic epidermis, and susceptibility to psoriasis is associated with high hBD genomic copy number [132]. In addition, a recent study found SNPs and the haplotype in the defensin gene DEFB1 are strongly associated with atopic dermatitis [133]. These studies suggest the level of AMP expression may be responsible for relatively low prevalence of microbial infections in psoriasis patients, in contrast to high infections observed in atopic dermatitis patients [24,134]. In healthy skin, LL-37 is secreted via sweat glands [135]. In a study reported by Kaus et al., the level of LL-37 mRNA expression in healthy versus burned skin was comparable, while the expression decreased by 10-fold in adjacent unburned skin [136]. The *in situ* hybridization shows the transcript of LL-37 in unburned skin is located in the stratum granulosum of the epidermis, while a few intact cells at the surface of burns express LL-37 mRNA [136]. On the other hand, the expression of hBD-2 and hBD-3 is highly upregulated (up to 380-fold) both in burned skin tissue and in the adjacent unburned area, compared to healthy skin [136–138]. All these studies underline the role AMPs play in inflammatory skin conditions.

Lichen sclerosus (LS), a chronic inflammatory sclerotic skin disease, frequently leads to skin barrier disruption, resulting in recruitment of AMPs at the site of inflammation. In LS patients, the expression of hBD-2 is significantly higher than in controls at the mRNA and protein levels, while hBD-3 and LL-37 expression is higher at the mRNA level, but not at the protein level [139]. Secondary bacterial infections are not a major cause of concern in LS patients, and spirochetes acquired by tick bites have been implicated in LS etiology [140]. Thus, upregulation of LL-37, which is shown to be effective against spirochetes, may provide innate antimicrobial defense for the host with LS [139,141].

Patients with diabetes mellitus (DM) often suffer from lower extremity ulcers and face increased risk of amputations [142,143]. Diabetic wounds in patients with DM are most commonly infected with *S. aureus*, and impaired would healing along with bacterial infections is the frequent cause of lower extremity amputations [144–146]. Wound infections can also lead to bacteremia or sepsis; thus, along with increased incidences of methicillin-resistant *S. aureus* (MRSA) seen in recent years, there is an urgent need to develop better options for treating and healing diabetic wounds. Both hBD-3 and hBD-4 have been shown to be effective against *S. aureus* and MRSA in *in vitro* studies [147,148]. The expression of hBD-3 induced by cutaneous wounds has been documented in epidermal keratinocytes (Figure 7.4) [149]. More recently, Hirsch et al. has shown that hBD-3 significantly promotes wound healing in *S. aureus*-infected diabetic wounds in porcine model [145], suggesting a possible role hBD-3 may play in diabetic wound healing and wound infections.

Normal skin, day 0   **Wound, day 4**

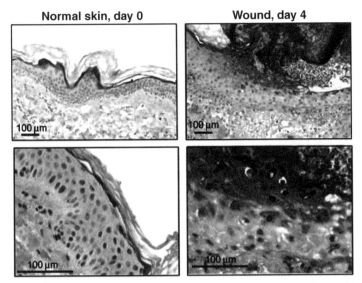

Figure 7.4   hBD-3 expression in a cutaneous wound. Samples of normal human skin and skin from a 4-day-old wound were immunostained for hBD-3. Color was developed with fast red chromogen, and Harris hematoxylin was used for counterstaining. (*See the color version of this figure in Color Plate section.*) Reproduced from Ref. [149] with permission from the American Society for Clinical Investigation.

7.6   THERAPEUTIC POTENTIAL OF ANTIMICROBIAL PEPTIDES

7.6.1   Human Defensins

The skin and the oral cavity are exposed to a wide range of microorganisms of different genetic origins. Generally, the physical and chemical barriers of the human skin and oral mucosa are capable of sustaining this enormous challenge by microorganisms [11]. Patients with compromised immune system, such as DM or AIDS, are highly susceptible to bacterial, viral, and/or fungal infections. For these patients, it is very important to successfully treat infections, making application of antibiotic drugs a crucial treatment procedure. Bacterial resistance to oral systemic antibiotics, such as methicillin or vancomycin, has emerged as an enormous problem in the treatment of inflammatory diseases in recent years. Since the application of antibiotics serves as a standard therapeutic procedure, the current research aims to find appropriate alternatives to replace or at least to support oral systemic antibiotic therapy [150,151]. The facts that AMPs exhibit a broad spectrum of antimicrobial activity and thereby show low risk for development of bacterial resistance make these peptides a promising target for therapeutic use [152,153].

AMPs are produced by a large number of organisms, including insects, fungi, bacteria, plants, and animals [6,11,154]. In humans, a number of different molecules show antimicrobial activity, including HNPs, hBDs, the cathelicidin LL-37, and some C–C and C–X–C chemokines [6,11,78,155]. These AMPs are synthesized at various locations of the human body and may act synergistically to fight infections caused by different microorganisms. While HNPs, hBDs, LL-37, C–C, and C–X–C chemokines show antimicrobial effects against Gram-positive and Gram-negative bacteria to various degrees [11,156,157], hBDs and HNPs are in particular very effective against viruses such as HIV [123–125,158–160]. Furthermore, hBDs and LL-37 exhibit distinct antifungal activity [6,84].

In a few animal studies, the effectiveness of human AMPs has been tested. One approach was to investigate the effect of HNP1 on *Mycobacterium tuberculosis*-infected mice [161,162]. The authors show that a subcutaneous administration of HNP1 significantly reduces *M. tuberculosis* infection in lung and spleen of the infected mice [162]. These results are very promising, especially considering the fact that tuberculosis is still one of the most prominent infectious diseases worldwide. Another study showed that hBD-2 may be protective against pneumonia and sepsis [163]. Prior to infection with *Pseudomonas aeruginosa* to induce pneumonia or cecal ligation to induce sepsis, rats received a recombinant adenovirus carrying rat beta-defensin-2 (BD-2), which is very similar to hBD-2. Overexpression of BD-2 led to significantly lower amounts of *P. aeruginosa* colony-forming units in the infected rats compared to the control rats. In rats with pneumonia and in those with sepsis, overexpression of BD-2 reduced general alveolar damage, intestinal edema, and infiltration of neutrophils. Furthermore, BD-2 significantly improved the survival of rats with sepsis compared to the control animals [163]. Although these animal studies suggest that human AMPs might be an attractive candidate for a new therapeutic approach, their effectiveness in human clinical studies is yet to be determined. Besides their antimicrobial capabilities, human AMPs also show multiple mediator-like functions leading to processes that may enhance immune reactions [6,164]. Therefore, the application of human AMPs might exhibit a certain distress to the human body, which possibly could result in unintentional side effects or more drastically in severe adverse events. Another therapeutic approach was the application of an AMP from saliva, histatin, in patients with *Candida* infection. Histatin was effective in reducing *Candida* infection and gingival bleeding, suggesting a potential use for histatin as an additive to artificial saliva [165–169].

In addition to their microbicidal activities, human AMPs, such as hBDs and antibacterial chemokines, also possess mediator-like function either by activating immature dendritic cells through the CCR6 receptor or by inducing the release of proinflammatory mediators from epithelial and other cells [64–66,73,157,170,171]. Here, human AMPs represent a possible link between the innate and the acquired immune system. Although these human AMPs appear to be suitable targets for a therapeutic approach, there is a certain risk for producing severe adverse side effects in patients. Therapeutic human AMPs may accelerate proinflammatory reactions and therefore cause harm not only to local sites but also to the patient's general health. Hence, AMPs produced by other organisms such as bacteria, fungi, plants, or animals may be of more value as new antimicrobial therapeutic alternatives. Peptides derived from other organisms have little influence on inflammatory responses in humans, and some of the very promising AMPs are discussed in the next sections.

7.6.2   Bacterial Defensins

Bacteriocins are bacterially produced, small, heat-stable peptides, which have been identified or believed to exist in every species of bacteria. Bacteriocins are produced for competition of one bacterium either against other bacteria of the same species or against bacteria of other genera [172,173]. Thus far, the most promising bacteriocins are produced by lactic acid bacteria (LAB) *Lactobacillus*. One application is the extensive use of LAB as probiotics in food processing and preservation [174,175]. While the bacteriocin nisin has been already approved for food processing and anti-infective bovine mastitis, other bacteriocins, such as lactinin 3147, mersacidin, and leucocin A, have been investigated for their effectiveness against antibiotic-resistant bacterial strains, such as MRSA and vancomycin-resistant enterococci (VRE). MRSA and VRE are a major cause for severe nosocomial infections of skin or mucosal wounds [153,172,175–177]. Therefore, these bacteriocins may represent a good lead to cure infections by multiresistant bacteria.

Furthermore, some bacteria have been shown to have an influence on the treatment outcome for periodontitis. After conventional biofilm removal by mechanical means, a new concept may be the replacement of periodontal pathogenic bacteria with oral commensal bacteria, such as *S. salivarius* and *S. sanguinis*, by simply applying them into the periodontal pocket [178,179]. A study reports a replacement treatment delayed and reduced recolonization of the periodontal pockets with pathogenic bacteria, such as *Prevotella intermedia* [178]. Also, the level of clinical gingival inflammation was significantly reduced. In another study, *Lactobacillus salivarius* was used following the same strategy. The study shows that dissolution of *L. salivarius*-containing tablets in the oral cavity provided a favorable clinical outcome in patients at higher risk (smokers) of periodontal disease [180]. Although no bacteriocin levels have been analyzed in these studies, it is conceivable that a "replacement therapy" for periodontitis can be successful only if bacteriocins are produced by nonpathogenic bacteria to combat pathogenic periodontal bacteria [178,179].

7.6.3   Plant and Insect Defensins

The plant defensin RsAFP2 from radish (*Raphanus sativus*) exhibits strong antifungal properties against *C. albicans* and *C. glabrata* by inducing endogenous reactive oxygen species (ROS) [181,182]. The induction of endogenous ROS is a phenotypic characteristic of apoptosis in yeast [183]. Therefore, the RsAFP2-induced ROS may be a direct link to the antifungal activity of RsAFP2 in yeast. The analysis of substitution variants of RsAFP2 (named RsAFP2(G9R) and RsAFP2(V39R)), in which a glycine and valine at positions 9 and 39, respectively, were replaced by an arginine showed even better antifungal activity [181,182,184].

Heliomicin is an insect defensin that also displays antifungal capabilities against *C. albicans* and *C. glabrata*. One of its variants EDT151 was used as a therapeutic agent to treat *Candida*- and *Aspergillus*-infected mice. Compared to the conventional antifungal therapy using amphotericin B, EDT151 performed well, while showing very low toxicity, even upon intravenous administration [184,185].

C. albicans infection of skin and/or oral mucosa is very common in patients under immunocompromised conditions (patients with DM or HIV/AIDS) or after radiotherapy. Plant and insect defensins, such as RsAFP2 or heliomicin, may serve as a new therapeutic strategy for patients with opportunistic infections. Also, plant and insect defensins may also be used for prevention of *Candida* infection. For instance, patients receiving radiotherapy carry intraoral splints for preventive fluoridation of teeth because caries is a common complication following radiotherapy. Both caries and *Candida* infection emerge from the lack of saliva (xerostomy), caused by radiologic damage of salivary glands [186]. Since preventive fluoridation of teeth has already been widely accepted, an additional application of plant and/or insect defensins may stand for a putative future preventive scheme for the treatment of radiotherapy-associated *Candida* infections.

7.6.4 Animal Defensins

Among the large number of animal defensins, some have been studied as therapeutics for human diseases. This section will discuss examples of AMPs from invertebrates and vertebrates that have, in some cases, been altered to exhibit better performance in humans. Tachyplesins (tachyplesin I, tachyplesin II, polyphemusin I, and polyphemusin II) are AMPs synthesized by leukocytes in horseshoe crabs. Studies on tachyplesins have shown that tachyplesin I is extremely stable and retains its antimicrobial activity even after boiling and acid treatment [187], whereas polyphemusin II is capable of inhibiting HIV-1 [188,189]. Since cytotoxicity by tachyplesins was noted, analogues of tachyplesins have been constructed, where the amino acids lysine or tyrosine were introduced to the sequence [188]. A markedly enhanced activity against HIV-1 along with an extensive reduction of cytotoxicity was noticed [188]. These potent and stable properties of tachyplesins may be desirable for treatment of viral infection in oral or dermal mucosa since both the skin and the oral cavity are exposed to environmental influences, including heat (sun exposure and hot drinks), chemicals (dermal creams, food, and acids), and more importantly microorganisms [190].

Magainin-2 is an AMP that has been discovered in *Xenopus laevis*, an African clawed frog, when wounds remained infection-free upon incisions on the frog skin. These frogs did not develop skin infection ever after they were placed in water containing high levels of microorganisms [191,192]. It was found that magainin-2 shows a broad-spectrum antimicrobial activity and was therefore considered to be a suitable candidate for therapeutic applications [193]. The amino acid sequences of magainin-2 were altered to improve the microbicidal activity, which resulted in the development of a magainin-2 analogue, pexiganan [193]. Phase III clinical trial revealed effectiveness of pexiganan against a broad microbial spectrum. In comparison to systemic antimicrobial therapy, mildly infected diabetic foot ulcers were treated with the topical application of a pexiganan cream [194]. It was shown that the topical application of pexiganan served as a good alternative compared to systemic antibiotics, especially since the risk of selecting an antimicrobial-resistant bacteria might be reduced [195]. *S. aureus* is known to quickly develop multiple resistances to antibiotics, such as methicillin and vancomycin, and was therefore tested for their ability to develop resistance against pexiganan. While the MIC for the systemic antimicrobial substance ofloxacin increased, the MIC for pexiganan remained constant in culture samples of *S. aureus* isolates from pexiganan-treated patients [194]. These findings may help alter current therapy strategies, especially in dermatology. The same may be true in dentistry in finding potential value of using pexiganan as a preventive approach to avoid dental complications such as peri-implantitis. A recent study observed that pexiganan acetate was helpful in preventing organisms from traversing the skin barrier around transcutaneous osseointegrated implants [196]. In dentistry, placement of transgingival implants is a common therapy for partly or totally edentulous jaws. Patients suffering from periodontitis are in particular considered to be more susceptible to develop peri-implantitis around osseointegrated implants. Here, a parallel administration of pexiganan along with implant placement may help prevent peri-implantitis in patients at high risk (patients with periodontitis or diabetes mellitus, smokers, etc.).

Another class of animal defensins, named protegrins, was initially discovered in pig leukocytes [197]. Protegrins and tachyplesins are structurally related antimicrobial peptides differing in the localization of their changed residues and their cysteine disulfides. The protegrins, PG-1, PG-2, and PG-3, exhibit a broad spectrum of microbicidal activity, which involves, very similar to other AMPs, the disruption of the membrane structure [190,197]. Miyasaki and Lehrer have studied the activity of protegrins against periodontal pathogenic bacteria, including *A. actinomycetemcomitans*, *Capnocytophaga* spp., *P. gingivalis*, *P. intermedia*, and *F. nucleatum*, and antimicrobial activity against all investigated periodontal pathogens was seen [190]. Protegrin analogues were constructed and developed to test the antimicrobial potency in humans. The protegrin analogue iseganan was tested for its impact on the treatment of ulcerative oral mucositis [198]. Iseganan is a new antimicrobial drug that reached phase III clinical testing [199]. The results, however, did not demonstrate a major positive effect of iseganan during treatment of ulcerative oral mucositis [198]. In another study, in which a possible preventive impact of iseganan on ventilator-associated pneumonia was tested, iseganan failed to improve the outcome in patients receiving prolonged mechanical ventilation [200].

Indolicidin has been isolated from cytoplasmic granules of bovine neutrophils, and this AMP exhibits a broad spectrum of antimicrobial activity against not only bacteria and fungi but also HIV-1 [201–204]. Although indolicidin shows promise as a potent AMP, it also shows cytotoxic effects on human T lymphocytes and erythrocytes [205]. Therefore, an attempt was made to develop indolicidin analogues, on the one hand, to improve the antimicrobial activity and, on the other hand, to eliminate cytotoxic properties. One indolicidin analogue, called omiganan, has shown to be very effective against a broad microbial spectrum [206]. A particularly effective antifungal activity was found when omiganan was tested both against a large number of different isolates of *Candida* spp., including *C. albicans*, *C. glabrata*, and *C. krusei*, and against *Aspergillus* spp. [207,208]. Furthermore, omiganan exhibits rapid microbicidal activity against *S. epidermidis* [206]. Therefore, omiganan is another promising candidate for new antimicrobial treatment procedures not only in dermatology but also in dentistry. Treatment of local opportunistic infections, such as

C. albicans infection, may be even more efficient when applying these naturally derived antimicrobials [207].

7.6.5 Application of Antimicrobial Peptides for Therapy

In general, there are multiple ways to administer an antimicrobial substance. One way is the local application of an AMP or a mixture of various AMPs in the form of solutions, gels, or cream [194,196]. Those locally applied AMPs may have the disadvantage of exhibiting only short-term effects because of the limited retention time at local sites. Also, AMPs as a topical agent are not applicable in every part of human body; thus, only the skin surface or the mucosal surface in the oral cavity can be easily reached and treated. All other areas may require invasive procedures, accompanied by known risks. On the other hand, topically applied AMPs might have less potential to cause unintentional side effects or adverse events related to general inflammatory reactions. The simple injection of synthetic AMPs may be another way to increase the concentration of AMPs locally (subcutaneous or intramuscular injection) or systemically (intravenous injection) [162]. Here, the risk to develop unintentional side effects may be higher compared to the topical local administration [194].

A new approach to increase the AMP synthesis and secretion has been described utilizing gene therapy [209]. Via transfection of cells with a viral vector, genes for AMPs can be incorporated into the human DNA. Thus, human cells exhibit genetic codes for AMPs and may thereby produce a higher quantity of AMPs to fight bacterial, fungal, or viral infections. Although first results from animal studies demonstrated promise [209], concerns should be raised regarding possible adverse events jeopardizing the patient's general health.

7.6.6 Summary

Both in dermatology and in dentistry, application of topical antimicrobial substances is a well-established therapy to treat local infections. But this treatment may sometimes be difficult, especially when microorganisms of different genera are the cause of a disease. Periodontitis is such a disease that is not caused only by one single bacterium but by a number of different bacterial species, organized in a complex biofilm and thereby exhibiting various properties [18]. Here, the topical application of a single antibiotic cream would not be very effective; hence a mixture of two different oral systemic antibiotics (metronidazole and amoxicillin) is usually necessary to eliminate those various bacterial species and to provide a successful supportive therapy for periodontitis [210–212]. Therefore, it is conceivable that a mixture of different AMPs, which all exhibit a broad spectrum of antimicrobial activity, but with slight differences regarding whether they are more potent against Gram-positives, Gram-negatives, fungi, yeast, and/or viruses, may be a good alternative for topical antimicrobial therapy [6]. This is particularly applicable both in dentistry and in dermatology, when considering the fact that the risk of selecting antimicrobial-resistant bacteria might be reduced after AMP treatment [194]. In addition, advancements in the creation and modification of some nonhuman AMPs indicate that adverse events or unintentional side effects of AMPs may be averted.

7.7 CONCLUSIONS

Many skin diseases have resulted in altered expression of AMPs, and these changes may play a role in ascertaining a patient's susceptibility to pathogens [139]. Two most common skin diseases, atopic dermatitis and psoriasis, both result in significant disruption of skin barrier, making the host susceptible to subsequent skin infections. However, there is a considerable difference in the prevalence of infections between atopic dermatitis patients (high) and psoriasis patients (low) [30,213]. A possible explanation for this difference is the levels of AMPs expressed between two groups of patients. The levels of hBD-2, hBD-3, and LL-37 expression are increased in psoriasis patients, whereas the expression of these AMPs is reduced in atopic dermatitis patients, underlining an important role these AMPs play in preventing cutaneous infection and in maintaining epidermal health [5,214,215]. In oral mucosa, expression levels of AMPs vary in different types of oral diseases, ranging from periodontitis and caries, to oral cancer [11,101,115,116]. As part of host innate immune system, AMPs are induced not only by various microorganism but also during tissue injury, thus serving as a primary innate immune defense mechanism. In addition, they function as a mediator of both innate and adaptive immunity. Further understanding the role AMPs play in epidermal and oral innate immunity will provide us with better insight into developing potential therapeutics against skin and oral inflammatory diseases, such as psoriasis, atopic dermatitis, caries and periodontitis.

ACKNOWLEDGMENTS

The authors thank Drs. Beverly A. Dale and Søren Jepsen for their kind support and guidance during former and ongoing research projects. Supported by grants from the US DHHS NIDCR R01 DE 16961 and R01 DE13573 (to WOC) and by grants from BONFOR, the German Society of Periodontology (DGP), and the German Research Foundation (DFG, clinical research unit: KFO 208) (to HD).

REFERENCES

1. Dale BA. Periodontal epithelium: a newly recognized role in health and disease. *Periodontol.* 2000, 2002;30:70–78.
2. Ganz T. Defensins: antimicrobial peptides of vertebrates. *C. R. Biol.* 2004;327(6):539–549.
3. Harder J, et al. A peptide antibiotic from human skin. *Nature* 1997;387(6636):861.
4. Harder J, et al. Isolation and characterization of human beta-defensin-3: a novel human inducible peptide antibiotic. *J. Biol. Chem.* 2001;276(8):5707–5713.
5. Ong PY, et al. Endogenous antimicrobial peptides and skin infections in atopic dermatitis. *N. Engl. J. Med.* 2002;347(15):1151–1160.
6. Lehrer RI. Primate defensins. *Nat. Rev. Microbiol.* 2004;2(9):727–738.

7. Premratanachai P, et al. Expression and regulation of novel human beta-defensins in gingival keratinocytes. *Oral Microbiol. Immunol.* 2004;19(2):111–117.
8. Abiko Y, et al. Role of beta-defensins in oral epithelial health and disease. *Med. Mol. Morphol.* 2007; 40(4):179–184.
9. Hancock RE, Scott MG. The role of antimicrobial peptides in animal defenses. *Proc. Natl. Acad. Sci. USA* 2000;97(16):8856–8861.
10. Selsted ME, Ouellette AJ. Mammalian defensins in the antimicrobial immune response. *Nat. Immunol.* 2005;6(6):551–557.
11. Chung WO, et al. Expression of defensins in gingiva and their role in periodontal health and disease. *Curr. Pharm. Des.* 2007;13(30):3073–3083.
12. Dale BA, Brown PS, Wells NJ. Picture talk: effective communication with participants as a critical element in oral health research. *J. Dent. Res.* 2003;82(9):669–670.
13. Buchmann R, et al. Amplified crevicular leukocyte activity in aggressive periodontal disease. *J. Dent. Res.* 2002;81(10):716–721.
14. Hatakeyama S, et al. Expression pattern of adhesion molecules in junctional epithelium differs from that in other gingival epithelia. *J. Periodontal. Res.* 2006;41(4):322–328.
15. Schroeder HE, Rossinsky K, Listgarten MA. Human junctional epithelium as a pathway for inflammatory exudation. *J. Biol. Buccale* 1989;17(3):147–157.
16. Armitage GC. Development of a classification system for periodontal diseases and conditions. *Ann. Periodontol.* 1999;4(1):1–6.
17. Socransky SS, Haffajee AD. Microbiology of periodontal disease. In: Lindhe J,editor. *Clinical Periodontology and Implant Dentistry.* Oxford: Blackwell, 2003.
18. Socransky SS, et al. Microbial complexes in subgingival plaque. *J. Clin. Periodontol.* 1998; 25(2):134–144.
19. Kinane DF, Hart TC. Genes and gene polymorphisms associated with periodontal disease. *Crit. Rev. Oral Biol. Med.* 2003;14(6):430–449.
20. Loos, BG, John RP, Laine ML. Identification of genetic risk factors for periodontitis and possible mechanisms of action. *J. Clin. Periodontol.* 2005;32(Suppl. 6):159–179.
21. Michalowicz BS, et al. Periodontal findings in adult twins. *J. Periodontol.* 1991;62(5):293–299.
22. Michalowicz BS, et al. Evidence of a substantial genetic basis for risk of adult periodontitis. *J. Periodontol.* 2000;71(11):1699–1707.
23. Pihlstrom BL, Michalowicz BS, Johnson NW. Periodontal diseases. *Lancet* 2005;366(9499): 1809–1820.
24. Jansen PA, et al. Beta-defensin-2 protein is a serum biomarker for disease activity in psoriasis and reaches biologically relevant concentrations in lesional skin. *PLoS One* 2009;4(3):e472–e475.
25. Wingens M, et al. Induction of SLPI (ALP/HUSI-I) in epidermal keratinocytes. *J. Invest. Dermatol.* 1998;111(6):996–1002.
26. Nonomura K, et al. Upregulation of elafin/SKALP gene expression in psoriatic epidermis. *J. Invest. Dermatol.* 1994;103(1):88–91.
27. Boguniewicz M, Leung DY. Atopic dermatitis. *J. Allergy Clin. Immunol.* 2006;117(2 Suppl. Mini-Primer):S475–S480.
28. Leung DY, et al. New insights into atopic dermatitis. *J. Clin. Invest.* 2004;113(5):651–657.
29. McGirt LY, Beck LA. Innate immune defects in atopic dermatitis. *J. Allergy Clin. Immunol.* 2006;118 (1):202–208.
30. Howell MD. The role of human beta-defensins and cathelicidins in atopic dermatitis. *Curr. Opin. Allergy Clin. Immunol.* 2007;7(5):413–417.
31. Chen X, et al. Synergistic effect of antibacterial agents human beta-defensins, cathelicidin LL-37 and lysozyme against *Staphylococcus aureus* and *Escherichia coli. J. Dermatol. Sci.* 2005; 40(2):123–132.
32. Lehrer RI, Ganz T. Defensins of vertebrate animals. *Curr. Opin. Immunol.* 2002;14(1):96–102.
33. van Wetering S, et al. Defensins: key players or bystanders in infection, injury, and repair in the lung? *J. Allergy Clin. Immunol.* 1999;104(6):1131–1138.
34. Lehrer RI, Lichtenstein AK, Ganz T. Defensins: antimicrobial and cytotoxic peptides of mammalian cells. *Annu. Rev. Immunol.* 1993;11:105–128.

35. Selsted ME, Miller SI, Henschen AH, Ouellette AJ. Enteric defensins: antibiotic peptide components of intestinal host defense. *J. Cell Biol.* 1992;118:929–936.

36. Ouellette AJ. Paneth cell antimicrobial peptides and the biology of the mucosal barrier. *Am. J. Physiol.* 1999;277:G257–G261.

37. Wilson CL, et al. Regulation of intestinal alpha-defensin activation by the metalloproteinase matrilysin in innate host defense. *Science* 1999;286(5437):113–117.

38. Rock FL, Hardiman G, Timans JC, Kastelein RA, Bazan JF. A family of human receptors structurally related to Drosophila Toll. *Proc. Natl. Acad. Sci. USA* 1998;95:588–593.

39. Dale BA, Krisanaprakornkit S. Defensin antimicrobial peptides in the oral cavity. *J. Oral. Pathol. Med.* 2001;30(6):321–327.

40. Liu L, et al. The human beta-defensin-1 and alpha-defensins are encoded by adjacent genes: two peptide families with differing disulfide topology share a common ancestry. *Genomics* 1997;43(3):316–320.

41. Friedrich CL, et al. Structure and mechanism of action of an indolicidin peptide derivative with improved activity against Gram-positive bacteria. *J. Biol. Chem.* 2001;276(26):24015–24022.

42. Valore EV, et al. Human beta-defensin-1: an antimicrobial peptide of urogenital tissues. *J. Clin. Invest.* 1998;101(8):1633–1642.

43. Cole AM, Dewan P, Ganz T. Innate antimicrobial activity of nasal secretions. *Infect. Immun.* 1999;67:3267–3275.

44. Sahasrabudhe KS, Kimball JR, Morton T, Weinberg W, Dale BA. Expression of the antimicrobial peptide, human b-defensin 1, in duct cells of minor salivary glands and detection in saliva. *J. Dental Res.* 2000;79:1669–1674.

45. Diamond DL, et al. Detection of beta-defensins secreted by human oral epithelial cells. *J. Immunol. Methods* 2001;256(1–2):65–76.

46. Diamond G, Russell JP, Bevins CL. Inducible expression of an antibiotic peptide gene in lipopolysaccharide-challenged tracheal epithelial cells. *Proc. Natl. Acad. Sci. USA* 1996;93(10): 5156–5160.

47. Krisanaprakornkit S, et al. Expression of the peptide antibiotic human beta-defensin 1 in cultured gingival epithelial cells and gingival tissue. *Infect. Immun.* 1998;66(9):4222–4228.

48. Zhao C, Wang I, Lehrer RI. Widespread expression of beta-defensin hBD-1 in human secretory glands and epithelial cells. *FEBS Lett.* 1996;396(2–3):319–322.

49. Mathews M, et al. Production of beta-defensin antimicrobial peptides by the oral mucosa and salivary glands. *Infect. Immun.* 1999;67(6):2740–2745.

50. O'Neil DA, et al. Expression and regulation of the human beta-defensins hBD-1 and hBD-2 in intestinal epithelium. *J. Immunol.* 1999;163(12):6718–6724.

51. Krisanaprakornkit S, et al. Inducible expression of human beta-defensin 2 by *Fusobacterium nucleatum* in oral epithelial cells: multiple signaling pathways and role of commensal bacteria in innate immunity and the epithelial barrier. *Infect. Immun.* 2000;68(5):2907–2915.

52. Harder J, et al. Mucoid *Pseudomonas aeruginosa*, TNF-alpha, and IL-1beta, but not IL6, induce human beta-defensin-2 in respiratory epithelia. *Am. J. Respir. Cell. Mol. Biol.* 2000;22(6):714–721.

53. Chung WO, Dale BA. Innate immune response of oral and foreskin keratinocytes: utilization of different signaling pathways by various bacterial species. *Infect. Immun.* 2004;72(1):352–358.

54. Dommisch H, et al. Protease-activated receptor 2 mediates human beta-defensin 2 and CC chemokine ligand 20 mRNA expression in response to proteases secreted by *Porphyromonas gingivalis*. *Infect. Immun.* 2007;75(9):4326–4333.

55. Dale BA, et al. Localized antimicrobial peptide expression in human gingiva. *J. Periodontal Res.* 2001;36(5):285–294.

56. Dommisch H, et al. Differential gene expression of human beta-defensins (hBD-1, -2, -3) in inflammatory gingival diseases. *Oral Microbiol. Immunol.* 2005;20(3):186–190.

57. Dunsche A, et al. The novel human beta-defensin-3 is widely expressed in oral tissues. *Eur. J. Oral Sci.* 2002;110(2):121–124.

58. Schutte BC, et al. Discovery of five conserved beta-defensin gene clusters using a computational search strategy. *Proc. Natl. Acad. Sci. USA* 2002;99(4):2129–2133.

59. Yang D, Chertov O, Oppenheim JJ. The role of mammalian antimicrobial peptides and proteins in awakening of innate host defenses and adaptive immunity. *Cell. Mol. Life Sci.* 2001;58(7):978–989.

60. Scott MG, et al. An alpha-helical cationic antimicrobial peptide selectively modulates macrophage responses to lipopolysaccharide and directly alters macrophage gene expression. *J. Immunol.* 2000;165(6):3358–3365.
61. Tani K, et al. Defensins act as potent adjuvants that promote cellular and humoral immune responses in mice to a lymphoma idiotype and carrier antigens. *Int. Immunol.* 2000;12(5):691–700.
62. Yang D, et al. Beta-defensins: linking innate and adaptive immunity through dendritic and T cell CCR6. *Science* 1999;286(5439):525–528.
63. Boniotto M, et al. Human beta-defensin 2 induces a vigorous cytokine response in peripheral blood mononuclear cells. *Antimicrob. Agents Chemother.* 2006;50(4):1433–1441.
64. Niyonsaba F, et al. Epithelial cell-derived antibacterial peptides human beta-defensins and cathelicidin: multifunctional activities on mast cells. *Curr. Drug Targets Inflamm. Allergy* 2003;2 (3):224–231.
65. Niyonsaba F, et al. The human beta-defensins (-1, -2, -3, -4) and cathelicidin LL-37 induce IL-18 secretion through p38 and ERK MAPK activation in primary human keratinocytes. *J. Immunol.* 2005;175(3):1776–1784.
66. Yang D, et al. Mammalian defensins in immunity: more than just microbicidal. *Trends Immunol.* 2002;23(6):291–296.
67. Dommisch H, et al. *P. gingivalis*-induced gene expression of MIP-3a/CCL20 in human oral keratinocytes is dependent on PLC, p38/MAPK, and NF-kB-mediated pathways. *Innate Immun.* 2010;16(4):226–34.
68. Chung WO, Dale BA. Differential utilization of NFκB signaling pathways for gingival epithelial cell responses to oral commensal and pathogenic bacteria. *Oral Microbiol. Immunol.* 2008;23:119–126.
69. Diamond G, et al. Transcriptional regulation of beta-defensin gene expression in tracheal epithelial cells. *Infect. Immun.* 2000;68(1):113–119.
70. Schroder NW, et al. Involvement of lipopolysaccharide binding protein, CD14, and Toll-like receptors in the initiation of innate immune responses by *Treponema* glycolipids. *J. Immunol.* 2000;165 (5):2683–2693.
71. Krisanaprakornkit S, Kimball JR, Dale BA. Regulation of human beta-defensin-2 in gingival epithelial cells: the involvement of mitogen-activated protein kinase pathways, but not the NF-kappaB transcription factor family. *J. Immunol.* 2002;168(1):316–324.
72. Chung WO, et al. Protease-activated receptor signaling increases epithelial antimicrobial peptide expression. *J. Immunol.* 2004;173(8):5165–5170.
73. Niyonsaba F, et al. Antimicrobial peptides human beta-defensins stimulate epidermal keratinocyte migration, proliferation and production of proinflammatory cytokines and chemokines. *J. Invest Dermatol.* 2007;127(3):594–604.
74. Zaiou M, Nizet V, Gallo RL. Antimicrobial and protease inhibitory functions of the human cathelicidin (hCAP18/LL-37) prosequence. *J. Invest. Dermatol.* 2003;120(5):810–816.
75. Zanetti M, et al. Structure and biology of cathelicidins. *Adv. Exp. Med. Biol.* 2000;479:203–218.
76. Kenshi Y, Gallo RL. Antimicrobial peptides in human skin disease. *Eur. J. Dermatol.* 2008; 18(1):11–21.
77. Frohm M, et al. The expression of the gene coding for the antibacterial peptide LL-37 is induced in human keratinocytes during inflammatory disorders. *J. Biol. Chem.* 1997;272(24):15258–15263.
78. Frohm Nilsson M, et al. The human cationic antimicrobial protein (hCAP18), a peptide antibiotic, is widely expressed in human squamous epithelia and colocalizes with interleukin-6. *Infect. Immun.* 1999;67(5):2561–2566.
79. Murakami M, et al. Cathelicidin antimicrobial peptides are expressed in salivary glands and saliva. *J. Dent. Res.* 2002;81(12):845–850.
80. Dale BA, Fredericks LP. Antimicrobial peptides in the oral environment: expression and function in health and disease. *Curr. Issues Mol. Biol.* 2005;7(2):119–133.
81. Tonetti MS, et al. Localized expression of mRNA for phagocyte-specific chemotactic cytokines in human periodontal infections. *Infect. Immun.* 1994;62(9):4005–4014.
82. Henzler Wildman KA, Lee DK, Ramamoorthy A. Mechanism of lipid bilayer disruption by the human antimicrobial peptide, LL-37. *Biochemistry* 2003;42(21):6545–6558.

83. Howell MD, et al. Selective killing of vaccinia virus by LL-37: implications for eczema vaccinatum. *J. Immunol.* 2004;172(3):1763–1767.

84. Lopez-Garcia B, et al. Antifungal activity of cathelicidins and their potential role in *Candida albicans* skin infection. *J. Invest. Dermatol.* 2005;125(1):108–115.

85. Nizet V, et al. Innate antimicrobial peptide protects the skin from invasive bacterial infection. *Nature* 2001;414(6862):454–457.

86. Altman H, et al. *In vitro* assessment of antimicrobial peptides as potential agents against several oral bacteria. *J. Antimicrob. Chemother.* 2006;58(1):198–201.

87. Braff MH, et al. Structure–function relationships among human cathelicidin peptides: dissociation of antimicrobial properties from host immunostimulatory activities. *J. Immunol.* 2005;174(7): 4271–4278.

88. Yang D, et al. Human neutrophil defensins selectively chemoattract naive T and immature dendritic cells. *J. Leukoc. Biol.* 2000;68(1):9–14.

89. Yang D, et al. LL-37, the neutrophil granule- and epithelial cell-derived cathelicidin, utilizes formyl peptide receptor-like 1 (FPRL1) as a receptor to chemoattract human peripheral blood neutrophils, monocytes, and T cells. *J. Exp. Med.* 2000;192(7):1069–1074.

90. Cunliffe RN. Alpha-defensins in the gastrointestinal tract. *Mol. Immunol.* 2003;40(7):463–467.

91. Ganz T, Lehrer RI. Defensins. *Curr. Opin. Immunol.* 1994;6(4):584–589.

92. Ganz T, et al. Defensins: natural peptide antibiotics of human neutrophils. *J. Clin. Invest.* 1985;76 (4):1427–1435.

93. Mizukawa N, et al. Levels of human defensin-1, an antimicrobial peptide, in saliva of patients with oral inflammation. *Oral Surg. Oral. Med. Oral Pathol. Oral Radiol. Endod.* 1999;87(5):539–543.

94. Goebel C, et al. Determination of defensin HNP-1, HNP-2, and HNP-3 in human saliva by using LC/ MS. *Peptides* 2000;21(6):757–765.

95. Lehrer RI, et al. Modulation of the *in vitro* candidacidal activity of human neutrophil defensins by target cell metabolism and divalent cations. *J. Clin. Invest.* 1988;81(6):1829–1835.

96. Chung WO, et al. Expression of defensins in gingiva and their role in periodontal health and disease. *Curr. Pharm. Design* 2007;13:3073–3083.

97. Kinane DF, et al. Human variability in innate immunity. *Periodontol 2000* 2007;45:14–34.

98. Ganz T, et al. Microbicidal/cytotoxic proteins of neutrophils are deficient in two disorders: Chediak–Higashi syndrome and "specific" granule deficiency. *J. Clin. Invest.* 1988;82(2):552–556.

99. Putsep K, et al. Deficiency of antibacterial peptides in patients with morbus Kostmann: an observation study. *Lancet* 2002;360(9340):1144–1149.

100. Carlsson G, et al. Periodontal disease in patients from the original Kostmann family with severe congenital neutropenia. *J. Periodontol.* 2006;77(4):744–751.

101. Tao R, et al. Salivary antimicrobial peptide expression and dental caries experience in children. *Antimicrob. Agents Chemother.* 2005;49(9):3883–3888.

102. Dale BA, et al. Oral antimicrobial peptides and biological control of caries. *BMC Oral Health* 2006; 6(Suppl. 1): S13.

103. Dork T, Stuhrmann M. Polymorphisms of the human beta-defensin-1 gene. *Mol. Cell. Probes*, 1998;12(3):171–173.

104. Jurevic RJ, et al. Single-nucleotide polymorphisms and haplotype analysis in betadefensin genes in different ethnic populations. *Genet. Test* 2002;6(4):261–269.

105. Vatta S, et al. Human beta-defensin 1 gene: six new variants. *Hum. Mutat.* 2000;15(6):582–583.

106. Jurevic RJ, et al. Single-nucleotide polymorphisms (SNPs) in human beta-defensin 1: high-throughput SNP assays and association with candida carriage in type i diabetics and nondiabetic controls. *J. Clin. Microbiol.* 2003;41(1):90–96.

107. Hollox EJ, Armour JA, Barber JC. Extensive normal copy number variation of a beta-defensin antimicrobial-gene cluster. *Am. J. Hum. Genet.* 2003;73(3):591–600.

108. Linzmeier RM, Ganz T. Human defensin gene copy number polymorphisms: comprehensive analysis of independent variation in alpha- and beta-defensin regions at 8p22-p23. *Genomics* 2005; 86(4):423–430.

109. Lu Q, et al. Expression of human beta-defensins-1 and -2 peptides in unresolved chronic periodontitis. *J. Periodontal Res.* 2004;39(4):221–227.

110. Lu Q, et al. Expression of human beta-defensin-3 in gingival epithelia. *J. Periodontal Res.* 2005; 40(6):474–481.

111. Bissell J, et al. Expression of beta-defensins in gingival health and in periodontal disease. *J. Oral Pathol. Med.* 2004;33(5):278–285.

112. Hosokawa I, et al. Innate immune peptide LL-37 displays distinct expression pattern from beta-defensins in inflamed gingival tissue. *Clin. Exp. Immunol.* 2006;146(2):218–225.

113. Vardar-Sengul S, et al. Human beta defensin-1 and -2 expression in the gingiva of patients with specific periodontal diseases. *J. Periodontal Res.* 2007;42(5):429–437.

114. Kesting MR, et al. Expression profile of human beta-defensin 3 in oral squamous cell carcinoma. *Cancer Invest.* 2009;27(5):575–581.

115. Wenghoefer M, et al. Decreased gene expression of human beta-defensin-1 in the development of squamous cell carcinoma of the oral cavity. *Int. J. Oral Maxillofac. Surg.* 2008;37(7):660–663.

116. Wenghoefer M, et al. Nuclear hBD-1 accumulation in malignant salivary gland tumours. *BMC Cancer* 2008;8:290.

117. Ouhara K, et al. Susceptibilities of periodontopathogenic and cariogenic bacteria to antibacterial peptides, beta-defensins and LL37, produced by human epithelial cells. *J. Antimicrob. Chemother.* 2005;55(6):888–896.

118. Joly S, et al. Human beta-defensins 2 and 3 demonstrate strain-selective activity against oral microorganisms. *J. Clin. Microbiol.* 2004;42(3):1024–1029.

119. Nishimura E, et al. Oral streptococci exhibit diverse susceptibility to human betadefensin-2: antimicrobial effects of hBD-2 on oral streptococci. *Curr. Microbiol.* 2004;48(2):85–87.

120. Guthmiller JM, et al. Susceptibilities of oral bacteria and yeast to mammalian cathelicidins. *Antimicrob. Agents Chemother.* 2001;45(11):3216–3219.

121. Feng Z, et al. Human beta-defensins: differential activity against candidal species and regulation by *Candida albicans. J. Dent. Res.* 2005;84(5):445–450.

122. Daher KA, Selsted ME, Lehrer RI. Direct inactivation of viruses by human granulocyte defensins. *J. Virol.* 1986;60(3):1068–1074.

123. Quinones-Mateu ME, et al. *Human epithelial beta-defensins 2 and 3 inhibit HIV-1 replication. AIDS* 2003;17(16):F39–F48.

124. Sun L, et al. Human beta-defensins suppress human immunodeficiency virus infection: potential role in mucosal protection. *J. Virol.* 2005;79(22):14318–14329.

125. Feng Z, et al. Cutting edge: human beta defensin 3: a novel antagonist of the HIV-1 coreceptor CXCR4. *J. Immunol.* 2006;177(2):782–786.

126. Maisetta G, et al. Activity of human beta-defensin 3 alone or combined with other antimicrobial agents against oral bacteria. *Antimicrob. Agents Chemother.* 2003;47(10):3349–3351.

127. Eckert RL, et al. S100 proteins in the epidermis. *J. Invest. Dermatol.* 2004;123(1):23–33.

128. Harder J, Schroder JM. Psoriatic scales: a promising source for the isolation of human skin-derived antimicrobial proteins. *J. Leukoc. Biol.* 2005;77(4):476–486.

129. Steinstraesser L, et al. Inhibition of early steps in the lentiviral replication cycle by cathelicidin host defense peptides. *Retrovirology* 2005;2:2.

130. Liu AY, et al. Human beta-defensin-2 production in keratinocytes is regulated by interleukin-1, bacteria, and the state of differentiation. *J. Invest. Dermatol.* 2002;118(2):275–281.

131. de Jongh GJ, et al. High expression levels of keratinocyte antimicrobial proteins in psoriasis compared with atopic dermatitis. *J. Invest. Dermatol.* 2005;125(6):1163–1173.

132. Hollox EJ, et al. Psoriasis is associated with increased beta-defensin genomic copy number. *Nat. Genet.* 2008;40(1):23–25.

133. Kim E, et al. Single nucleotide polymorphisms and the haplotype in the DEFB1 gene are associated with atopic dermatitis in a Korean population. *J. Dermatol. Sci.* 2009;54(1):25–30.

134. Henseler T, Christophers E. Disease concomitance in psoriasis. *J. Am. Acad. Dermatol.* 1995;32 (6):982–986.

135. Murakami M, et al. Cathelicidin anti-microbial peptide expression in sweat, an innate defense system for the skin. *J. Invest. Dermatol.* 2002;119(5):1090–1095.

136. Kaus A, et al. Host defence peptides in human burns. *Burns* 2008;34(1):32–40.

137. Milner SM, et al. Expression of human beta defensin 2 in thermal injury. *Burns* 2004;30(7):649–654.

138. Poindexter BJ, et al. Localization of antimicrobial peptides in normal and burned skin. *Burns* 2006; 32(4):402–407.

139. Gambichler T, et al. Significant upregulation of antimicrobial peptides and proteins in lichen sclerosus. *Br. J. Dermatol.* 2009;161(5):1136–1142.

140. Eisendle K, et al. Possible role of *Borrelia burgdorferi sensu lato* infection in lichen sclerosus. *Arch. Dermatol.* 2008;144(5):591–598.

141. Lusitani D, Malawista SE, Montgomery RR. *Borrelia burgdorferi* are susceptible to killing by a variety of human polymorphonuclear leukocyte components. *J. Infect. Dis.* 2002;185(6): 797–804.

142. Moss SE, Klein R, Klein BE. The prevalence and incidence of lower extremity amputation in a diabetic population. *Arch. Intern. Med.* 1992;152(3):610–616.

143. Pecoraro RE, Reiber GE, Burgess EM. Pathways to diabetic limb amputation: basis for prevention. *Diabetes Care* 1990;13(5):513–521.

144. Apelqvist J, Larsson J. What is the most effective way to reduce incidence of amputation in the diabetic foot? *Diabetes Metab. Res. Rev.* 2000;16(Suppl. 1):S75–S83.

145. Hirsch T, et al. Human beta-defensin-3 promotes wound healing in infected diabetic wounds. *J. Gene Med.* 2009;11(3):220–228.

146. Goldstein EJ, Citron DM, Nesbit CA. Diabetic foot infections: bacteriology and activity of 10 oral antimicrobial agents against bacteria isolated from consecutive cases. *Diabetes Care* 1996;19 (6):638–641.

147. Maisetta G, et al. *In vitro* bactericidal activity of human beta-defensin 3 against multidrug-resistant nosocomial strains. *Antimicrob. Agents Chemother.* 2006;50(2):806–809.

148. Supp DM, et al. Antibiotic resistance in clinical isolates of *Acinetobacter baumannii, Pseudomonas aeruginosa,* and *Staphylococcus aureus* does not impact sensitivity to human beta-defensin-4. *Burns* 2009;35(7):949–955.

149. Sorensen OE, et al. Injury-induced innate immune response in human skin mediated by transactivation of the epidermal growth factor receptor. *J. Clin. Invest.* 2006;116(7):1878–1885.

150. Gordon YJ, Romanowski EG, McDermott AM. A review of antimicrobial peptides and their therapeutic potential as anti-infective drugs. *Curr. Eye Res.* 2005;30(7):505–515.

151. McPhee JB, Hancock RE. Function and therapeutic potential of host defence peptides. *J. Pept. Sci.* 2005;11(11):677–687.

152. Boman HG. Antibacterial peptides: basic facts and emerging concepts. *J. Intern. Med.* 2003; 254(3):197–215.

153. Hancock RE, Sahl HG. Antimicrobial and host-defense peptides as new anti-infective therapeutic strategies. *Nat. Biotechnol.* 2006;24(12):1551–1557.

154. Sang Y, Blecha F. Antimicrobial peptides and bacteriocins: alternatives to traditional antibiotics. *Anim. Health Res. Rev.* 2008;9(2):227–235.

155. Yang D, et al. Multiple roles of antimicrobial defensins, cathelicidins, and eosinophil-derived neurotoxin in host defense. *Annu. Rev. Immunol.* 2004;22:181–215.

156. Puklo M, et al. Analysis of neutrophil-derived antimicrobial peptides in gingival crevicular fluid suggests importance of cathelicidin LL-37 in the innate immune response against periodontogenic bacteria. *Oral Microbiol. Immunol.* 2008;23(4):328–335.

157. Yang D, et al. Many chemokines including CCL20/MIP-3alpha display antimicrobial activity. *J. Leukoc. Biol.* 2003;74(3):448–455.

158. Chang TL, et al. Dual role of alpha-defensin-1 in anti-HIV-1 innate immunity. *J. Clin. Invest.* 2005;115(3):765–773.

159. Wang W, et al. Activity of alpha- and theta-defensins against primary isolates of HIV1. *J. Immunol.* 2004;173(1):515–520.

160. Zhang L, et al. Contribution of human alpha-defensin-1, -2, and -3 to the anti-HIV-1 activity of CD8 antiviral factor. *Science* 2002;98(5595):995–1000.

161. Fu LM. The potential of human neutrophil peptides in tuberculosis therapy. *Int. J. Tuberc. Lung Dis.*, 2003;7(11):1027–1032.

162. Sharma S, Verma I, Khuller GK. Therapeutic potential of human neutrophil peptide 1 against experimental tuberculosis. *Antimicrob. Agents Chemother.* 2001;45(2):639–640.

163. Shu Q, et al. Protection against *Pseudomonas aeruginosa* pneumonia and sepsis-induced lung injury by overexpression of beta-defensin-2 in rats. *Shock* 2006;26(4):365–371.

164. Oppenheim JJ, et al. Roles of antimicrobial peptides such as defensins in innate and adaptive immunity. *Ann. Rheum. Dis.* 2003;62(Suppl. 2):ii17–ii21.

165. Mickels N, et al. Clinical and microbial evaluation of a histatin-containing mouthrinse in humans with experimental gingivitis. *J. Clin. Periodontol.* 2001;28(5):404–410.

166. Reddy KV, Yedery RD, Aranha C. Antimicrobial peptides: premises and promises. *Int. J. Antimicrob. Agents* 2004;24(6):536–547.

167. Rothstein DM, et al. Histatin-derived peptides: potential agents to treat localised infections. *Expert Opin. Emerg. Drugs* 2002;7(1):47–59.

168. Tsai H, Bobek LA. Human salivary histatins: promising anti-fungal therapeutic agents. *Crit. Rev. Oral Biol. Med.* 1998;9(4):480–497.

169. Van Dyke T, et al. Clinical and microbial evaluation of a histatin-containing mouthrinse in humans with experimental gingivitis: a phase-2 multi-center study. *J. Clin. Periodontol.* 2002;9(2):168–176.

170. Dommisch H, et al. Immune regulatory functions of human beta-defensin-2 in odontoblast-like cells. *Int. Endod. J.* 2007;40(4):300–307.

171. Niyonsaba F, Ogawa H, Nagaoka I. Human beta-defensin-2 functions as a chemotactic agent for tumour necrosis factor-alpha-treated human neutrophils. *Immunology* 2004;111(3):273–281.

172. Cotter PD, Hill C, Ross RP. Bacteriocins: developing innate immunity for food. *Nat. Rev. Microbiol.* 2005;3(10):777–788.

173. Willey JM, van der Donk WA. Lantibiotics: peptides of diverse structure and function. *Annu. Rev. Microbiol.* 2007;61:477–501.

174. De Vuyst L, Leroy F. Bacteriocins from lactic acid bacteria: production, purification, and food applications. *J. Mol. Microbiol. Biotechnol.* 2007;13(4):194–199.

175. Sit CS, Vederas JC. Approaches to the discovery of new antibacterial agents based on bacteriocins. *Biochem. Cell. Biol.* 2008;86(2):116–123.

176. Dufour A, et al. The biology of lantibiotics from the lacticin 481 group is coming of age. *FEMS Microbiol. Rev.* 2007;31(2):134–167.

177. Kruszewska D, et al. Mersacidin eradicates methicillin-resistant *Staphylococcus aureus* (MRSA) in a mouse rhinitis model. *J. Antimicrob. Chemother.* 2004;54(3):648–653.

178. Nackaerts O, et al. Replacement therapy for periodontitis: pilot radiographic evaluation in a dog model. *J. Clin. Periodontol.* 2008;35(12):1048–1052.

179. Teughels W, et al. Guiding periodontal pocket recolonization: a proof of concept. *J. Dent. Res.* 2007;86(11):1078–1082.

180. Shimauchi H, et al. Improvement of periodontal condition by probiotics with *Lactobacillus salivarius* WB21: a randomized, double-blind, placebo-controlled study. *J. Clin. Periodontol.* 2008;35(10): 897–905.

181. Aerts AM, et al. The antifungal activity of RsAFP2, a plant defensin from *Raphanus sativus,* involves the induction of reactive oxygen species in *Candida albicans*. *J. Mol. Microbiol. Biotechnol.* 2007; 13(4):243–247.

182. De Samblanx GW, et al. Mutational analysis of a plant defensin from radish (*Raphanus sativus* L.) reveals two adjacent sites important for antifungal activity. *J. Biol. Chem.* 1997;272(2): 1171–1179.

183. Madeo F, Frohlich E, Frohlich KU. A yeast mutant showing diagnostic markers of early and late apoptosis. *J. Cell. Biol.* 1997;139(3):729–734.

184. Thevissen K, et al. Therapeutic potential of antifungal plant and insect defensins. *Drug Discov. Today* 2007;12(21–22):966–971.

185. Andres E, Dimarcq JL. Cationic anti-microbial peptides: from innate immunity study to drug development. *Rev. Med. Interne* 2004;25(9):629–635.

186. Aguiar GP, et al. A Review of the biological and clinical aspects of radiation caries. *J. Contemp. Dent. Pract.* 2009;10(4):83–89.

187. Muta T, et al. Tachyplesins isolated from hemocytes of Southeast Asian horseshoe crabs (*Carcinoscorpius rotundicauda* and *Tachypleus gigas*): identification of a new tachyplesin, tachyplesin III, and a processing intermediate of its precursor. *J. Biochem.* 1990;108(2): 261–266.

188. Masuda M, et al. A novel anti-HIV synthetic peptide, T-22 ([Tyr5,12, Lys7]polyphemusin II). *Biochem. Biophys. Res. Commun.* 1992;189(2):845–850.

189. Tamamura H, et al. Antimicrobial activity and conformation of tachyplesin I and its analogs. *Chem. Pharm. Bull. (Tokyo)* 1993;41(5):978–980.

190. Miyasaki KT, Lehrer RI. Beta-sheet antibiotic peptides as potential dental therapeutics. *Int. J. Antimicrob. Agents.* 1998;9(4):269–280.

191. Giovannini MG, et al. Biosynthesis and degradation of peptides derived from *Xenopus laevis* prohormones. *Biochem. J.* 1987;243(1):113–120.

192. Zasloff M. Magainins: a class of antimicrobial peptides from Xenopus skin: isolation, characterization of two active forms, and partial cDNA sequence of a precursor. *Proc. Natl. Acad. Sci. USA* 1987;84 (15):5449–5453.

193. Gottler LM, Ramamoorthy A. Structure, membrane orientation, mechanism, and function of pexiganan: a highly potent antimicrobial peptide designed from magainin. *Biochim. Biophys. Acta.* 2009;1788(8):1680–1686.

194. Lipsky BA, Holroyd KJ, Zasloff M. Topical versus systemic antimicrobial therapy for treating mildly infected diabetic foot ulcers: a randomized, controlled, double-blinded, multicenter trial of pexiganan cream. *Clin. Infect. Dis.* 2008;47(12):1537–1545.

195. Ge Y, et al. *In vitro* antibacterial properties of pexiganan: an analog of magainin. *Antimicrob. Agents Chemother.*, 1999;43(4):782–788.

196. Chou TG, et al. Evaluating antimicrobials and implant materials for infection prevention around transcutaneous osseointegrated implants in a rabbit model. *J. Biomed. Mater. Res. A* 2010;92(3): 942–952.

197. Cole AM, Waring AJ. The role of defensins in lung biology and therapy. *Am. J. Respir. Med.* 2002;1 (4):249–259.

198. Stokman MA, et al. Preventive intervention possibilities in radiotherapy—and chemotherapy-induced oral mucositis: results of meta-analyses. *J. Dent. Res.* 2006;85(8):690–700.

199. Giles FJ, et al. A phase III, randomized, double-blind, placebo-controlled, study of iseganan for the reduction of stomatitis in patients receiving stomatotoxic chemotherapy. *Leuk. Res.* 2004;28 (6):559–565.

200. Kollef M, et al. A randomized double-blind trial of iseganan in prevention of ventilator-associated pneumonia. *Am. J. Respir. Crit. Care Med.* 2006;173(1):91–97.

201. Kim SM, et al. Indolicidin-derived antimicrobial peptide analogs with greater bacterial selectivity and requirements for antibacterial and hemolytic activities. *Biochim. Biophys. Acta* 2009;1794(2):185–192.

202. Lee DG, et al. Fungicidal effect of indolicidin and its interaction with phospholipid membranes. *Biochem. Biophys. Res. Commun.* 2003;305(2):305–310.

203. Robinson WE, Jr., et al. Anti-HIV-1 activity of indolicidin: an antimicrobial peptide from neutrophils. *J. Leukoc. Biol.* 1998;63(1):94–100.

204. Selsted ME, et al. Indolicidin, a novel bactericidal tridecapeptide amide from neutrophils. *J. Biol. Chem.* 1992;267(7):4292–4295.

205. Schluesener HJ, et al. Leukocytic antimicrobial peptides kill autoimmune T cells. *J. Neuroimmunol.* 1993;47(2):199–202.

206. Rubinchik E, et al. Antimicrobial and antifungal activities of a novel cationic antimicrobial peptide, omiganan, in experimental skin colonisation models. *Int. J. Antimicrob. Agents* 2009;34(5):457–461.

207. Fritsche TR, et al. Antimicrobial activity of omiganan pentahydrochloride against contemporary fungal pathogens responsible for catheter-associated infections. *Antimicrob. Agents Chemother.* 2008;52(3):1187–1189.

208. Kamysz W, et al. *In vitro* activity of synthetic antimicrobial peptides against *Candida. Pol. J. Microbiol.* 2006;55(4):303–307.

209. Zhang C, et al. A gene delivery approach for antimicrobials: expression of defensins. *J. Drug Target* 2006;14(9):646–651.

210. Pavicic MJ, van Winkelhoff AJ, de Graaff J. Synergistic effects between amoxicillin, metronidazole, and the hydroxymetabolite of metronidazole against *Actinobacillus actinomycetemcomitans. Antimicrob. Agents Chemother.* 1991;35(5):961–966.

211. van Winkelhoff AJ, Tijhof CJ, de Graaff J. Microbiological and clinical results of metronidazole plus amoxicillin therapy in *Actinobacillus actinomycetemcomitans* associated periodontitis. *J. Periodontol.* 1992;63(1):52–57.

212. van Winkelhoff AJ, Winkel EG. Systemic antibiotic therapy in severe periodontitis. *Curr. Opin. Periodontol.* 1997;4:35–40.

213. Christophers E, Henseler T. Contrasting disease patterns in psoriasis and atopic dermatitis. *Arch. Dermatol. Res.* 1987;279 (Suppl): S48–S51.

214. Fulton C, et al. Expression of natural peptide antibiotics in human skin. *Lancet* 1997;350 (9093):1750–1751.

215. Nomura I, et al. Cytokine milieu of atopic dermatitis: as compared to psoriasis, skin prevents induction of innate immune response genes. *J. Immunol.* 2003;171(6):326–329.

CHAPTER 8

VERNIX CASEOSA AND INNATE IMMUNITY

Steven B. Hoath, Vivek Narendran, and Marty O. Visscher

Cincinnati Children's Hospital Medical Center, Department of Pediatrics, Division of Neonatology and Pulmonary Biology, Skin Sciences Institute, University of Cincinnati, Cincinnati, OH

8.1 INTRODUCTION

In classical immunology, the primary function of the immune system is discrimination of self from nonself with the goal of protecting the organism from the threats of a hostile environment [1]. The evolutionarily older innate immune system consists of structurally coherent physical barriers such as the stratum corneum, chemical defenses such as lipids, lectins, and mucins, and antimicrobial peptides often synthesized *in situ* at specific epithelial surfaces. The adaptive immune system, a more recently acquired evolutionary modification found in vertebrates, consists of lymphocyte-based memory responses to foreign antigens with B-cell antibody production and T-cell stimulation. Nonspecific cellular elements with tissue mobility such as neutrophils, macrophages, and antigen-presenting cells constitute a connecting link between the simpler structural components of the innate immune system and the more sophisticated system of adaptive immune response.

Over the past 15 years, Matzinger and others have offered an alternative to the classical self–nonself model [2–4]. The Matzinger model proposes that immune responses are triggered by endogenous mechanisms derived from local tissue damage. Thus, tissue-derived danger signals evoke an alarm response to which the body responds with the ultimate goal of tissue repair and restoration of homeostasis. A rigid distinction between the self and nonself in this model is not only blurred but also unnecessary. There is no required distinction between the body of the organism proper, for example, and the superficial population of commensal microorganisms that comprise the outermost environmental interface of the skin and gut. The primary function of the immune system in the danger model is communication and maintenance of integrity of the organism.

Innate Immune System of Skin and Oral Mucosa: Properties and Impact in Pharmaceutics, Cosmetics, and Personal Care Products, First Edition. Nava Dayan and Philip W. Wertz.

8.2   FETAL AND NEONATAL IMMUNITY

The fetus and newborn provide an instructive focus for investigating the complex interplay between innate and adaptive immunity [5,6]. Traditionally, the fetus and newborn are considered disadvantaged with diminished innate and adaptive immune responses. Moreover, immunological naiveté is considered necessary for fetal survival insofar as the mother is "foreign" and maternal immune responses can be deleterious to the fetus, as illustrated by Rh incompatibility disease [7]. Adding to the complexity of the fetal environment is the recently recognized fact that evocation of a systemic inflammatory response in the fetus may have long-term detrimental effects leading to induction of preterm labor, an increased rate of premature birth, neurodevelopmental delay, and death [8–11]. The fetus must traverse a fine line during gestation: avoiding immunological "rejection" by the mother while participating in its own defense by marshaling and controlling its comparatively meager immunological resources.

Figure 8.1 gives a developmental overview of some of the immunological changes occurring during the fetal and neonatal period. The central ontogenetic notion is that the fetus occupies an increasingly complex "privileged" space *in utero*; that is, the amniotic fluid compartment. Innate immune responses are deemed particularly important in this space insofar as a robust inflammatory response by the mother or the fetus may be life-threatening with induction of labor, expulsion of the fetus, and potential injury with long-term consequences such as white matter damage [8–10,12,13]. A similar "privileged" space with diminished immune response has been described for the eye [14].

Significant differences exist between the early and late fetal life. Early in gestation, that is, before the so-called border of viability at 23–25 weeks, the fetoplacental unit develops in an environment separated from the mother's genito-

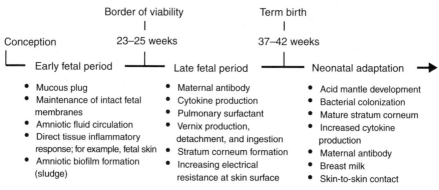

Figure 8.1   Ontogeny of fetal and neonatal innate immunity. Events are selected with relevance to the biology of vernix caseosa and are divided into three main time periods: the early fetal period before the border of viability at 23–25 weeks, the late fetal period extending until the time of birth, and the period after birth of neonatal adaptation that involves bacterial colonization and maternal–infant bonding.

urinary tract and potentially harmful microbial invasion by a physical and antimicrobial barrier called the "mucous plug" [15]. Production of amniotic fluid by the fetus in part via urine formation and swallowing with reabsorption results in a sequestered space in which the outermost fetal epidermal layer (periderm) is in direct contact with the amniotic fluid. Not surprisingly, microbial invasion of the amniotic cavity results in fetal dermatitis with activation of Toll-like receptors in epidermal keratinocytes [16]. As gestation progresses, the periderm is shed and direct exposure of living, nucleated epidermal keratinocytes to the amniotic cavity is blocked by production of a superficial film of vernix caseosa that overlies the nascent stratum corneum [17].

The origin of the vernix lipids and contained corneocytes is unclear and may derive from several sources. Analyses of the lipid constituents of vernix have been previously reviewed [18–24]. Vernix contains triglycerides, wax and sterol esters, squalene, and phospholipids as well as ceramides and cholesterol. The former are components of sebum, whereas ceramides and cholesterol are generally considered prominent epidermal barrier lipids present in the stratum corneum. These findings support the concept that vernix lipids are derived from both the sebaceous gland and the stratum corneum. Recently, Ran-Ressler et al. studied the branched chain fatty acid (BCFA) component of vernix in comparison to meconium (fetal stool) and noted presumptive catabolism and disappearance of BCFAs in the gut [25]. The authors suggested that vernix-derived BCFA may play a role in gut colonization postnatally and should be considered a nutritional component for the fetus/newborn. Absence of vernix and BCFA in the gut of formula-fed preterm infants might predispose this vulnerable population to necrotizing enterocolitis [25]. Rissmann et al. also demonstrated lipids bound to vernix corneocytes with lower levels of barrier lipids compared to previous reports [22]. The method by which lipid is obtained following delivery may be an important variable governing lipid composition insofar as scraping the stratum corneum surface may increase the concentration of barrier lipids.

The origin of the fetal corneocytes in vernix is intriguing. Hyperplasia of sebaceous glands is a common finding in the third trimester of pregnancy, although this phenomenon has been little investigated [17]. A hypothetical endocrine-based mechanism for vernix production and epidermal barrier maturation has been proposed [26–29]. It is well known that the adrenal glands are hyperplastic in the human fetus with increased production of dehydroepiandrosterone (DHEA) that can subsequently be converted in the sebaceous gland to active androgens [28]. The sebaceous gland produces not only a superficial lipid film (sebum) but also the lining of the upper portion of the pilosebaceous unit that undergoes progressive keratinization, particularly during periods of hyperplastic growth such as adolescence [30]. It is proposed that bacterial biofilms in acne may lead to adhesion of shed corneocytes leading to microcomedone production [31]. Thus, the intriguing possibility exists that the fetal sebaceous gland is actively involved in production of *both* vernix lipids and corneocytes. The role of this superficial barrier film in innate immune protection of the fetus deserves investigation and may shed unexpected light on the mechanisms underlying the pathogenesis of adolescent acne.

Recently, investigators have used intrapartum ultrasound to identify free-floating hyperechogenic material within the amniotic fluid [32–34]. This material is often localized to the area of the uterine cervix above the mucous plug. Upon needle aspiration, this material, called "amniotic fluid sludge," consists of a viscous mix of fetal epithelial cells, neutrophils, and bacteria [35]. The authors propose that the presence of amniotic fluid sludge indicates microbial contamination of the amniotic cavity and the onset of an inflammatory response. One unanswered question is whether the bacteria in amniotic fluid are in planktonic form (single cells) or are organized in biofilms or both. The authors suggest that the ability to form biofilms makes antimicrobial eradication difficult despite antibiotic treatment of the mother. The formation of biofilms upon epithelial cells of fetal origin may also represent one method of sequestering and controlling intrauterine infections. This hypothesis, if verified, would indicate a potentially important and novel innate immune mechanism protecting the fetus *in utero*. Whether the fetal epithelial cells, for example, periderm, or vernix corneocytes participate as substrates for bacterial biofilm production is unknown. This process, however, would represent an intriguing intrauterine innate immune response with potential relevance for understanding bacterial adherence and colonization following birth [36,37].

Adding to the complexity of fetal immune function is the fact that the placenta, the fetal membranes (amnion and chorion), the umbilical cord, and the amniotic fluid are all of fetal origin in much the same way as a cocoon forms the immediate environment for the developing butterfly or earthworm. In this view, mammalian gestation and birth are akin to a morphogenetic process. The distinction of self and nonself in such a "manufactured" environment is difficult and a facile anthropomorphic description may obscure or make fetal organ functions difficult to discern. The developing fetal environment is multilayered consisting not only of the direct placental–maternal interface but also the more immediate interface between the amniotic fluid and the developing fetus *per se* [38]. It is this latter interface where vernix and the nascent stratum corneum are intimately positioned. This surface undergoes dramatic structural changes precisely at the border of viability between 23 and 25 weeks gestation [39].

Thus, the synthesis and spread of vernix at the fetal skin–amniotic fluid interface *in utero* sets the stage for subsequent bacterial colonization and postnatal acclimation to a dry, cool, oxygen-rich environment. The fact that vernix detaches *in utero* during the third trimester of gestation [40] and is swallowed by the fetus suggests additional functions of vernix caseosa on the oral mucosa, esophagus, and foregut (Figure 8.2). Before the infant swallows breast milk, the fetus actively swallows amniotic fluid and its contents [41]. Finally, the rheological mixing of vernix with pulmonary surfactant *in utero* [40] and the importance of antimicrobial peptides in both vernix and pulmonary surfactant support the presence of an intraamniotic innate immune system protecting the fetus from microbial assault and a potentially harmful fetal systemic inflammatory response [42–46]. Thus, vernix participates as one of the components of a complex innate immune system established *in utero* with critical gatekeeper functions that are at present poorly understood.

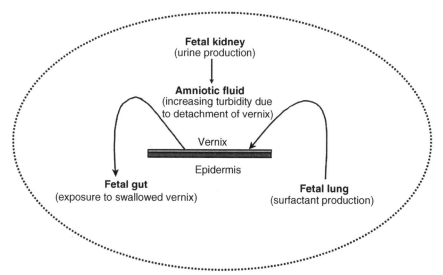

Figure 8.2   Interaction of fetal organs producing the "privileged space" of the amniotic fluid compartment indicated by the sum total of processes within the dotted oval. During the third trimester of human pregnancy, the fetal kidney produces copious amounts of urine that contributes to the amniotic fluid volume surrounding the developing fetus. Concomitantly, the fetal lung synthesizes increasing amounts of pulmonary surfactant in the form of lamellar bodies that are translocated into the amniotic fluid via the trachea and fetal breathing movements. On the fetal skin surface, sebaceous gland hyperplasia occurs simultaneously with loss of periderm, spreading of vernix over the skin surface, and steady formation of the underlying stratum corneum over the viable nucleated epidermis. The vernix on the skin surface builds up and detaches into the surrounding milieu resulting in increasing amniotic fluid turbidity. Recent data indicate a role for pulmonary surfactant to emulsify vernix and aide in the detachment mechanism [40]. Vernix within the amniotic fluid is subsequently swallowed by the fetus with potential effects on the fetal foregut and systemic absorption of vernix components (modified from Ref. 26).

8.3   INFLAMMATION AND PRETERM BIRTH: CLINICAL SIGNIFICANCE OF THE FETAL INFLAMMATORY RESPONSE SYNDROME

Worldwide, preterm birth is the leading cause of perinatal morbidity and mortality, particularly in the developed world. Infants are considered preterm if birth occurs at less than 37 weeks of gestation. Preterm birth occurs at a frequency of approximately 12–13% in the United States and 5–9% in many other developed countries [47]. Although only 1% of preterm births occur before 28 weeks gestation, this group constitutes 50–70% of neonatal deaths [48,49]. Of concern, the rate of preterm birth is increasing in many locations in part secondary to *indicated* preterm delivery following maternal preeclampsia, intrauterine growth restriction, or following artificially conceived multiple pregnancies. Preterm birth may also result from preterm labor associated with infection or intrauterine inflammation resulting in premature rupture of membranes and/or onset of uterine contractions with subsequent preterm delivery. Considerable effort has been expended over the past decade to understand and prevent preterm births particularly resulting from infection and inflammation.

In general, inflammation is clinically assessed postnatally by the presence of five classical signs; that is, swelling, pain, redness, heat, and loss of function. The induction of inflammation is a regulated process by which the body responds to potentially harmful physiological, chemotactic, or gene modulatory effects in an attempt to decrease tissue damage and induce regeneration of affected tissues [50]. *In utero* inflammation has a clear causal association with the onset of preterm labor [51]. Elevated levels of IL-6 and other proinflammatory cytokines in the amniotic fluid are predictive of preterm birth [52–54]. Invasion of the fetal membranes (chorioamnionitis) and umbilical cord (funisitis) is strongly associated with the onset of preterm labor and subsequent delivery [55]. Even normal spontaneous term delivery in the absence of detectable infection has been reported to exhibit a number of features commonly ascribed to the inflammatory process [56]. A better understanding of intrauterine inflammation and the differential effects of the adaptive and innate arms of the immune system in mediating the inflammatory response may be important in preventing preterm delivery and associated morbidities and in better understanding the normal process of term labor induction and spontaneous vaginal birth.

Although inflammation is typically an essential and desired response to tissue injury and microbiological assault, the excessive or inappropriate induction of a heightened inflammatory response may be the cause of morbidity and mortality. Over a decade ago, Gomez et al. described a fetal inflammatory response syndrome (FIRS) that had similarities to the adult systemic inflammatory response syndrome (SIRS) and was characterized by elevated levels of cord blood IL-6 [12]. The authors proposed that the onset of preterm labor had survival value for the fetus insofar as it was initiated when the intrauterine environment was so hostile that it threatened survival of both the mother and the fetus.

Recent data, however, strongly implicate the induction of an inflammatory cascade in the fetus as causally associated with the postnatal development of cerebral palsy [9,10,13,57–59]. This is particularly important insofar as major advances have been made in other areas of neonatology with resultant reduction in preterm deaths, but the overall incidence of cerebral palsy has not been significantly decreased [60]. It is a reasonable hypothesis supported by both human and animal data that the development of the fetal inflammatory response is an evolving process progressing from chorioamnionitis to frank intraamniotic fluid infection and subsequently to systemic invasion with elevated cord blood IL-6 and funisitis [13]. The prevention of FIRS would be aided by a robust innate immune mechanism *in utero* serving to "sequester" intraamniotic infection to the fetal membranes, amniotic fluid, and fetal surfaces of the skin and gut lumen.

This proposed innate immune mechanism is well situated to involve vernix caseosa along with other developing organs important for the innate immune response such as the lung and gut. This hypothesis supports the notion that the fetal period

(a)   (b)

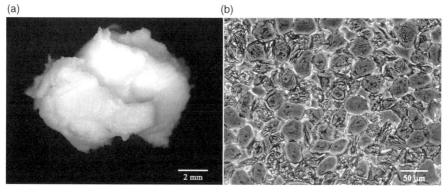

Figure 8.3   Appearance of vernix caseosa. In (a), the macroscopic appearance of vernix is a thick, viscous, white paste. The phase contrast image of native vernix (b) reveals a dense packing of fetal corneocytes surrounded by a thin lipid matrix. The cells are heterogeneous in size and structure and are smaller than corneocytes from infant skin or adults. Many nuclear ghosts are evident. Scale bars are shown in the figures (after Ref. 27).

preceding vernix synthesis, stratum corneum formation, and pulmonary surfactant production *in utero*, that is, the period prior to the edge of viability at 23–25 weeks, represents a time of extreme vulnerability to intrauterine infection in large part due to deficient innate immune mechanisms. The elaboration of the innate immune properties associated with vernix caseosa, therefore, is intimately connected with a broader system of immune response aimed at preventing fetal infection and the fetal inflammatory response syndrome.

8.4   INNATE IMMUNE PROPERTIES OF VERNIX CASEOSA

Table 8.1 lists a number of biophysical functions of vernix related to innate immunity with the latter defined as mechanisms protecting the organism from danger, damage, dissolution, and death. The macroscopic and microscopic appearance of native vernix caseosa is shown in Figure 8.3.

8.4.1   Water Handling Properties

The epidermal barrier is strongly involved in innate immunity and appears to have evolved as a mechanism to limit evaporative water transport to enable terrestrial life while simultaneously using water as its chief plasticizing agent [61]. Hypothetically, vernix *in utero* participates in controlling both the water transport and gradients of nutrients and calcium across the developing epidermal barrier and the water content of the stratum corneum after birth. This dual requirement at birth to function in both aqueous and dry environments imposes special constraints upon the epidermal barrier. Animals such as rodents possess a terminally differentiated hydrophobic cell layer on the skin surface, the periderm, which presumably

TABLE 8.1 Biophysical Functions of Vernix Related to Innate Immunity

Function	Evidence	Reference
Water handling properties Hydrophobicity/waterproofing Hydrophilicity/moisturization	Newborn animals exhibit hydrophobic surface, surface-free energy of vernix indicates hydrophobic material, postnatal temperature control	[62,72,75,154]
	High water content of corneocytes, *in vivo* and *in vitro* evidence of hydrating ability, slow release of endogenous water, osmoregulation	[63,73,75,76,98]
Protectant/physical barrier	Barrier film to passage of chymotrypsin and methylene blue, mechanical barrier to bacterial passage, structural composition similar to stratum corneum (spreadable corneocytes embedded in complex barrier lipid matrix)	[27,90,155]
Temperature regulation/acid mantle	Forms hydrophobic barrier on newborn skin surface, effects on slowing evaporative heat loss, conflicting effects on temperature control, facilitates acid mantle production in newborn infants	[73,97–100]
Wound healing/maturation	Increases skin metabolism *in vitro*, high glutamine content, effect on trophic ulcers, wound healing efficacy in barrier deficient mouse models	[108–109, 157,158]
Anti-infective	Contains multiple diverse antimicrobial peptides in particulate form; reports of barrier properties to bacterial passage	[42–46,88,155]
Antioxidant	Contains alpha-tocopherol and melanin, human sebum high in vitamin E	[73,130–135]
Cleansing	Possesses both hydrophilic and hydrophobic domains, comparable efficacy to commercial cleansers	[72,138]
Electrical isolation	Increased skin surface electrical resistance due to developing vernix caseosa and stratum corneum	[139,140]
Psychosensory	Provides direct tactile, visual, and potential olfactory cues to mother at birth, derived in part from sebaceous secretions, forms major component of amniotic fluid in last trimester with ingestion by fetus, many constituents similar to breast milk, sensory evidence for feeding behavior in newborns due to cues in amniotic fluid and breast milk	[144–150]

facilitates perinatal transition and minimizes evaporative heat loss [62]. A spreadable stratum corneum-like material such as vernix has thus far only been described in humans.

Compositionally, vernix has the appearance of a complex water-in-oil emollient in which the major bulk constituent is water. Approximately 80–81% (w/w) of vernix is volatile and analysis by Karl–Fischer titration demonstrates that this volatility is exclusively due to its water content [63]. The water in vernix consists in at least two discrete particulate forms, that is, within the fetal corneocytes where it is responsive to the external osmotic environment [27,64] and within the hydrated relatively amorphous granules containing hydrophilic antimicrobial peptides embedded in the hydrophobic lipid matrix [42].

Seong and Matzinger have proposed that hydrophobic portions of biological molecules are exposed by tissue-derived danger/alarm signals and act to initiate an innate immune response [65]. Vernix presents the unusual physicochemical challenge of a naturally produced hydrophobic film containing structured internal domains with high water content. The strategic location of vernix on the fetal skin surface *in utero* or upon the skin following birth ideally mediates multiple innate immune responses associated with potential danger and environmental transitions. The location is important insofar as vernix itself can be immunogenic when present in a noncompatible biological site; hence, there are multiple reports of vernix peritonitis following Caesarian section in which fetal vernix has contaminated the maternal peritoneal cavity and elicited an inflammatory reaction [66–70].

An unusual aspect of equilibrium water binding in vernix is the relatively slow release of water at room temperature and the ability of vernix to demonstrate full recovery of water content in both native vernix and isolated vernix corneocytes supporting a structured internal domain [71]. In contrast, water-in-oil emollients release water but show no significant water resorption indicating the lack of an internal structured domain. Thus, vernix hydrophobicity supports a role in expelling exogenous water [72], whereas its high internal water content may maintain stratum corneum moisturization and slow controlled drying after birth [73]. Scott and Harding demonstrated that natural moisturizing factor (NMF) production following birth is optimal at relative humidities of 80–95% [74]. Hypothetically, the high water content of vernix facilities slow water loss from the skin surface leading to retention of a high humidity microenvironment and stratum corneum plasticization.

In contrast, Saijo and Tagami have reported that term infants exhibit marked drying of the skin surface with impaired stratum corneum water holding capacity occurring shortly after birth [75]. It is possible that vernix left in place after birth will diminish desquamation associated with postnatal drying, radiant warmer use, and exposure to soaps and surfactants with bathing. Retention of vernix has been demonstrated to result in a significantly more hydrated skin surface as evidenced by a higher moisture accumulation rate and higher baseline hydration compared to infants where vernix is removed at birth [73]. The application of vernix to freshly bathed human skin results in significant emolliency and moisturization [76]. The ability to control surface hydration may facilitate acid mantle formation and hydrolysis of triglycerides to free fatty acids, production of solutes such as lactic acid, and establishment of surface colonization with commensal bacteria. All these processes improve innate immune function in the newborn infant and would be lacking in the very low birth weight preterm infant.

Of interest, the percent of the skin surface visibly covered by vernix at birth is maximal between 33 and 37 weeks gestation and falls off at term reaching a low point in postterm infants [73]. This finding is consistent with the notion that pulmonary surfactant mediates vernix dislodgement from the skin surface *in utero* with subsequent swallowing by the fetus. The extremely low birth weight preterm infants, for example, 23–25 weeks gestation, are considered disadvantaged with no significant vernix coverage and minimal stratum corneum formation.

8.4.2 Physical Barrier

The multifunctionality of the skin barrier as an innate immune organ has been addressed by Elias [61]. Many of the defensive (barrier) functions of the epidermis localize to the stratum corneum. Formation of the stratum corneum *in utero* occurs in intimate physical juxtaposition to the overlying vernix caseosa. As early as week 5 of gestation, the embryo is covered by a single-cell epithelium derived from ectoderm [17]. By the end of the second trimester, a stratified epidermal structure can be detected but terminal differentiation and stratum corneum formation are scant. Vernix caseosa is a viscous, whitish material that coats the fetal skin surface during the last trimester (Figure 8.3b).

Agorastos et al. first reported a cellular component of vernix that was characterized in part by acid phosphatase activity within intracellular granules and within amorphous material deposited between the cellular components [77–80]. Lanugo hairs were also frequently seen within vernix and exhibited strong acid phosphatase activity especially within the papillae. More extensive characterization of the cells within vernix caseosa reveals that the fetal cells have many of the characteristics of corneocytes found in mature stratum corneum but lack intercellular desmosomal attachments [22,63]. Ultrastructural analysis of vernix corneocytes by transmission electron microscopy shows a sparse network of keratin filaments and little evidence of tonofilament organization [63]. The vernix corneocytes are smaller than corneocytes derived from infant or adult stratum corneum [27]. Vernix corneocytes will swell or contract in response to changes in their osmotic environment [27,64]. These corneocytes are surrounded by a hydrophobic mantle of amorphous lipids that lack the typical lamellar architecture present in the stratum corneum [22,63]. The lack of corneodesmosomes and lipid lamellae imparts a different dynamic architecture to vernix compared to stratum corneum. Vernix appears to be a sort of mobile or fluidic (spreadable) stratum corneum possessing a more permeable barrier to the passage of water and other small molecules [73,81,82]. Parenthetically, regulation of the transepidermal water gradient is an apparent effector of DNA synthesis and epidermal barrier lipid biosynthesis [83–85].

Of potential heuristic interest is the finding that the outermost layer of the stratum corneum is similarly devoid of lipid lamellae and corneodesmosomes [27,86]. The concept advanced here is that in its oldest (outermost) layer, the adult stratum corneum reverts to a form characteristic of the fetus, that is, the morphology of vernix, just prior to desquamation to the environment. Unlike the stratum corneum whose structure is ideally suited to act as a physical barrier conferring innate immune properties on the body surface, the structure of vernix is much more malleable and permeable to substances such as water [71,81,82,87]. *In utero,* the production of vernix coincides with the presence of epidermal terminal differentiation and formation of the stratum corneum [17,26]. These findings support a possible facilitating role of vernix in the process of fetal skin barrier formation, although the mechanism is not clearly understood. Early reports suggest that vernix acts as a physical barrier to the passage of pathogenic bacteria such as *Escherichia coli* [88]. Penetration of exogenous methylene blue dye is also blocked by vernix [27]. This latter finding is consistent with Hardman et al. who demonstrated the presence of a physical barrier to human dye penetration in developing human fetal skin, particularly in the vicinity of the pilosebaceous apparatus [89]. An intriguing report by Tansirikongkol et al. demonstrates the ability of vernix caseosa to act as a physical barrier to passage of chymotryptic enzyme (SCCE) [90]. SCCE is a major enzyme contributing to the process of desquamation by catalyzing degradation of intercellular cohesive structures, that is, desmosomes at the stratum corneum surface [91]. Chymotryptic enzymes have been identified in amniotic fluid during midgestation, although their source is unknown [92]. Pancreatic chymotrypsin is a normal constituent of fetal feces (meconium) and in combination with other lipolytic and proteolytic enzymes present in meconium it has been reported to possess barrier irritation potential *in vivo* [93–96].

Thus, the thin films of vernix caseosa offer a protective barrier to penetration of potentially injurious substances such as SCCE either prenatally in the form of meconium or postnatally in the form of stool in the diaper region [90]. This property appears to be due to mechanical obstruction rather than enzyme inhibition insofar as native vernix contains no detectable enzyme activity or inhibitory function. A film of vernix *in utero*, therefore, may function to prevent loss of endogenous chymotrypsin from the underlying epidermis while preserving the microstructure of the developing stratum corneum and protecting the epidermal barrier from noxious chemicals in the amniotic fluid. This role of vernix as a physical barrier is consistent with the function of an innate immune structure protecting the organism from potential harm.

8.4.3 Temperature Regulation/Acid Mantle

The definition of innate immunity as the sum of those processes that allow the organism to respond to potential danger or loss of tissue integrity allows the inclusion of surface mechanisms as diverse as the regulation of evaporative heat loss and bacterial colonization. Saunders reported that vernix removal in preterm infants resulted in subnormal body temperature [97], whereas other authors have linked vernix removal to decreased evaporative heat loss [98]. Shulak noted that vernix could provide some thermal stability, but it was not a primary factor in temperature regulation at birth [99]. In a more recent clinical study, the retention of vernix in term infants was compared with a cohort of infants with vernix removed following birth [73]. No effect of vernix on thermal regulation was seen in this population, although the infants were maintained in a modern delivery room setting and, thus, not subjected to cold stress. This study, however, did demonstrate a more rapid development of the skin surface acid mantle in infants with vernix retained after birth [73]. Factors facilitating a decrease in skin surface pH after birth are multiple and may include a contribution of vernix caseosa. Fox et al. have shown that skin surface acid mantle formation is delayed in very low birth weight preterm infants [100]. In summary, skin surface acidification appears to occur earlier in the presence of vernix and the presence of an acidic stratum corneum is putatively involved in the antimicrobial function and the inhibition of growth of pathogenic bacteria [61].

8.4.4 Wound Healing Properties

The interrelationship of tissue repair, wound healing, and specific immune responses mediating inflammation is complex [101–103]. Not surprisingly, the innate immune system, with its overriding role to protect normal tissues from infection and to maintain homeostasis, is called upon during times of wounding or when there is a need for tissue regeneration. The literature contains reports of vernix as a potential wound healing ointment when used with lower extremity trophic ulcers [104]. Vernix is presumably easily transferred to the mother's perineum during the process of vaginal birth. This anatomical area is subject to tearing or surgical episiotomy. It is, therefore, not unreasonable to anticipate a beneficial effect of vernix on epidermal wound healing. Other barrier creams, such as Aquaphor and natural oils like sunflower or safflower oil, have been reported to reduce nosocomial infections in preterm infants [105–107]. Recently, a murine model has been utilized to demonstrate an effect of vernix caseosa on skin barrier recovery following disruption by tape stripping [108,109]. The application of vernix caseosa in this model promoted formation of the stratum corneum and prevented epidermal thickening. These findings support the efficacy of vernix caseosa as a wound healing ointment with the ability to enhance epidermal barrier recovery following superficial disruption of the stratum corneum. Endogenous innate immune molecules such as antimicrobial peptides would presumably act synergistically with wound healing mechanisms.

8.4.5 Antimicrobial Peptides

One of the more intriguing aspects of fetal and neonatal innate immunity is the panoply of antimicrobial peptides in vernix caseosa that has been identified by direct extraction or proteome analysis [38,42–46,110,111]. These peptides, listed in Table 8.2, are putatively part of an ancient evolutionary system found in multicellular organisms that are particularly important in innate immune protection of epithelial surfaces [112–114]. Peptide/protein extracts of vernix have been demonstrated to have direct antimicrobial activity against a variety of perinatal pathogens, including Group B *streptococcus*, *E. coli*, *Bacillus megaterium*, and *Candida albicans* [43]. Both amniotic fluid and soluble extracts of vernix exhibit muramidase (lysozyme) activity [42]. Earlier studies have suggested a direct anti-infective role of amniotic

TABLE 8.2   Antimicrobial Peptides in Vernix Caseosa [42–46]

Lysozyme

Lactoferrin

SLPI

Mucin 7

Histone H2A and B

[Alpha]-defensins (human neutrophil peptide) [1–3]

Cathelicidins (LL-37)

Psoriasin

Ubiquitin

Neutrophil gelatinase-associated lipocalin (NGAL)

Ribonuclease-7

Annexin 1

Secretory leukocyte protease inhibitors

Calgranulin A and Calgranulin B (Calprotectin)

fluid in protecting the fetus [115–118]. The mucous plug protecting the cervical os contains multiple antimicrobial peptides in normal pregnancy [15,119]. Many of the innate immune molecules in vernix are similar to those found in breast milk [120,121]. Vernix, in part a glandular secretion of sebaceous origin, detaches from the skin surface *in utero* and is swallowed by the fetus [40]. Pulmonary surfactant, another source of intraamniotic antimicrobial peptides such as collectins [122], increases in amniotic fluid toward term.

Thus, there are a plethora of potential sources for antimicrobial peptides *in utero* and interactions between tissues and secretions are likely in producing a robust innate immune response. Tollin et al. recently demonstrated that free fatty acids extracted from vernix caseosa showed synergism with the peptide LL-37 in bacterial inhibition assays [43]. Akinbi et al. identified multiple antimicrobial peptides in vernix, but LL-37 was not identified in vernix samples obtained from mothers with no evidence of chorioamnionitis or intrauterine infection [42]. The possibility of an inducible cohort of peptides is intriguing whereby amniotic fluid, pulmonary surfactant, and vernix caseosa may have augmented peptide concentrations in the face of intraamniotic microbial assault. Protecting the fetus from a systemic inflammatory response by sequestration of the infection to the amniotic fluid compartment is teleologically desirable.

Adding to the complexity of the intrauterine innate immune system is the report by Akinbi of discrete, organized, acellular granules embedded in the nonlamellar lipid matrix of vernix caseosa (Figure 8.4) [42]. These granules measuring 50–100 μm in diameter showed consistent immunostaining for lysozyme, lactoferrin, SLPI, and HNP 1–3. Thus, the peptides are not randomly distributed in vernix but colocalize to discrete granular islands within the vernix. Whether this asymmetric morphological distribution offers a quick release form of bioavailable innate immune molecules remains to be determined. Similarly, whether infection upregulates the levels of antimicrobial peptides is unclear. Reduced levels of specific antimicrobial peptides and proteins have been reported in human cord blood from preterm infants compared

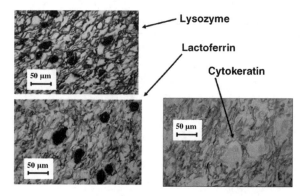

Figure 8.4 Spatial distribution of antimicrobial peptides in vernix. Paraffin sections of vernix were immunostained for lysozyme, lactoferrin, and pan-cytokeratin (control). Antimicrobial peptides are sequestrated in inclusion bodies (arrows) that are distributed throughout the vernix within the lipid matrix. Scale bar: 50 μm.

to from term infants. Whether circulating levels of peptides are inducible with prenatal infection is a promising area for future investigation.

Increased cord levels of cytokines such as IL-6 and other inflammatory molecules such as C-reactive protein have been implicated as markers of the fetal inflammatory response syndrome [12,51,123]. Both antimicrobial peptides and inflammatory cytokines can be detected on the newborn skin surface shortly after birth [111,124]. Of interest, proinflammatory cytokines such as IL-6 and IL-8 are elevated on the skin surface of preterm infants compared to adults, term newborns, or in vernix samples from normal term pregnancies without chorioamnionitis (Figure 8.5) [111]. Whether the biomarkers are elevated in the preterm cohort as a consequence of premature delivery secondary to chorioamnionitis is unknown but is a reasonable and testable hypothesis. The finding that other molecular mediators of inflammation such as cortisol can be measured from the skin surface and are elevated in preterm infants points to a fascinating road for future investigation [111].

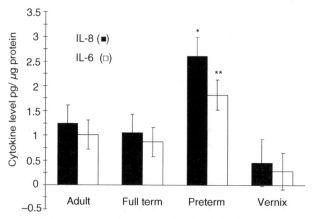

Figure 8.5 Ontogeny of cytokines (IL-6 and IL-8) in vernix and on the skin surface. IL-8 (■) was higher in preterms versus all others (*) ($p = 0.003$). IL-6 (□) was higher in preterms than full terms and vernix, but not different from adults (**) ($p = 0.02$). Individual pairs did not show significant differences (data from Ref. 111).

The fact that the human hair follicle possesses the enzymatic machinery of the hypothalamic–pituitary–adrenal axis and can synthesize cortisol *de novo* requires rethinking the importance of the skin surface as a stress response organ and invites comparison with the common embryological origin of the epidermis and brain as ectodermal derivatives [125–127]. In interpreting these results, it may prove useful to bear in mind that the epithelial surfaces forming the boundary of the amniotic fluid compartment, that is, the amnion and epidermis, are both of ectodermal origin. Embryologically, the skin is the surface of the brain and the privileged and dynamic space of amniotic fluid circulation may be usefully compared with the other ectodermal fluid compartments such as the aqueous humor [14] or cerebrospinal fluid [128].

8.4.6 Antioxidation

Although not widely recognized, the fetal environment is one of the extremely low oxygen tensions forming what the famed fetal physiologist Joseph Barcroft called "Mount Everest *in utero*" [129]. Thus, birth marks a time of abrupt passage into an environment replete not only with pathological and commensal microorganisms but also with exposure to high oxidative stress. Thiele et al. have clearly shown that human stratum corneum and sebum are rich in antioxidant properties secondary to high levels of alpha tocopherol [130–132]. Alpha tocopherol or vitamin E has also been detected in vernix [133,134]. This finding was recently corroborated with detection of mean vitamin E levels of 13–19 µg/g wet weight of vernix (0.03–0.04 µmol/g wet weight) [73,135]. Thus, when the skin surface is exposed to a pro-oxidant environment at birth, vernix may function as an antioxidant. Prenatal chorioamnionitis may also lead to the production of oxygen radicals and a potential protective (innate immune) role for vitamin E *in utero*.

8.4.7 Skin Cleansing

Skin cleansing is not typically considered a property of the innate immune system. Nevertheless, an instructive analogy can be drawn linking endogenous mechanisms of skin cleansing with exogenous mechanisms associated with bathing, hand hygiene, alcohol disinfection, and so on (Table 8.3). This concept is particularly useful in relation to the hygiene hypothesis whereby excessive cleansing or lack of

TABLE 8.3 Mechanisms of Skin Cleansing in Relation to Innate Immune Function

Endogenous	Exogenous
Immersion in continuously circulating amniotic fluid	Water submersion (bathing or showering)
Detachment of vernix from fetal skin; for example, following exposure to pulmonary surfactant	Commercial surfactant application to skin; for example, soaps and shampoos
Desquamation of stratum corneum corneocytes to the environment	Mechanical disruption; for example, toweling or abrasive brushing of skin

childhood exposure to infectious agents, including symbiotic microorganisms of the skin and gut, lead to future susceptibility to allergic disease and impaired development of adaptive immunity [136,137]. The biology of vernix caseosa offers a particularly useful example of normal skin cleansing mechanisms. The replacement of normal endogenous mechanisms of skin cleansing with excessive man-made exogenous surfactant exposure, for example, may result in a weakening of innate immune function and subsequent deleterious effects on the adaptive immune system.

Controlled skin cleansing experiments using uniform fine carbon particles as a typical "soil" demonstrated that vernix has comparable efficacy to standard commercial skin cleansers [138]. In fact, vernix was in some cases superior in removing residual carbon particles from soiled skin, particularly in cleaning of skin furrows, crevices, pores, and other microdermatoglyphic features. These results are consistent with the idea that the human infant is born covered with a material possessing both emollient and endogenous cleansing capabilities (Table 8.3). Unlike soaps, vernix is composed of biologically compatible lipids derived in part from sebaceous glands that will presumably integrate seamlessly with the skin surface and pores. Any residual material remaining after cleansing would have secondary beneficial effects in the form of emolliency, infection control, antioxidation, and so on. In this view, vernix has a strong analogy to the self-cleaning properties of the stratum corneum in which desquamation results in continual dynamic renewal and cleaning of the organism's skin surface. Again, the morphological comparison of vernix with the outermost layer of the stratum corneum lacking desmosomes or a lamellar lipid matrix is instructive [27,86]. Moreover, the colonization of the skin surface with normal microflora is presumably facilitated by materials present on the skin surface at birth.

8.4.8 Electrical Isolation (Increased Skin Surface Resistance)

The combination of vernix and stratum corneum contribute to increased electrical resistance at the surface of the body [139,140] and the resultant difficulty in detecting the fetal heart rate by routine electrocardiography [141,142]; hence, the need for Doppler measurements [143]. The role of vernix and stratum corneum in electrically isolating the fetus and increasing fetal autonomy as a form of innate immune protection has not been investigated.

8.4.9 Psychosensory

If innate immunity is defined according to the danger hypothesis as the provision of "cues" protecting biological tissue or the organism from harm, then innate immunity can be considered to include olfactory, tactile, or visual cues that elicit oriented behaviors in the neonate with survival advantage. Similarly, the ability of the newborn to elicit oriented caregiving behavior in the mother resulting in the provision of breast milk, warmth, tactile stimuli, or other sustenance will improve newborn survival and decrease danger. Accumulating evidence has shown that human newborns as well as other species such as rabbits demonstrate an orienting, head turning preference toward the source of familiar odors derived from amniotic fluid [144–147]. Similarly, breast milk will elicit head turning and orienting behaviors presumably secondary to release of a pheromone acting as an olfactory cue [148–150]. These data are consistent with the hypothesis that the fetus and newborn respond to familiar chemical cues present in the intrauterine environment and these cues play an important role in early food seeking behavior in infants. Whether vernix caseosa contributes to this intriguing neurobehavioral reflex pattern is unknown, but is consistent with the fact that many pheromones are derived from glandular skin secretions. Also, as mentioned, vernix is swallowed by the third trimester fetus long before the infant has access to breast milk [27,40,41,86]. The participation of vernix as a potential source for olfactory pheromones is an intriguing area for future research that dovetails with the broader goal of elucidating those tactile, visual, and olfactory cues that target the mother and elicit increased acceptance and maternal bonding. These "innate" cues clearly improve survival by removing the newborn infant from potentially dangerous situations; for example, hypothermia, dehydration, starvation, and so on. These cues can, therefore, legitimately be classified within the purview of the innate immune system.

8.5 SUMMARY AND FUTURE IMPLICATIONS

A discussion of the innate immune properties of vernix caseosa sheds light on complex biological areas such as immune tolerance of the fetus by the mother, the interplay of multiple fetal organs with essentially unknown or poorly understood intrauterine functions (skin, lung, and gut), and the critical transitional physiology associated with birth. The fact that other species lack a vernix equivalent makes its experimental study more difficult insofar as other materials such as pulmonary surfactant and breast milk have natural analogues in other species. Vernix provides a neat prototype for a potential platform technology leading to development of a natural multifunctional skin cream (Figure 8.6) [151–153]. Many of the functions listed in this figure relate immediately to innate immunity, including "cosmetic" aspects such as psychosensory cues and pheromonal attraction that may promote maternal/infant bonding and survival at birth. All these functions, therefore, can be subsumed under the broad category of innate immunity.

Multiple intriguing questions persist with respect to vernix biology and its role in innate immune function. Does vernix contribute to an increasingly robust innate immune system *in utero* protecting the fetus from systemic fetal inflammatory response and premature birth? To what extent do sebaceous glands contribute to vernix lipids and corneocytes? What is the source of antimicrobial peptides in vernix and are they present in bioavailable form due to their particulate morphology within the vernix lipid matrix? Does the increasing content of pulmonary surfactant in amniotic fluid emulsify skin surface vernix leading to a combination of pulmonary surfactant/vernix mixture that is swallowed by the fetus? Does this mixture have biological effects on the fetal foregut in anticipation of birth? Does vernix contribute or facilitate bacterial colonization of the foregut and skin surface with commensal microorganisms? How does vernix function biophysically as a skin surface

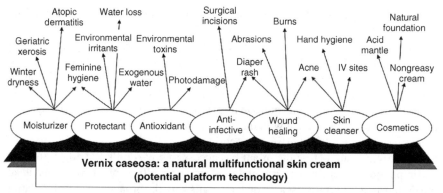

Figure 8.6   Multiple functions and potential applications of vernix caseosa. Vernix is a uniquely human skin cream synthesized *in utero* that combines a plethora of properties related to innate immune function prenatally and after birth. The combination of a continuous hydrophobic matrix containing discrete hydrophilic domains offers a challenging platform technology for the synthesis of natural or synthetic skin creams exhibiting similar combinatorial functionality. Evidence in support of each area is cited in text.

cleanser? Does vernix control water gradients *in utero* or function to sequester drugs or deleterious molecules within the amniotic fluid resulting in a unique fetal water purification system? Does vernix postnatally contribute to stratum corneum plasticization and formation of natural moisturizing factors? Does vernix contain pheromones similar to amniotic fluid and breast milk that promote infant feeding behavior and may lead to caregiver attraction and maternal bonding with subsequent benefits of long-term survival?

These questions indicate an active and exciting field of biological research with practical implications for the clinician and commercial applications for consumer care.

REFERENCES

1. Janeway CA, Jr. The immune system evolved to discriminate infectious nonself from noninfectious self. *Immunol. Today* 1992;13:11–16.
2. Matzinger P. Tolerance, danger, and the extended family. *Annu. Rev. Immunol.* 1994;12:991–1045.
3. Matzinger P. The danger model: a renewed sense of self. *Science* 2002;296:301–305.
4. Matzinger P. Friendly and dangerous signals: Is the tissue in control? *Nat. Immunol.* 2007;8:11–13.
5. Kvell K, Cooper EL, Engelmann P, Bovari J, Nemeth P. Blurring borders: innate immunity with adaptive features. *Clin. Dev. Immunol.* 2007;2007:83671.
6. Levy O. Innate immunity of the newborn: basic mechanisms and clinical correlates. *Nat. Rev. Immunol.* 2007;7:379–390.
7. Minon JM, Gerard C, Schaaps JP, Foidart JM. Rh D foeto-maternal alloimmunization prophylaxis with anti-D immunoglobulins reviewed in the era of foetal RHD genotyping. *Acta Clin. Belg.* 2009;64:195–202.
8. Bashiri A, Burstein E, Mazor M. Cerebral palsy and fetal inflammatory response syndrome: a review. *J. Perinat. Med.* 2006;34:5–12.
9. Dammann O, Leviton A. Inflammation, brain damage and visual dysfunction in preterm infants. *Semin. Fetal Neonatal Med.* 2006;11:363–368.

10. Polin RA. Systemic infection and brain injury in the preterm infant. *J. Pediatr. (Rio J.)* 2008;84:188–191.

11. Wolfberg AJ, Dammann O, Gressens P. Anti-inflammatory and immunomodulatory strategies to protect the perinatal brain. *Semin. Fetal Neonatal Med.* 2007;12:296–302.

12. Gomez R, Romero R, Ghezzi F, Yoon BH, Mazor M, Berry SM. The fetal inflammatory response syndrome. *Am. J. Obstet. Gynecol.* 1998;179:194–202.

13. Hermansen MC, Hermansen MG. Perinatal infections and cerebral palsy. *Clin. Perinatol.* 2006;33:315–333.

14. Niederkorn JY, Wang S. Immune privilege of the eye and fetus: parallel universes? *Transplantation* 2005;80:1139–1144.

15. Hein M, Helmig RB, Schonheyder HC, Ganz T, Uldbjerg N. An *in vitro* study of antibacterial properties of the cervical mucus plug in pregnancy. *Am. J. Obstet. Gynecol.* 2001;185:586–592.

16. Kim YM, Romero R, Chaiworapongsa T, Espinoza J, Mor G, Kim CJ. Dermatitis as a component of the fetal inflammatory response syndrome is associated with activation of Toll-like receptors in epidermal keratinocytes. *Histopathology* 2006;49:506–514.

17. Holbrook KA. Structural and biochemical organogenesis of skin and cutaneous appendages in the fetus and newborn. In: Polin RA, Fox WW, editors. *Fetal and Neonatal Physiology*. Philadelphia: W. B. Saunders Co., 1998.

18. Hoeger PH, Schreiner V, Klaassen IA, Enzmann CC, Friedrichs K, Bleck O. Epidermal barrier lipids in human vernix caseosa: corresponding ceramide pattern in vernix and fetal skin. *Br. J. Dermatol.* 2002;146:194–201.

19. Nicolaides N. The structures of the branched fatty acids in the wax esters of vernix caseosa. *Lipids* 1971;6:901–905.

20. Nicolaides N, Apon J. Further studies of the saturated methyl branched fatty acids of vernix caseosa lipid. *Lipids* 1976;11:781–790.

21. Nicolaides N, Fu HC, Ansari MN, Rice G.R. The fatty acids of wax esters and sterol esters from vernix caseosa and from human skin surface lipid. *Lipids* 1972;7:506–517.

22. Rissmann R, Groenink HW, Weerheim AM, Hoath SB, Ponec M, Bouwstra JA. New insights into ultrastructure, lipid composition and organization of vernix caseosa. *J. Invest. Dermatol.* 2006;126:1823–1833.

23. Sumida Y, Yakumaru M, Tokitsu Y, Iwamato Y, Ikemoto T, Mimura K. Studies on the function of vernix caseosa: the secrecy of baby's skin. International Federation of the Societies of Cosmetic Chemists 20th International Conference, Cannes, France, 1998. pp. 1–7.

24. Downing DT, Greene RS. Double bond positions in the unsaturated fatty acids of vernix caseosa. *J. Invest. Dermatol.* 1968;50:380–386.

25. Ran-Ressler RR, Devapatla S, Lawrence P, Brenna JT. Branched chain fatty acids are constituents of the normal healthy newborn gastrointestinal tract. *Pediatr. Res.* 2008;64:605–609.

26. Hoath S, Narendran V. Role and biology of vernix. *Neonat. Infant Nurs. Rev.* 2001;1:53–58.

27. Hoath SB, Pickens WL, Visscher MO. The biology of vernix caseosa. *Int. J. Cosmet. Sci.* 2006;28:319–333.

28. Zouboulis C, Fimmel S, Ortmann J, Turnbull J, Boschnakow A. Sebaceous glands. In: Hoath SB, Maibach H, (editors) *Neonatal Skin: Structure and Function*. New York: Marcel Dekker, 2003. pp. 59–88.

29. Zouboulis CC, Baron JM, Bohm M, Kippenberger S, Kurzen H, Reichrath J, Thielitz A. Frontiers in sebaceous gland biology and pathology. *Exp. Dermatol.* 2008;17:542–551.

30. Zaenglein AL, Thiboutot CM. Acne vulgaris and related disorders. In: Bolognia JL, Jorizzo JL, Rapini RP, (editors) *Dermatology*. Edinburgh: Mosby, 2003. pp. 531–544.

31. Burkhart CG, Burkhart CN. Expanding the microcomedone theory and acne therapeutics: propionibacterium acnes biofilm produces biological glue that holds corneocytes together to form plug. *J. Am. Acad. Dermatol.* 2007;57:722–724.

32. Espinoza J, Goncalves LF, Romero R, Nien JK, Stites S, Kim YM, Hassan S, Gomez R, Yoon BH, Chaiworapongsa T, Lee W, Mazor M. The prevalence and clinical significance of amniotic fluid 'sludge' in patients with preterm labor and intact membranes. *Ultrasound Obstet. Gynecol.* 2005;25:346–352.

33. Kusanovic JP, Espinoza J, Romero R, Goncalves LF, Nien JK, Soto E, Khalek N, Camacho N, Hendler I, Mittal P, Friel LA, Gotsch F, Erez O, Than NG, Mazaki-Tovi S, Schoen ML, Hassan SS. Clinical significance of the presence of amniotic fluid 'sludge' in asymptomatic patients at high risk for spontaneous preterm delivery. *Ultrasound Obstet. Gynecol.* 2007;30:706–714.

34. Romero R, Schaudinn C, Kusanovic JP, Gorur A, Gotsch F, Webster P, Nhan-Chang CL, Erez O, Kim CJ, Espinoza J, Goncalves LF, Vaisbuch E, Mazaki-Tovi S, Hassan SS, Costerton JW. Detection of a microbial biofilm in intraamniotic infection. *Am. J. Obstet. Gynecol.* 2008;198:135:e131–e135.

35. Romero R, Kusanovic JP, Espinoza J, Gotsch F, Nhan-Chang CL, Erez O, Kim CJ, Khalek N, Mittal P, Goncalves LF, Schaudinn C, Hassan SS, Costerton JW. What is amniotic fluid 'sludge'? *Ultrasound Obstet. Gynecol.* 2007;30:793–798.

36. Grice EA, Kong HH, Conlan S, Deming CB, Davis J, Young AC, Bouffard GG, Blakesley RW, Murray PR, Green ED, Turner ML, Segre JA. Topographical and temporal diversity of the human skin microbiome. *Science* 2009;324:1190–1192.

37. Grice EA, Kong HH, Renaud G, Young AC, Bouffard GG, Blakesley RW, Wolfsberg TG, Turner ML, Segre JA. A diversity profile of the human skin microbiota. *Genome Res.* 2008;18:1043–1050.

38. Zasloff M. Vernix, the newborn, and innate defense. *Pediatr. Res.* 2003;53:203–204.

39. Higgins RD, Delivoria-Papadopoulos M, Raju TN. Executive summary of the workshop on the border of viability. *Pediatrics* 2005;115:1392–1396.

40. Narendran V, Pickens W, Wickett R, Hoath S. Interaction between pulmonary surfactant and vernix: a potential mechanism for induction of amniotic fluid turbidity. *Pediatr. Res.* 2000;48:120–124.

41. Ross MG, Nijland MJ. Development of ingestive behavior. *Am. J. Physiol.* 1998;274:R879–R893.

42. Akinbi HT, Narendran V, Pass AK, Markart P, Hoath SB. Host defense proteins in vernix caseosa and amniotic fluid. *Am. J. Obstet. Gynecol.* 2004;191:2090–2096.

43. Tollin M, Bergsson G, Kai-Larsen Y, Lengqvist J, Sjovall J, Griffiths W, Skuladottir GV, Haraldsson A, Jornvall H, Gudmundsson GH, Agerberth B. Vernix caseosa as a multi-component defence system based on polypeptides, lipids and their interactions. *Cell Mol. Life Sci.* 2005;62:2390–2399.

44. Tollin M, Jagerbrink T, Haraldsson A, Agerberth B, Jornvall H. Proteome analysis of vernix caseosa. *Pediatr. Res.* 2006;60:430–434.

45. Yoshio H, Lagercrantz H, Gudmundsson GH, Agerberth B. First line of defense in early human life. *Semin. Perinatol.* 2004;28:304–311.

46. Yoshio H, Tollin M, Gudmundsson GH, Lagercrantz H, Jornvall H, Marchini G, Agerberth B. Antimicrobial polypeptides of human vernix caseosa and amniotic fluid: implications for newborn innate defense. *Pediatr. Res.* 2003;53:211–216.

47. Goldenberg RL, Culhane JF, Iams JD, Romero R. Epidemiology and causes of preterm birth. *Lancet* 2008;371:75–84.

48. Hack M, Fanaroff AA. Outcomes of children of extremely low birthweight and gestational age in the 1990s. *Semin. Neonatol.* 2000;5:89–106.

49. Lemons JA, Bauer CR, Oh W, Korones SB, Papile LA, Stoll BJ, Verter J, Temprosa M, Wright LL, Ehrenkranz RA, Fanaroff AA, Stark A, Carlo W, Tyson JE, Donovan EF, Shankaran S, Stevenson DK. Very low birth weight outcomes of the National Institute of Child health and human development neonatal research network, January 1995 through December 1996. NICHD Neonatal Research Network. *Pediatrics* 2001;107:E1.

50. Medzhitov R. Origin and physiological roles of inflammation. *Nature* 2008;454:428–435.

51. Romero R, Espinoza J, Goncalves LF, Kusanovic JP, Friel LA, Nien JK. Inflammation in preterm and term labour and delivery. *Semin. Fetal Neonatal Med.* 2006;11:317–326.

52. El-Bastawissi AY, Williams MA, Riley DE, Hitti J, Krieger JN. Amniotic fluid interleukin-6 and preterm delivery: a review. *Obstet. Gynecol.* 2000;95:1056–1064.

53. Keelan JA, Marvin KW, Sato TA, Coleman M, McCowan LM, Mitchell MD. Cytokine abundance in placental tissues: evidence of inflammatory activation in gestational membranes with term and preterm parturition. *Am. J. Obstet. Gynecol.* 1999;181:1530–1536.

54. Saji F, Samejima Y, Kamiura S, Sawai K, Shimoya K, Kimura T. Cytokine production in chorioamnionitis. *J. Reprod. Immunol.* 2000;47:185–196.

55. Andrews WW, Goldenberg RL, Faye-Petersen O, Cliver S, Goepfert AR, Hauth JC. The Alabama Preterm Birth study: polymorphonuclear and mononuclear cell placental infiltrations, other markers

of inflammation, and outcomes in 23- to 32-week preterm newborn infants. *Am. J. Obstet. Gynecol.* 2006;195:803–808.

56. Osman I, Young A, Ledingham MA, Thomson AJ, Jordan F, Greer IA, Norman JE. Leukocyte density and pro-inflammatory cytokine expression in human fetal membranes, decidua, cervix and myometrium before and during labour at term. *Mol. Hum. Reprod.* 2003;9:41–45.
57. Dalitz P, Harding R, Rees SM, Cock ML. Prolonged reductions in placental blood flow and cerebral oxygen delivery in preterm fetal sheep exposed to endotoxin: possible factors in white matter injury after acute infection. *J. Soc. Gynecol. Investig.* 2003;10:283–290.
58. Nitsos I, Rees SM, Duncan J, Kramer BW, Harding R, Newnham JP, Moss TJ. Chronic exposure to intra-amniotic lipopolysaccharide affects the ovine fetal brain. *J. Soc. Gynecol. Investig.* 2006;13:239–247.
59. Rezaie P, Dean A. Periventricular leukomalacia, inflammation and white matter lesions within the developing nervous system. *Neuropathology* 2002;22:106–132.
60. Roberts G, Anderson PJ, Doyle LW. Neurosensory disabilities at school age in geographic cohorts of extremely low birth weight children born between the 1970s and the 1990s. *J. Pediatr.* 2009;154:829–834; e821.
61. Elias PM. The skin barrier as an innate immune element. *Semin. Immunopathol.* 2007;29:3–14.
62. Wickett RR, Mutschelknaus JL, Hoath SB. Ontogeny of water sorption–desorption in the perinatal rat. *J. Invest. Dermatol.* 1993;100:407–411.
63. Pickens WL. Warner RR, Boissy YL, Boissy RE, Hoath SB. Characterization of vernix caseosa: water content, morphology, and elemental analysis. *J. Invest. Dermatol.* 2000;115:875–881.
64. Hoath SB, Pickens WL, Scarborough TE, Kasting GB, Visscher MO. Characterization of vernix caseosa: relevance to stratum corneum. In: Marks R, (editor) *Stratum Corneum IV*. Paris, 2004.
65. Seong SY, Matzinger P. Hydrophobicity: an ancient damage-associated molecular pattern that initiates innate immune responses. *Nat. Rev. Immunol.* 2004;4:469–478.
66. George E, Leyser S, Zimmer HL, Simonowitz DA, Agress RL, Nordin DD. Vernix caseosa peritonitis. An infrequent complication of cesarean section with distinctive histopathologic features. *Am. J. Clin. Pathol.* 1995;103:681–684.
67. Nunez C. Vernix caseosa peritonitis. *Am. J. Clin. Pathol.* 1996;105:657.
68. Schwartz IS, Bello GV, Feigin G, Sherman DH. Maternal vernix caseosa peritonitis following premature rupture of fetal membranes. *JAMA* 1985;254:948–950.
69. Selo-Ojeme D, Donkor P, Francis D. Vernix caseosa peritonitis: an unusual and rare complication of caesarean section. *J. Obstet. Gynaecol.* 2007;27:190–191.
70. Stuart OA, Morris AR, Baber RJ. Vernix caseosa peritonitis: no longer rare or innocent: a case series. *J. Med. Case Reports* 2009;3:60.
71. Tansirikongkol A, Hoath SB, Pickens WL, Visscher MO, Wickett RR. Equilibrium water content in native vernix and its cellular component. *J. Pharm. Sci.* 2008;97:985–994.
72. Youssef W, Wickett R, Hoath S. Surface free energy characterization of vernix caseosa: role in waterproofing the newborn infant. *Skin Res. Technol.* 2001;7:10–17.
73. Visscher MO, Narendran V, Pickens WL, LaRuffa AA, Meinzen-Derr J, Allen K, Hoath SB. Vernix caseosa in neonatal adaptation. *J. Perinatol.* 2005;25:440–446.
74. Scott I, Harding C. Filaggrin breakdown to water binding compounds during development of the rat stratum corneum is controlled by the water activity of the environment. *Dev. Biol.* 1986;115:84–92.
75. Saijo S, Tagami H. Dry skin of newborn infants: functional analysis of the stratum corneum. *Pediatr. Dermatol.* 1991;8:155–159.
76. Bautista MI, Wickett RR, Visscher MO, Pickens WL, Hoath SB. Characterization of vernix caseosa as a natural biofilm: comparison to standard oil-based ointments. *Pediatr. Dermatol.* 2000;17:253–260.
77. Agorastos T, Bar T, Grussendorf EI, Liedtke B, Lamberti G. Ultrastructural aspects of amniotic-fluid cells: A. Non-vital cells. III. Large squamous cells (author's translation). *Z. Geburtshilfe Perinatol.* 1981;185:231–235.
78. Agorastos T, Hollweg G, Grussendorf EI, Papaloucas A. Features of vernix caseosa cells. *Am. J. Perinatol.* 1988;5:253–259.
79. Agorastos T, Lamberti G, Vlassis G, Zournatzi B, Papaloucas A. Methods of prenatal determination of fetal maturity based on differentiation of the fetal skin during the last weeks of pregnancy. *Eur. J. Obstet. Gynecol. Reprod. Biol.* 1986;22:29–40.

80. Agorastos T, Vlassis G, Zournatzi B, Papaloukas A. Fetal lung maturity and skin maturity: 2 distinct concepts and the clinical significance of their differences. *Z. Geburtshilfe Perinatol.* 1983;187:146–150.
81. Gunt HB. Masters Thesis. Water Handling Properties of Vernix Caseosa, University of Cincinnati, 2002.
82. Utturkar RS. Masters Thesis. Vernix caseosa: a source of natural moisturizing factors and its possible role in neonatal infant skin hydration, University of Cincinnati, 2005.
83. Denda M, Sato J, Masuda Y, Tsuchiya T, Koyama J, Kuramoto M, Elias P, Feingold K. Exposure to a dry environment enhances epidermal permeability barrier function. *J. Invest. Dermatol.* 1998;111:858–863.
84. Denda M, Sato J, Tsuchiya T, Elias P, Feingold K. Low humidity stimulates epidermal DNA synthesis and amplifies the hyperproliferative response to barrier disruption: implication for seasonal exacerbations of inflammatory dermatoses. *J. Invest. Dermatol.* 1998;111:873–878.
85. Proksch E, Holleran W, Menon G, Elias P, Feingold K. Barrier function regulates epidermal lipid and DNA synthesis. *Br. J. Dermatol.* 1993;128:473–482.
86. Rawlings AV, Watkinson A, Rogers J. Abnormalities in stratum corneum structure lipid composition and desmosome degradation in soap-induced winter xerosis. *J. Soc. Cosmet. Chem.* 1994;45:203–220.
87. Tansirikongkol A, Visscher MO, Wickett RR. Water-handling properties of vernix caseosa and a synthetic analogue. *J. Cosmet. Sci.* 2007;58:651–662.
88. Kitzmiller JL, Highby S, Lucas WE. Retarded growth of *E. coli* in amniotic fluid. *Obstet. Gynecol.* 1973;41:38–42.
89. Hardman MJ, Moore L, Ferguson MW, Byrne C. Barrier formation in the human fetus is patterned. *J. Invest. Dermatol.* 1999;113:1106–1113.
90. Tansirikongkol A, Wickett RR, Visscher MO, Hoath SB. Effect of vernix caseosa on the penetration of chymotryptic enzyme: potential role in epidermal barrier development. *Pediatr. Res.* 2007;62:49–53.
91. Horikoshi T, Igarashi S, Uchiwa H, Brysk H, Brysk MM. Role of endogenous cathepsin D-like and chymotrypsin-like proteolysis in human epidermal desquamation. *Br. J. Dermatol.* 1999;141:453–459.
92. Carrere J, Figarella C, Guy O, Thouvenot JP. Human pancreatic chymotrypsinogen A: a non-competitive enzyme immunoassay, and molecular forms in serum and amniotic fluid. *Biochim. Biophys. Acta* 1986;883:46–53.
93. Andersen PH, Bucher AP, Saeed I, Lee PC, Davis JA, Maibach HI. Faecal enzymes: *in vivo* human skin irritation. *Contact Dermatitis* 1994;30:152–158.
94. Berg RW. Etiology and pathophysiology of diaper dermatitis. *Adv. Dermatol.* 1988;3:75–98.
95. Scott A. A study of the action of chymotrypsin on the skin. *J. Invest. Dermatol.* 1958;30:201–205.
96. Visscher MO, Hoath SB. Diaper dermatitis. In: Maibach H, (editor) *Handbook of Irritant Dermatitis.* Berlin: Springer, 2003. pp. 37–51.
97. Saunders C. The vernix caseosa and subnormal temperature in premature infants. *Br. J. Obstet. Gynaecol.* 1948;55:442–444.
98. Riesenfeld B, Stromberg B, Sedin G. The influence of vernix caseosa on water transport through semipermeable membranes and the skin of full-term infants. In: Rolfe P, editor. *Neonatal Physiological Measurements: Proceedings of the Second International Conference on Fetal and Neonatal Physiological Measurements.* Butterworth-Heinemann, 1986. pp. 3–6.
99. Shulak B. The antibacterial action of vernix caseosa. *Harper Hosp. Bull.* 1963;21:111–117.
100. Fox C, Nelson D, Wareham J. The timing of skin acidification in very low birth weight infants. *J. Perinatol.* 1998;18:272–275.
101. Eming SA, Hammerschmidt M, Krieg T, Roers A. Interrelation of immunity and tissue repair or regeneration. *Semin. Cell Dev. Biol.* 2009;20:517–527.
102. Mescher AL, Neff AW. Regenerative capacity and the developing immune system. *Adv. Biochem. Eng. Biotechnol.* 2005;93:39–66.
103. Steinstraesser L, Koehler T, Jacobsen F, Daigeler A, Goertz O, Langer S, Kesting M, Steinau H, Eriksson E, Hirsch T. Host defense peptides in wound healing. *Mol. Med.* 2008;14:528–537.
104. Zhukov B, Neverova E, Nikitin K. A comparative evaluation of the use of vernix caseosa and solcoseryl in treating patients with trophic ulcers of the lower extremities. *Vestn. Khir. Im. I. I. Grek.* 1992;148:339–341.

105. Darmstadt GL. Badrawi N. Law PA. Ahmed S. Bashir M. Iskander I. Al Said D. El Kholy A. Husein MH, Alam A, Winch PJ, Gipson R, Santosham M. Topically applied sunflower seed oil prevents invasive bacterial infections in preterm infants in Egypt: a randomized, controlled clinical trial. *Pediatr. Infect. Dis. J.* 2004;23:719–725.
106. Darmstadt GL, Mao-Qiang M, Chi E, Saha SK, Ziboh VA, Black RE, Santosham M, Elias PM. Impact of topical oils on the skin barrier: possible implications for neonatal health in developing countries. *Acta Paediatr.* 2002;91:546–554.
107. Darmstadt GL, Saha SK, Ahmed AS, Chowdhury MA, Law PA, Ahmed S, Alam MA, Black RE, Santosham M. Effect of topical treatment with skin barrier-enhancing emollients on nosocomial infections in preterm infants in Bangladesh: a randomised controlled trial. *Lancet* 2005;365:1039–1045.
108. Oudshoorn MH, Rissmann R, van der Coelen D, Hennink WE, Ponec M, Bouwstra JA. Effect of synthetic vernix biofilms on barrier recovery of damaged mouse skin. *Exp. Dermatol.* 2009;18:695–703.
109. Oudshoorn MH, Rissmann R, van der Coelen D, Hennink WE, Ponec M, Bouwstra JA. Development of a murine model to evaluate the effect of vernix caseosa on skin barrier recovery. *Exp. Dermatol.* 2009;18:178–184.
110. Marchini G, Lindow S, Brismar H, Stabi B, Berggren V, Ulfgren AK, Lonne-Rahm S, Agerberth B, Gudmundsson GH. The newborn infant is protected by an innate antimicrobial barrier: peptide antibiotics are present in the skin and vernix caseosa. *Br. J. Dermatol.* 2002;147:1127–1134.
111. Narendran V, Visscher MO, Abril I, Hendrix SW, Hoath SB. Biomarkers of epidermal innate immunity in premature and full-term infants. *Pediatr. Res.* 2009;67(4):382–386.
112. Hoffmann JA, Kafatos FC, Janeway CA, Ezekowitz RA. Phylogenetic perspectives in innate immunity. *Science* 1999;284:1313–1318.
113. Huttner KM, Bevins CL. Antimicrobial peptides as mediators of epithelial host defense. *Pediatr. Res.* 1999;45:785–794.
114. Zasloff M. Antimicrobial peptides of multicellular organisms. *Nature* 2002;415:389–395.
115. Galask RP, Snyder IS. Antimicrobial factors in amniotic fluid. *Am. J. Obstet. Gynecol.* 1970;106:59–65.
116. Otsuki K, Yoda A, Saito H, Mitsuhashi Y, Toma Y, Shimizu Y, Yanaihara T. Amniotic fluid lactoferrin in intrauterine infection. *Placenta* 1999;20:175–179.
117. Sachs BP, Stern CM. Activity and characterization of a low molecular fraction present in human amniotic fluid with broad spectrum antibacterial activity. *Br. J. Obstet. Gynaecol.* 1979;86:81–86.
118. Thadepalli H, Gangopadhyay PK, Maidman JE. Amniotic fluid analysis for antimicrobial factors. *Int. J. Gynaecol. Obstet.* 1982;20:65–72.
119. Hein M, Valore EV, Helmig RB, Uldbjerg N, Ganz T. Antimicrobial factors in the cervical mucus plug. *Am. J. Obstet. Gynecol.* 2002;187:137–144.
120. Goldman AS. Evolution of the mammary gland defense system and the ontogeny of the immune system. *J. Mammary Gland Biol. Neoplasia* 2002;7:277–289.
121. Oftedal OT. The mammary gland and its origin during synapsid evolution. *J. Mammary Gland Biol. Neoplasia* 2002;7:225–252.
122. Narendran V, Hull W, Akinbi H, Whitsett J, Pickens W, Lambers D, Hoath SB. Vernix caseosa contains surfactant proteins: potential role in innate immune function in the fetus. *Pediatr. Res.* 2000;47:420A.
123. Yoon BH, Romero R, Park JS. Kim M, Oh SY, Kim CJ, Jun JK. The relationship among inflammatory lesions of the umbilical cord (funisitis), umbilical cord plasma interleukin 6 concentration, amniotic fluid infection, and neonatal sepsis. *Am. J. Obstet. Gynecol.* 2000;183:1124–1129.
124. Walker VP, Akinbi HT, Meinzen-Derr J, Narendran V, Visscher M, Hoath SB. Host defense proteins on the surface of neonatal skin: implications for innate immunity. *J. Pediatr.* 2008;152:777–781.
125. Arck PC, Slominski A, Theoharides TC, Peters EM, Paus R. Neuroimmunology of stress: skin takes center stage. *J. Invest. Dermatol.* 2006;126:1697–1704.
126. Ito N, Ito T, Kromminga A, Bettermann A, Takigawa M, Kees F, Straub RH, Paus R. Human hair follicles display a functional equivalent of the hypothalamic-pituitary–adrenal axis and synthesize cortisol. *FASEB J.* 2005;19:1332–1334.

127. Paus R, Theoharides TC, Arck PC. Neuroimmunoendocrine circuitry of the 'brain–skin connection'. *Trends Immunol.* 2006;27:32–39.

128. Hu S, Loo JA, Wong DT. Human body fluid proteome analysis. *Proteomics* 2006;6:6326–6353.

129. Raju TNK. Historical perspectives: perinatal profiles: Sir Joseph Barcroft: the 20th century's renaissance perinatal physiologist. *NeoReviews* 2007;8:e311–e312.

130. Thiele JJ, Packer L. Noninvasive measurement of alpha-tocopherol gradients in human stratum corneum by high-performance liquid chromatography analysis of sequential tape strippings. *Methods Enzymol.* 1999;300:413–419.

131. Thiele JJ, Schroeter C, Hsieh SN, Podda M, Packer L. The antioxidant network of the stratum corneum. *Curr. Probl. Dermatol.* 2001;29:26–42.

132. Thiele JJ, Weber SU, Packer L. Sebaceous gland secretion is a major physiologic route of vitamin E delivery to skin. *J. Invest. Dermatol.* 1999;113:1006–1010.

133. Gerloczy F, Bencze B, Ivanyi K. Demonstration of a new biologically active substance vitamin E, in the vernix caseosa. *Int. Z. Vitaminforsch.* 1961;32:1–4.

134. Gerloczy F, Bencze B, Ivanyi K. Demonstration of vitamin E, a new biologically active substrate, in the vernix caseosa. *Magy. Noorv. Lapja* 1963;26:21–22.

135. Pickens W, Zhou Y, Wickett R, Visscher M, Hoath S. Antioxidant defense mechanisms in vernix caseosa: potential role of endogenous vitamin E. *Pediatr. Res.* 2000;47:425A.

136. Sublett JL. The environment and risk factors for atopy. *Curr. Allergy Asthma Rep.* 2005;5:445–450.

137. Vassallo MF, Walker WA. Neonatal microbial flora and disease outcome. *Nestle Nutr. Workshop Ser. Pediatr. Program.* 2008;61:211–224.

138. Moraille R, Pickens WL, Visscher MO, Hoath SB. A novel role for vernix caseosa as a skin cleanser. *Biol. Neonate* 2005;87:8–14.

139. Wakai R, Lengle J, Leuthold A. Transmission of electric and magnetic foetal cardiac signals in a case of ectopia cordis: the dominant role of the vernix caseosa. *Phys. Med. Biol.* 2000;45:1989–1995.

140. Shivanand P. PhD Thesis. Electrical and transport properties of neonatal rat skin, University of Cincinnati, 1995.

141. Graatsma EM, Jacod BC, van Egmond LA, Mulder EJ, Visser GH. Fetal electrocardiography: feasibility of long-term fetal heart rate recordings. *BJOG* 2009;116:334–337; discussion 337–338.

142. Pieri JF, Crowe JA, Hayes-Gill BR, Spencer CJ, Bhogal K, James DK. Compact long-term recorder for the transabdominal foetal and maternal electrocardiogram. *Med. Biol. Eng. Comput.* 2001;39:118–125.

143. Shakespeare SA, Crowe JA, Hayes-Gill BR, Bhogal K, James DK. The information content of Doppler ultrasound signals from the fetal heart. *Med. Biol. Eng. Comput.* 2001;39:619–626.

144. Marlier L, Schaal B, Soussignan R. Orientation responses to biological odours in the human newborn. Initial pattern and postnatal plasticity. *C. R. Acad. Sci. III* 1997;320:999–1005.

145. Marlier L, Schaal B, Soussignan R. Bottle-fed neonates prefer an odor experienced *in utero* to an odor experienced postnatally in the feeding context. *Dev. Psychobiol.* 1998;33:133–145.

146. Schaal B, Marlier L, Soussignan R. Olfactory function in the human fetus: evidence from selective neonatal responsiveness to the odor of amniotic fluid. *Behav. Neurosci.* 1998;112:1438–1449.

147. Varendi H, Christensson K, Porter RH, Winberg J. Soothing effect of amniotic fluid smell in newborn infants. *Early Hum. Dev.* 1998;51:47–55.

148. Marlier L, Schaal B. Human newborns prefer human milk: conspecific milk odor is attractive without postnatal exposure. *Child Dev.* 2005;76:155–168.

149. Nishitani S, Miyamura T, Tagawa M, Sumi M, Takase R, Doi H, Moriuchi H, Shinohara K. The calming effect of a maternal breast milk odor on the human newborn infant. *Neurosci. Res.* 2009;63:66–71.

150. Schaal B, Coureaud G, Doucet S, Delaunay-El Allam M, Moncomble AS, Montigny D, Patris B, Holley A. Mammary olfactory signalisation in females and odor processing in neonates: ways evolved by rabbits and humans. *Behav. Brain Res.* 2009;200:346–358.

151. Rissmann R, Oudshoorn MH, Kocks E, Hennink WE, Ponec M, Bouwstra JA. Lanolin-derived lipid mixtures mimic closely the lipid composition and organization of vernix caseosa lipids. *Biochim. Biophys. Acta* 2008;1778:2350–2360.

152. Rissmann R, Oudshoorn MH, Zwier R, Ponec M, Bouwstra JA, Hennink WE. Mimicking vernix caseosa: preparation and characterization of synthetic biofilms. *Int. J. Pharm.* 2009;372:59–65.

153. Wiechers JW, Gabard B. Vernix caseosa: the ultimate natural cosmetic? *Cosmet. Toiletries* 2009; 124(9):36–55.

154. Okah FA, Wickett RR, Pompa K, Hoath SB. Human newborn skin: the effect of isopropanol on skin surface hydrophobicity. *Pediatr. Res.* 1994;35:443–446.

155. Joglekar V. Barrier properties of vernix caseosa. *Arch. Dis. Child.* 1980;55:817–819.

156. Baker SM, Balo NN, Abdel Aziz FT. Is vernix caseosa a protective material to the newborn? A biochemical approach. *Indian J. Pediatr.* 1995;62:237–239.

157. Barai N. PhD Thesis. Effect of vernix caseosa on epidermal barrier maturation and repair: implications in wound healing, University of Cincinnati, 2005.

158. Zhukov B, Neverova E, Nikitin K. A comparative evaluation of the use of vernix caseosa and solcoseryl in treating patients with trophic ulcers of the lower extremities. *Vestn. Khir. Im. I. I. Grek.* 1992;148:339–341.

PART III

HOST CELLULAR COMPONENTS OF INNATE IMMUNITY

CHAPTER 9

SENTINEL ROLE OF MAST CELLS IN INNATE IMMUNITY

Zhenping Wang and Anna Di Nardo

Department of Medicine, University of California, San Diego, La Jolla, CA

9.1 BASICS OF MAST CELLS

Paul Ehrlich, who received the Nobel Prize for discoveries in immunology in 1908, discovered mast cells in 1878. He describes mast cells in his doctoral thesis as "granular cells of the connective tissue." The typical aspect of these "granular cells" is characterized by an "undetermined chemical substance" in the protoplasm with which the aniline dye reacts to give a typical metachromasia [1]. To this day, mast cells are still recognized by the presence of metachromatic granules with toluidine blue staining. As resident cells, mast cells have strategic locations. They are within the tissues that are mostly exposed to the external environment, such as the skin, airways, and intestine, where they can initiate and enhance early responses to a variety of challenges. In addition, mast cells are close to blood vessels, nerve, or lymphatic vessels where they can regulate vascular permeability and effector cell recruitment by releasing mediators. Estimated concentrations of mast cells range from 500 to 4000/mm^3 in the lungs, 7000 to 12,000/mm^3 in the skin, and 20,000/mm^3 in the gastrointestinal tract [2]. Mast cells are bone marrow-derived hematopoietic cells, and the main *in vivo* mast cell growth factors in rodents are interleukin-3 (IL-3) and stem cell factor (SCF, also known as KIT ligand) [3–5]. In humans, stem cell factor with IL-6 supports mast cell growth *in vitro* [6,7]. Mast cells have a long half-life in tissues, for example, 40 days in rodent intestinal mast cells [8]. They express the high-affinity receptor for IgE (FcεRI) that can be occupied by IgE following *in vivo* sensitization and restimulated *ex vivo* with antigen. In a typical allergic reaction, the antigen/allergen cross-links two IgE molecules occupying FcεRI, resulting in a cascade of rapid sequence signaling events and leading to degranulation and elaboration of mediators [9]. There are two mast cell subtypes in tissue—the mucosal (MC_T) or connective tissue (MC_{TC}) mast cell—based on structural, biochemical, and functional differences [10–12]. They have been implicated in a variety of diseases such as allergy, asthma, rheumatoid arthritis, atherosclerosis, interstitial cystitis, inflammatory bowel disease, progressive systemic sclerosis, chronic graft-versus-host disease, fibrotic

Innate Immune System of Skin and Oral Mucosa: Properties and Impact in Pharmaceutics, Cosmetics, and Personal Care Products, First Edition. Nava Dayan and Philip W. Wertz.

diseases, sarcoidosis, asbestosis, ischemic heart disease, keloid scars, and malignancy [10]. However, mast cells play important roles in wound repair-remodeling responses and in host defense against infectious pathogens [13–15]. They have a unique "armamentarium" of receptor systems and mediators for responding to pathogen-associated signals [16]. Here, we will present an overview on the crucial sentinel role of these fascinating and multifunctional cells in innate immunity.

9.2 MAST CELLS RESPONSES TO PARASITES

In the past 30 years, there have been many studies showing that mast cells get activated during parasite infection by increasing their number, releasing granule, producing proteases and cytokines, recruiting other effector cells, and regulating inflammation to control infection, and promote parasite expulsion.

Daily injections of phospholipid preparations from the nematode *Ascaris suum* or cysts of *Echinococcus granulosus* (hydatid cysts) induced peritoneal eosinophilia accompanied by blood eosinophilia, mast cell granule lysis, and mast cell hyperplasia [17]. Primary infections with the protozoan parasite, *Eimeria nieschulzi* induced systemic secretion of rat mucosal mast cell protease, a major product of rat mucosal mast cells (MMCs) [18], and mast cells are predominant cells containing IgE in the intestinal mucosa of mice infected with the nematode parasite *Trichinella spiralis* [19]. Pentastomid parasite *Porocephalus crotali* can selectively recruit MMCs to a variety of tissue sites, most of which are nonmucosal [20]. However, MMCs that accumulate in the small intestine in response to parasite infection may not be functionally involved in the rejection mechanism [21–25]. Miller et al. believed systemic release of rat mast cell protease II (RMCPII) in primed rats challenged with *Nippostrongylus brasiliensis* (*Nb*) demonstrated that MMCs are activated in response to *Nb* challenge infection or to parasite antigens [26], and the numbers of MMCs and concentrations of RMCPII increased in the heterozygotes but not in nude rats [18]. Depletion of mucosal mast cell protease by corticosteroids abolished systemic anaphylactic shock induced by injecting intravenously with soluble whole-worm antigen in rats primed by infection with the intestinal nematode *Nb* [27]. During infection of *Toxoplasma gondii*, there was a significant increase in the number of mast cells and in the influx of neutrophils after mast cells' degranulation, suggesting that mast cells are deeply involved in the host inflammatory response after infection with *T. gondii* [28,29]. Mast cells play a role in protecting against disseminated parasitic disease by increasing MMC numbers and releasing histamine in the intestines not only of rodents but also of higher primates [30]. However, epithelial injury at the villus tips in intestine, during infection with the nematode parasite, may be related to activation of MMC [31]. The activation of sensitized peritoneal mast cells obtained from rats infected with the parasite *Nb* can be inhibited by interferon-alpha/beta [32]. In addition to the T helper 2 cell-mediated regulation of MMC hyperplasia during nematode infection, the c-kit ligand, stem cell factor, plays a key role in the early development of the MMC response in protection against certain nematodes that enter the mucosa, but not against lumen-dwelling nematodes [33]. Newlands et al. reported SCF contributes to intestinal MMC hyperplasia in rats infected with *Nb* or *T. spiralis*, but anti-SCF treatment decreases parasite egg production during *Nb* infection, which raises the interesting possibility that certain activities of intestinal MMCs may contribute to parasite fecundity during infection with this nematode [34].

During infection with *Schistosoma mansoni*, a pronounced hepatic masto-cytosis occurs in the rat and this is concomitant with the demise of the parasite. The majority of recruited hepatic mast cells contain the highly soluble granule chymase, rat mast cell protease-II, which is released systemically into blood during the period of parasite elimination. Therefore, in rat, infection is terminated in the liver before egg laying commences, whereas the parasite completes its life cycle in mice because very few mast cells are found in the liver of parasitized mice and none contains the soluble granule chymase and mouse mast cell protease-1 [35]. Furthermore, direct cell–parasite contact between mouse bone marrow-derived mast cells (BMMCs) and *Leishmania major* or *L. infantum*-induced TNF-alpha synthesis and release of preformed mediators such as beta-hexosaminidase and TNF-alpha by mast cells within minutes, which suggests that mast cell can parti-cipate in the first line of innate immunity, during local cutaneous infection with *Leishmania* parasites [36,37]. However, parasite expulsion and mast cell develop-ment are impaired severely in IL-3-deficient mice. These mice also show a marked reduction in signaling by stem cell factor receptor, c-kit; in fact, IL-3 is particularly critical for the development, survival, and function of tissue mast cells, and host defense against infection [38]. Immunosuppressive treatment with cyclosporin A (CsA) prevented *Hymenolepis diminuta* worm expulsion, permitting some indivi-duals to reach maturity, and abrogated mast cell proliferation and mast cell protease-I production and release [39].

Mast cell capacity to fight parasites or pathogens at large seems to be more related to their capacity to release the granules than to increase in their number. Mast cell-deficient WBB6F1-W/Wv mice are more susceptible to *Trichuris muris* infection than their wild-type littermates; however, no MMC responses were induced in either infected W/Wv or wild-type mice [40]. Moreover, FcRgamma (−/−) mice had significantly higher egg counts and number of adult worms of *Strongyloides venezuelensis* than FcRgamma(+/+) mice, but mastocytosis and serum mast cell protease-I release were comparable. The delay in worm expulsion in the FcRgamma(−/−) mice might be related to inability of the MMC to degranulate and release effector molecules other than mast cell protease-I since FcRgamma deletion abrogates mast cell degranulative responses [41]. Urban et al. find that Stat6 activation by IL-4/IL-13 is required in *T. spiralis*-infected mice both for the mast cell responses that induce worm expulsion and for the cytokine responses that induce intestinal mastocytosis [42]. Sasaki et al. used STAT6(−/−), IL-18(−/−), or IL-18Ralpha(−/−) mice to show that collaboration between IL-18-dependent and Th2 cell-dependent mastocytosis is important for prompt parasite *S. venezuelensis* expulsion [43]. Furthermore, analysis of gene expression in MMCs by using DNA microarray technology suggests that IL-18 may contribute to mast cell-influenced Th2 responses by inducing Ccl1 (I-309, TCA-3) production in MMCs primarily via the activation of NF-κB [44]. Blockage of either alpha-4 or beta-7 integrins, expressed at high levels in mast cells, selectively inhibits intestinal mast cell hyperplasia and worm expulsion in response to *N. brasiliensis* infection [45]. McDermott et al. demonstrated using anti-c-kit antibody and IL-9 transgenic mice that mast cells are directly responsible for increasing epithelial paracellular permeability. Mice deficient in a mast cell-specific protease fail to increase intestinal permeability and fail to expel their parasite burden, providing the mechanism whereby mucosal mast cells mediate parasite expulsion from the intestine [46]. The splenic mastocytosis observed in BALB/c mice following infection with *T. spiralis* was significantly diminished in IgE(−/−) mice, and serum levels of mouse mast cell protease-1 also were lower in parasite-infected IgE(−/−) animals and these animals were slower to eliminate the adult worms from the small intestine, suggesting IgE enhances parasite clearance and regulates mast cell responses [47]. Anti-c-kit-treated C57BL/6 mice lacked mast cell responses, had reduced IL-6 mRNA in the small intestine, and failed to control the infection of *Giardia lamblia*. Interestingly, IL-6-deficient mice had enhanced mast cell responses, yet failed to control the infection, indicating mast cell production of IL-6 is important for control of *G. lamblia* infection [48]. MMCs in FcRgamma-knockout mice failed to release sufficient amount of sulfated proteoglycans into the gut lumen, which prevented expulsion of adult *S. venezuelensis* from the gut [49]. Pennock et al. reported that during *T. spiralis* infection, the bone marrow environment generates mast cells destined for the intestinal mucosa before their exit into the periphery, indicating a clear interplay between infection site and hematopoietic tissue [50]. During *G. intestinalis* infection, cholecystokinin release triggers mast cell degranulation, leading to increase in smooth muscle contractility coupled with nitric oxide-mediated muscle relaxation, which promotes intestinal transit and parasite elimination [51]. By using WBB6F1-KitW/KitW-v (W/W(v)) mice reconstituted with wild-type, TNF-alpha(−/−), or IL-4(−/−) bone marrow prior to infection with *T. spiralis*, Ierna et al. reported mast cell-derived IL-4 and TNF-alpha may regulate the induction of protective Th2 responses and intestinal inflammation associated with the expulsion of *T. spiralis* [52]. The regulatory effect of mast cells on parasite infections seems to depend on the genetic background of the host: mast cells of BALB/c mice facilitate disease progression due to an augmented inflammatory response early in the infection, whereas mast cells of C57BL/6 mice produce cytokines that regulate inflammation and maintain an elevated number of immune cells in the lesions, promoting disease control [53]. Romao et al. reported that pharmacological inactivation of mast cells before infection may be a new field of study for strategies to control the parasite dissemination. They found that mast cell degranulation, before the animal infection with *L. major*, induces more resistance to infection, as measured by decrease in lesion size and lower parasite loads. Mast cell preemptive degranulation reduced IL-4 production and enhanced mRNA expression for IFN-gamma, inducible nitric oxide, CCL2, and CCL5 in response to infection [54].

In mast cells and parasite infections, it has been uncertain if mast cells are also involved in the effectory phase of the immune cell response. Recently, Blum et al. reported data against a role for mast cells in the mechanism underlying the effector phase of protective immunity against *T. spiralis* in rats. Their results indicate that during secondary infection, rapid expulsion of 90–99% of *T. spiralis* first-stage larvae can occur in rats in the absence of either intestinal mastocytosis or RMCPII release, though primary intestinal infection by *T. spiralis* induces mastocytosis and mast cell degranulation [55].

In summary, mast cells have strong association with parasite infection that induces mastocytosis depending on the presence of type 2 cytokines such as IL-4, IL-9, IL-10, and IL-13 [56]. Although the role of mast cells in the mechanism of worm expulsion is yet to be fully defined, it is now evident that mast cells can both amplify protective responses against parasite in innate immunity and play a conflicting role in inflammation and pathology at the sites of infection.

9.3 MAST CELLS RESPONSES TO BACTERIA

Due to the strategic location of mast cells at the host–environment interface, mast cells also play an important role in innate immunity against bacteria by their ability to phagocytose bacteria, process and present bacterial antigens to T cells, recruit phagocytic cells, release mediators and cytokines, and produce cathelicidin antimicrobial peptides [16,57–60].

As early as 1979, Sher et al. demonstrated that phagocytosis of bacteria by rat peritoneal mast cells can be promoted by complement receptors [61]. Complement C3-deficient mice also exhibited reductions in peritoneal mast cell degranulation, production of TNF-alpha, neutrophil infiltration, and clearance of bacteria. Treating the C3-deficient mice with purified C3 protein enhanced activation of peritoneal mast cells, TNF-alpha production, neutrophil recruitment, opsonin phagocytosis of bacteria, and resistance to cecal ligation and puncture, confirming that complement activation is essential for the full expression of innate immunity in this mast cell-dependent model of bacterial infection [62]. In jejunal biopsy from untreated patient with Whipple's disease, Whipple's bacilli were often seen within the cytoplasm of mast cells, enclosed within vacuoles; mast cells were in intimate contact with macrophages containing bacteria, which suggests a cooperation between mast cell and macrophage in the defense against Whipple's bacillus [63]. Formalin-killed bacteria such as *Escherichia coli*, *Enterobacter cloacae*, *Staphylococcus epidermidis*, *Proteus vulgaris*, *Klebsiella oxytoca*, and *K. pneumoniae*, bacterial antigens such as hemolysin, and collagen degradation products by bacteria have the ability to release histamine from mast cells [64–69]. Live, but not heat-killed, *Streptococcus pneumoniae* can induce mast cell degranulation in a dose- and time-dependent manner, only partially controlled by cytosolic calcium, with no production of TNF-alpha and IL-6 [70]. Human intestinal mast cells interact with hemolysin-producing *E. coli* strains, but not *Shigella flexneri* and several hemolysin-negative *E. coli* strains, suggesting *E. coli* hemolysin is a factor regulating mast cell functions [71]. However, high doses of nonpathogenic commensal *E. coli* bacteria can function as a strong, direct inhibitor of mast cell degranulation [72]. *Helicobacter pylori* can cause inhibition of histamine release from rat mast cells, which contributes to its persistence within the gastric mucosa [73]. Mast cells are actively involved in the pathogenesis of *Helicobacter pylori*-infected gastritis through degranulation and secreted mediators to induce inflammatory cells to infiltrate the site of edema, and may act both to maintain gastritis and to repair tissue damage in *H. pylori*-infected gastritis [74]. During middle ear inflammation, mast cells account for a substantial proportion of the innate immune response to bacteria in the middle ear [75]. Although mast cell-deficient mice exhibited more susceptibility to *Salmonella typhimurium*, and died more rapidly after infection, adoptive transfer of mast cells does not enhance the impaired survival of mast cell-deficient mice. This suggests that mast cells which have a significant role in enhancing survival during bacterial infections, may depend on the details of the particular experimental systems examined [76]. Mast cells protect the host from systemic infection by reducing the bacterial load and preventing dissemination of the bacterium from the colon following infection with *Citrobacter rodentium* [77]. During the early phase of listeriosis, mast cells control infection not via direct bacterial uptake, but by initiating neutrophils influx to the site of infection [78]. Mast cells are also important for innate immune containment of and recovery from respiratory mycoplasma infection [79]. Interestingly, Carvalho et al. reported that in a polymicrobial sepsis model in mice, where mast cells were depleted by compound 48/80 or lyzed by distilled water, neutrophil migration failed. This phenomenon was accompanied by reduction of bacteria in the peritoneal cavity and blood, serum TNF-alpha, IL-1beta, and nitrate (NO_3) and by an increase in mice survival rate, suggesting that mast cells play a key role in the genesis of neutrophil migration failure, and, consequently, contribute to the systemic inflammatory response and mortality in severe sepsis [80].

In 1994, Malaviya et al. was the first to report that mast cells can specifically bind FimH, a mannose binding subunit on type 1 fimbriae expressed by *E. coli* and other enterobacteria. This interaction triggers mast cell phagocytosis and killing of the bacteria within vacuoles and through the release of superoxide anions, and mast cells have the capacity to release inflammatory mediators and are particularly abundant in the skin, mucosal surfaces, and around blood vessels, which suggests that these cells play an important role in host defense against microbial infection [57,81–84]. In addition, *in vivo* study with mast cell-deficient mouse model demonstrated that FimH was the necessary enterobacterial component for mast cell to release TNF-alpha and to recruit neutrophil at sites of infection [85]. FimH expressed by bacteria-induced murine bone marrow-derived mast cells to produce protective modest amounts of TNF-alpha via a pathway that is distinct from that used by IgE/antigen [86]. Both human mast cell line HMC-1 5C6 and human cord blood-derived mast cell can internalize significant numbers of FimH + *E. coli*, but not its isogenic FimH− mutant, and protein kinase C (PKC) may be a critical intracellular mediator of this function [87]. Again Malaviya et al. proved CD48, a glycosylphosphatidylinositol-anchored molecule in rodent mast cell membrane fractions, to be a functionally relevant microbial receptor binding FimH expressed by bacteria, which plays a role in triggering phagocytosis and TNF-alpha release [88]. Furthermore, Shin et al. reported CD48 was specifically localized to plasmalemmal caveolae in mouse BMMCs, indicating the involvement of caveolae in bacterial entry into mast cells because caveolae-disrupting and -usurping agents specifically blocked FimH + *E. coli* entry, and markers of caveolae were actively recruited to sites of bacterial entry [89]. In experimental cystitis induced by type 1 fimbriated *E. coli*, the mast cells are activated by FimH-expressing *E. coli* and release large amount of histamine in the urinary bladder, and play a protective role to clear bacteria [90]. In addition to phagocytosis, mast cells can kill bacteria by entrapping them in extracellular structures composed of DNA, histones, tryptase, and cathelicidin antimicrobial peptides, which are similar to the extracellular traps described for neutrophils (NETs) [91]. However, *S. aureus* can overcome mast cell phagocytosis and survive within mast cell, though human cord blood-derived mast cells (CBMCs) release TNF-alpha and IL-8 and express increased TLR2 and CD48 [92].

High-density oligonucleotide probe arrays (GeneChip) analysis indicated that human mast cells might modulate the immune system in a receptor-specific manner by releasing cytokines in quantitatively and qualitatively different ways [93]. Human intestinal mast cells express the proinflammatory cytokines TNF-alpha, IL-1beta, IL-6, IL-8, IL-16, and IL-18 without further stimulation. Both IgE-dependent and IgE-independent agonists (e.g., Gram-negative bacteria) enhanced expression of TNF-alpha [94]. But addition of IL-4 to the culture medium induces the expression of Th2-type cytokines (IL-3, IL-5, and IL-13), and a downregulation of proinflammatory cytokines, namely, IL-6 [95,96]. Mast cell-derived TNF-alpha plays a critical role in host defense against Gram-negative bacterial infections by the recruitment of neutrophils to the sites of infection. And mast cells are an important source of TNF-alpha in the human intestinal mucosa. Expression of TNF-alpha mRNA and release of TNF-alpha protein were substantially enhanced by IgE receptor cross-linking and by coculture of mast cells with intestinal bacteria [97]. Cord blood-derived human mast cells also phagocytozed and killed various Gram-negative and Gram-positive bacteria and simultaneously released considerable amounts of TNF-alpha [98]. Expression of IL-1, IL-8, and CCL4 was increased by human mast cells after *Pseudomonas aeruginosa* infection [99]. Another important chemotactic factor released by mast cell is leukotriene (LT). Mast cells release significant amounts of LTB4 and LTC4 in response to exposure to FimH-expressing type 1 fimbriated *E. coli in vitro*, and LT synthesis inhibitor, A-63162, reduced neutrophil influx and bacterial clearance in the peritoneal cavities of mast cell-sufficient but not cell-deficient mice [100]. Lipoteichoic acids (LTAs) from the major components of cell walls of most Gram-positive bacteria are important bacterial antigens involved in mast cell activation during bacterial infections. LTAs from *S. aureus* and *Bacillus subtilis* induced mast cell generation and release of significant levels of LT [101]. In addition, LTAs can increase complement receptor 3 expression and enhance the uptake of opsonized bacteria, suggesting LTA increases the capability of mast cell as a sentinel in innate immune response [102]. VacA, the virulent *H. pylori* cytotoxin, directly bound and showed a chemotactic activity to the mast cell, and induced BMMCs to produce TNF-alpha, macrophage inflammatory protein-1alpha, IL-1beta, IL-6, IL-10, and IL-13 in a dose-dependent manner without causing degranulation [103]. Both *Moraxella catarrhalis* and *Neisseria cinerea* can directly make contact with mast cells and induce mast cell activation and selective secretion of two key inflammatory cytokines, IL-6 and monocyte chemotactic protein-1 (MCP-1), accompanied by NF-κB activation [104]. Mast cell IL-6 is a critical mediator of survival following *K. pneumoniae* infection and sepsis, which protects from death by augmenting neutrophil killing of bacteria [105]. Mouse mast cells express both constitutive and lipopolysaccharide-inducible IL-15 and store it intracellular. Deletion of IL-15 in mice markedly increases chymase activities, leading to greater mast cell bactericidal responses, increased processing and activation of neutrophil-recruiting chemokines, and significantly higher survival rates of mice after septic peritonitis [106].

Moreover, mast cells can process bacterial Ags for presentation through class I MHC molecules to T-cell hybridomas after phagocytic uptake of live bacteria such as Gram-negative enterobacteria including *S. typhimurium* and *E. coli*, and parallel assays show that processing of the model Ag from enterobacteria by mast cells is similar in efficiency to processing by peritoneal macrophages [107].

Murine mast cells express CD28 costimulatory molecule, which has functions similar to those of T-cell CD28 and can be modulated by lipopolysaccharide (LPS) and outer surface protein A lipoprotein from *Borrelia burgdorferi* [108]. In addition, mast cells express MHC class II antigens, ICAM-1 and -3, CD43, CD80, CD86, and CD40L, which allow them to interact with T and B lymphocytes [15]. Mast cells are able to process and present *Bordetella pertussis* antigens to T lymphocytes and *B. pertussis* also induced mast cell to release proinflammatory cytokines TNF-alpha and IL-6 [109].

Mast cells make and secrete an abundance of peptidases such as tryptases and chymases, which are important and even critical for host defense and homeostasis [110]. Human pulmonary mast cells express tryptases alpha and beta I. Huang et al. reported that only tryptase beta I-treated mast cell-deficient mice had fewer viable *K. pneumoniae* in their lungs relative to inactive zymogen-treated mast cell-deficient mice. Their data indicated mast cell tryptase beta I plays a critical role in the antibacterial host defenses of the lung by recruiting neutrophils in a manner that does not alter airway reactivity [111]. Mouse mast cell protease 6 is a tetramer-forming tryptase that is abundant in the secretory granules and is exocytozed upon bacterial challenge, and mice lacking this neutral protease cannot efficiently clear *K. pneumoniae* from their peritoneal cavities, which reveal an essential role for this serine protease in innate immunity [112].

Janus kinase 3 (JAK3), a tyrosine kinase that belongs to the Janus family, is predominantly expressed in immune cells and transduces a signal in response to its activation via tyrosine phosphorylation by interleukin receptors. Malaviya et al. reported the neutrophil influx, bacterial clearance, and survival outcome in mast cell-deficient mice reconstituted with JAK3($+/+$) mast cells were better than in mast cell-deficient mice reconstituted with JAK3($-/-$) mast cells, providing evidence that JAK3 is a key regulator of mast cell-mediated innate immunity against Gram-negative bacteria [113]. Smad3, a major signal transducer of TGF-beta, also regulates innate immune response by mast cells. BMMCs obtained from Smad3 null mutant mice showed augmented capacity to produce proinflammatory cytokines upon stimulation with LPS. In acute septic peritonitis model induced by cecal ligation and puncture, mast cell-deficient mice reconstituted with Smad3 null BMMC had significantly higher survival rate associated with higher production of proinflammatory cytokines in the peritoneal cavity, suggesting that Smad3 deficiency in mast cells provides efficient host protection against acute septic peritonitis [114].

Toll-like receptors (TLRs) are mammalian homologues of the Drosophila Toll receptors and play key role in the innate immune system. They are single membrane-spanning noncatalytic receptors that recognize structurally conserved molecules derived from microbes. Once these microbes have breached physical barriers such as the skin or intestinal tract mucosa, they are recognized by TLRs that activate immune cell responses [115,116]. In humans, TLR1, 2, 4, 5, and 6 are outer membrane associated and TLR3, 7, 8, and 9 are found on the surface of endosomes. And it is interesting to note that the expression of TLRs in humans is highly variable and this has been linked to susceptibility to infections [117]. TLRs are primarily found on macrophages, mast cells, and dendritic cells, the three sentinel cells of the innate immunity. Mast cells express all TLRs though there are some important species-specific differences in the expression and function of TLRs on mast cells from different sources or exposed to different cytokine environments [16,118–120]. The core pathway utilized by most TLRs leads to activation of the transcription factor NF-κB and the MAPKs (mitogen-activated protein kinases) p38 and JNK (c-Jun N-terminal kinase). However, the activation of TLRs on these cells begins a complex set of signaling cascades that are not yet completely understood. TLR2 and TLR4 play important roles in the different innate immune responses of mast cells against bacteria. Live *S. equi* infection of mast cells causes a TLR2- and cell–cell contact-dependent cytokine and chemokine response [121]. TLR4 was required for a full responsiveness of BMMCs to produce IL-1beta, TNF-alpha, IL-6, and IL-13 by *E. coli* LPS stimulation, and in the cecal ligation and puncture-induced acute septic peritonitis model, higher mortality of TLR4-mutated BMMC-reconstituted mast cell-deficient mice was well correlated with defective neutrophil recruitment and production of proinflammatory cytokines in the peritoneal cavity [122], whereas peptidoglycan (PGN) from *S. aureus* stimulated mast cells in a TLR2-dependent manner to produce TNF-alpha, IL-4, IL-5, IL-6, and IL-13, but not IL-1beta. Intradermal injection of PGN led to increased vasodilatation and inflammation through TLR2-dependent activation of mast cells in the skin [123]. Both LPS and PGN enhanced expression of promatrix metalloproteinase-9 (pro-MMP-9) in a dose-dependent manner, and DNA fragmentation was induced by LPS but not by PGN [124]. PGN from Gram-positive bacteria-induced lymph node (LN) hypertrophy and migration of Langerhans cells (LCs) to draining LNs were dependent on the presence of mast cells, which did not require TLR2, TLR4, or MYD88. TNF-deficient mice exhibited normal increases in LN cellularity, but significantly reduced LC migration, demonstrating a critical role for mast cells in LN responses to PGN and illustrating a novel TNF-independent mechanism whereby mast cells participate in the initiation of immunity [125].

The cysteine protease dipeptidyl peptidase I (DPPI) activates granule-associated serine proteases, several of which play important roles in host responses to bacterial infection. Mallen-St Clair et al. reported that the absence of DPPI in mast cells, rather than in other cell types, is responsible for the survival advantage in cecal ligation and puncture model, but deleting IL-6 expression in DPPI(−/−) mice eliminates the survival advantage, indicating that mast cell DPPI harms the septic host and that DPPI is a novel potential therapeutic target for treatment of sepsis [126].

Although cathelicidin antimicrobial peptides are originally found in neutrophils, they have also been found in many other cells including epithelial cells and macrophages after activation by bacteria, viruses, fungi, or the hormone 1,25-vitamin D [127]. Cathelicidins serve a critical role in innate immune defense against invasive bacterial infection [128]. LL-37, human cathelicidin antimicrobial peptide, has at least two classes of receptors, namely, high- and low-affinity receptors, on mast cells. LL-37 induces mast cell degranulation and chemotaxis through a Gi protein-phospholipase C signaling pathway, indicating that besides its antibacterial activities, LL-37 may have the potential to recruit mast cells to inflammation foci [129]. LL-37 can increase the level of TLR4 and induce the release of IL-4, IL-5, and IL-1beta from mast cells. LL-37 coexisting with the bacterial component switches mast cell function and directs human mast cells toward innate immunity [130]. Di Nardo et al. were the first to report that cathelicidins are also expressed in cultured murine or human skin mast cells and this expression is necessary for efficient bacterial killing, suggesting that the presence of cathelicidins is vital to the ability of mast cells to participate in antimicrobial defense [131]. Furthermore, using mast cell-deficient mice and cathelicidin-deficient mice, Di Nardo et al. demonstrated that mast cells help protect against invasive group A *Streptococcus* infection of the skin through the expression of cathelicidin that was purified from mast cells and defined as a unique 28-aa peptide by surface-enhanced laser desorption/ionization time-of-flight mass spectrometry (SELDI-TOF-MS) analysis [132].

In summary, interaction between bacteria and mast cell results in mast cell activation and mediator release eliciting an inflammatory response or direct killing leading to bacterial clearance [133,134]. The *in vivo* relevance of these *in vitro* observations has been demonstrated by the use of mast cell-deficient and mast cell-reconstituted mice [135]. Although it is uncertain whether mast cells participate in innate immune responses in human against bacteria, mast cells do play a role in innate immunity in animal models of bacterial infection.

9.4 MAST CELLS RESPONSES TO FUNGI

Fungi are one of the four major groups of microorganisms (bacteria, viruses, parasites, and fungi). Fungal infections range from superficial, localized skin conditions to deeper tissue infections to serious lung, blood (septicemia), or systemic diseases. Most fungal infections occur when there is a break or deficiency in the host defenses such as organ transplantation, HIV infection, chemotherapy, diabetes, or lung disease [136]. However, our knowledge of mast cell and fungi is very limited.

Early in 1960, Sheldon et al. histologically studied the role of the tissue mast cells in relation to the acute inflammatory reaction to experimental cutaneous mucormycosis in rats. They found in normal rats that the function of tissue mast cell response to fungi, is releasing granules and initiating the rapid onset of acute inflammation. In animals whose tissue mast cells had been depleted of their cytoplasmic granules prior to infection, the onset of inflammation was briefly delayed and the fungus growth in the early lesions was increased. However, the infection did not spread and the lesions were well localized. The tissue mast cells in the diabetic and acidotic rats completely failed to discharge their cytoplasmic granules, the onset and intensity of the acute inflammatory response were markedly delayed and decreased, and the infection progressed rapidly with massive fungus growth invading adjacent tissues, suggesting that a severe metabolic disorder inhibits the normal function of mast cells and contributes to the greatly increased susceptibility of the host to infection [137].

Since then, there have been only a few studies on mast cell and fungi. Gliotoxin, one of the fungal secondary metabolites, has suppressive effects on mast cell degranulation, leukotriene C4 secretion, and TNF-alpha and IL-13 production, by a calcium- and superoxide-dependent mechanism, indicating that suppression of mast cell activation might contribute to the establishment of gliotoxin-producing fungal infections [138]. However, fungal zymosan induces significant amounts of LTB4 and LTC4 production by human mast cells through a coreceptor dectin-1-dependent mechanism [139].

Thus, interactions between mast cell and fungi are very poorly understood. How mast cells participate in innate immune responses against fungi remains unclear, and mast cell's role in fungi infection need to be proved with mast cell-deficient and mast cell-reconstituted animal models.

9.5 MAST CELLS RESPONSES TO VIRUSES

Most virus infections eventually result in the death of the host cell. The causes of death include cell lysis, alterations to the cell's surface membrane, and apoptosis. The ability of viruses to cause devastating epidemics in human societies has led to the concern that viruses could be weaponized for biological warfare. Since innate immune system is the first line of defense against viruses and mast cell has very important role in innate immunity [15,133], more and more research endeavors focused on the interaction between mast cell and virus, though mast cell's role in viral infection has not yet been fully elucidated.

Many research works demonstrated that mast cells can be activated by viruses to increase numbers [140–144] and release contents of the granules [145]. Sendai virus generates permeability lesions in the membrane of rat mast cells and induces histamine [146] and beta-N-acetylglucosaminidase release by a normal exocytotic secretory mechanism [147]. Sindbis virus induces vasoactive amines release by mast cells in the central nervous system, which plays a facilitating role in the development of the inflammatory response [148]. Parainfluenza-3 virus induces enhancement of histamine release from calf lung mast cells [149]. There is a significant increase in mast cell density in the tissues of patients with chronic hepatitis C virus (HCV) infection [150]. During respiratory syncytial virus (RSV) infection, mast cell degranulation occurred only in coculture with RSV-infected A549 airway epithelial cells, with upregulation of TNF-alpha secretion; however, direct RSV infection into mast cells or incubation with RSV-infected A549 cell culture medium failed to induce mast cell degranulation, suggesting that RSV-infected cells are critical for degranulation [151]. Interestingly, lactic dehydrogenase virus infection can suppress lung mastocytosis induced by nematode *N. brasiliensis*, which enhances parasite egg production [152].

Mast cells are susceptible to antibody-enhanced dengue virus infection, degranulating, producing histamine, IL-1, IL-6, and CCL5 [153–155]. In addition, antibody-enhanced dengue virus results in a massive induction of caspase-dependent apoptosis in mast cells [156]. Specific FcgammaRII blockade can significantly abrogate dengue virus binding to mast cells and inhibit dengue virus infection and the production of CCL5 by mast cells [157].

Murine and human mast cells produce type I IFNs after exposure to double-stranded RNA and/or virus, the former via specific interactions with TLR3, suggesting that mast cells contribute to innate immune responses to viral infection via the production of type I IFNs [119].

Both mast cell progenitors (c-kit(+) CD13(+) cells with chloroacetate esterase activity) and mast cells are susceptible to infection with retrovirus, macrophagetropic (M-tropic) human immunodeficiency virus type 1 (HIV-1) due to their surface expression of CD4 and the chemokine receptors CCR3, CCR5, and CXCR4. HIV-1 glycoprotein gp120 acts as a viral superantigen to induce cytokine release from mast cells. And the trafficking of mast cell progenitors to multiple tissues, combined with the long lifespan of mature mast cells, suggests that they provide a widespread and persistent HIV reservoir in AIDS [158–161]. Furthermore, *in vivo* evidence also indicates that tissue mast cells, developed from infected circulating progenitor mast cells, comprise a long-lived inducible reservoir of persistent HIV in infected persons [162]. IgE-FcepsilonRI interactions significantly increase expression of CXCR4 mRNA, enhance mast cell progenitor susceptibility to X4 and R5X4 HIV, but have no significant effect on CD4, CCR3, or CCR5 expression, susceptibility to R5 HIV, or degranulation [163]. Because IL-16 is a ligand for CD4 and/or an undefined CD4-associated protein, IL-16-treated mast cells are less susceptible to infection by an M/R5-tropic strain of HIV-1 [164]. Stimulation by ligands for TLR2, TLR4, or TLR9 significantly enhanced viral replication in both HIV-1-infected mast cell progenitor and latently infected mature mast cells, without promoting degranulation, apoptosis, cellular proliferation, or dysregulation of TLR agonist-induced cytokine production in infected mast cells [165]. However, Nelson et al. reported that tissue mast cells do not show evidence for active HIV replication by immunohistochemistry analysis of various tissue sites of HIV patients, which challenges the hypothesis that mast cell population is a significant reservoir for persistent HIV infection [166].

Mast cells can recruit granulocytes and monocytes in allergic disease and bacterial infection [58,167], but their ability to recruit antiviral effector cells such as natural killer (NK) cells and T cells has not been fully elucidated. Burke et al. reported that human cord blood-derived mast cells can produce significant amounts of CXCL8 in response to low levels of reovirus infection, and supernatants from CBMCs infected with reovirus-induced substantial NK cell chemotaxis that was highly dependent on CXCL8 and CXCR1, suggesting a role of mast cells in the recruitment of human NK cells to sites of early viral infection via CXCL8 [168].

Mast cells can protect against bacterial infection through the expression of cathelicidin antimicrobial peptides [131,132]; however, it is not clear whether they can also use these antimicrobial peptides to fight viruses. Recently, by using cathelicidin-deficient mice, mast cell-deficient mice, and mast cell-reconstituted mice, Wang et al. found that cathelicidin-deficient BMMCs are more susceptible to vaccinia virus infection than wild-type BMMCs, and mast cells play a role in defense against vaccinia virus by expression of cathelicidin antimicrobial peptides via TLR2 [169].

Therefore, mast cells may play both negative and positive roles in response to different types of viruses. Although mechanisms involved in interaction between mast cell and virus have not been fully understood and the roles of mast cell in virus infection in human still remain unclear, mast cells do play a role in innate immunity against virus in animal model.

9.6 CONCLUSIONS

As discussed in this chapter, hundreds of research studies provide compelling evidence that mast cells have a crucial role in innate immunity though little is known on this role in humans. But in clinic, mast cells are ignored as effector cells that can benefit the host defense and are still regarded as harmful cells initiating allergic and inflammatory diseases, which need to be treated with corticosteroids, antihistamines, and mast cell stabilizing agents to inhibit mast cell function that is necessary for them to perform their sentinel task in innate immunity. Thus, the opinion about mast cells needs to be updated, and more studies are required to fully demonstrate the role and mechanism of mast cell involved in host defense. Moreover, the strategic locations of mast cells and their selective production of potent immunomodulatory mediators provide us opportunities to develop novel effective therapies for treatment of infectious diseases and immune-related disorders.

REFERENCES

1. Crivellato E, Beltrami C, Mallardi F, Ribatti D. Paul Ehrlich's doctoral thesis: a milestone in the study of mast cells. *Br. J. Haematol.* 2003;123:19–21.
2. Wasserman SI. Mast cell-mediated inflammation in asthma. *Ann. Allergy* 1989;63:546–550.
3. Tsai M, Shih LS, Newlands GF, Takeishi T, Langley KE, Zsebo KM, Miller HR, Geissler EN, Galli SJ. The rat c-kit ligand, stem cell factor, induces the development of connective tissue-type and mucosal mast cells in vivo. Analysis by anatomical distribution, histochemistry, and protease phenotype. *J. Exp. Med.* 1991;174:125–131.
4. Schrader JW, Lewis SJ, Clark-Lewis I, Culvenor JG. The persisting (P) cell: histamine content, regulation by a T cell-derived factor, origin from a bone marrow precursor, and relationship to mast cells. *Proc. Natl. Acad. Sci. USA* 1981;78:323–327.
5. Ihle JN, Keller J, Oroszlan S, Henderson LE, Copeland TD, Fitch F, Prystowsky MB, Goldwasser E, Schrader JW, Palaszynski E, Dy M, Lebel B. Biologic properties of homogeneous interleukin 3. I. Demonstration of WEHI-3 growth factor activity, mast cell growth factor activity, p cell-stimulating factor activity, colony-stimulating factor activity, and histamine-producing cell-stimulating factor activity. *J. Immunol.* 1983;131:282–287.
6. Saito H, Ebisawa M, Tachimoto H, Shichijo M, Fukagawa K, Matsumoto K, Iikura Y, Awaji T, Tsujimoto G, Yanagida M, Uzumaki H, Takahashi G, Tsuji K, Nakahata T. Selective growth of human mast cells induced by Steel factor, IL-6, and prostaglandin E2 from cord blood mononuclear cells. *J. Immunol.* 1996;157:343–350.

7. Costa JJ, Demetri GD, Harrist TJ, Dvorak AM, Hayes DF, Merica EA, Menchaca DM, Gringeri AJ, Schwartz LB, Galli SJ. Recombinant human stem cell factor (kit ligand) promotes human mast cell and melanocyte hyperplasia and functional activation *in vivo*. *J. Exp. Med.* 1996;183:2681–2686.

8. Enerback L, Lowhagen GB. Long term increase of mucosal mast cells in the rat induced by administration of compound 48/80. *Cell Tissue Res.* 1979;198:209–215.

9. Marone G, Casolaro V, Patella V, Florio G, Triggiani M. Molecular and cellular biology of mast cells and basophils. *Int. Arch. Allergy Immunol.* 1997;114:207–217.

10. Church MK, Levi-Schaffer F. The human mast cell. *J. Allergy Clin. Immunol.* 1997;99:155–160.

11. Schwartz LB, Irani AM, Roller K, Castells MC, Schechter NM. Quantitation of histamine, tryptase, and chymase in dispersed human T and TC mast cells. *J. Immunol.* 1987;138:2611–2615.

12. Kraemer R. Mechanisms of allergic reactions and potential therapeutic approach in childhood bronchial asthma. *Schweiz. Rundsch. Med. Prax.* 1987;76:581–585.

13. Galli SJ, Maurer M, Lantz CS. Mast cells as sentinels of innate immunity. *Curr. Opin. Immunol.* 1999;11:53–59.

14. Abraham SN, Thankavel K, Malaviya R. Mast cells as modulators of host defense in the lung. *Front. Biosci.* 1997;2:d78–d87.

15. Henz BM, Maurer M, Lippert U, Worm M, Babina M. Mast cells as initiators of immunity and host defense. *Exp. Dermatol.* 2001;10:1–10.

16. Marshall JS. Mast-cell responses to pathogens. *Nat. Rev. Immunol.* 2004;4:787–799.

17. Archer GT, Robson JE, Thompson AR. Eosinophilia and mast cell hyperplasia induced by parasite phospholipid. *Pathology* 1977;9:137–153.

18. Huntley JF, Newlands GF, Miller HR, McLauchlan M, Rose ME, Hesketh P. Systemic release of mucosal mast cell protease during infection with the intestinal protozoal parasite, *Eimeria nieschulzi*. Studies in normal and nude rats. *Parasite Immunol.* 1985;7:489–501.

19. Alizadeh H, Urban JF, Jr., Katona IM, Finkelman FD. Cells containing IgE in the intestinal mucosa of mice infected with the nematode parasite *Trichinella spiralis* are predominantly of a mast cell lineage. *J. Immunol.* 1986;137:2555–2560.

20. McHardy P, Riley J, Huntley JF. The recruitment of mast cells, exclusively of the mucosal phenotype, into granulomatous lesions caused by the pentastomid parasite *Porocephalus crotali*: recruitment is irrespective of site. *Parasitology*. 1993;106(Pt 1):47–54.

21. Uber CL, Roth RL, Levy DA. Expulsion of *Nippostrongylus brasiliensis* by mice deficient in mast cells. *Nature* 1980;287:226–228.

22. Crowle PK, Reed ND. Rejection of the intestinal parasite *Nippostrongylus brasiliensis* by mast cell-deficient W/Wv anemic mice. *Infect. Immun.* 1981;33:54–58.

23. Lee TD, Wakelin D. The use of host strain variation to assess the significance of mucosal mast cells in the spontaneous cure response of mice to the nematode *Trichuris muris*. *Int. Arch. Allergy Appl. Immunol.* 1982;67:302–305.

24. Crowle PK. Mucosal mast cell reconstitution and *Nippostrongylus brasiliensis* rejection by W/Wv mice. *J. Parasitol.* 1983;69:66–69.

25. Levy DA, Frondoza C. Immunity to intestinal parasites: role of mast cells and goblet cells. *Fed. Proc.* 1983;42:1750–1755.

26. Miller HR, Woodbury RG, Huntley JF, Newlands G. Systemic release of mucosal mast-cell protease in primed rats challenged with *Nippostrongylus brasiliensis*. *Immunology* 1983;49:471–479.

27. King SJ, Miller HR, Newlands GF, Woodbury RG. Depletion of mucosal mast cell protease by corticosteroids: effect on intestinal anaphylaxis in the rat. *Proc. Natl. Acad. Sci. USA* 1985;82:1214–1218.

28. Gil CD, Mineo JR, Smith RL, Oliani SM. Mast cells in the eyes of *Calomys callosus* (Rodentia: Cricetidae) infected by *Toxoplasma gondii*. *Parasitol. Res.* 2002;88:557–562.

29. Ferreira GLS, Mineo JR, Oliveira JG, Ferro EAV, Souza MA, Santos AAD. *Toxoplasma gondii* and mast cell interactions *in vivo* and *in vitro*: experimental infection approaches in *Calomys callosus* (Rodentia, Cricetidae). *Microbes Infect.* 2004;6:172–181.

30. Barrett KE, Neva FA, Gam AA, Cicmanec J, London WT, Phillips JM, Metcalfe DD. The immune response to nematode parasites: modulation of mast cell numbers and function during *Strongyloides stercoralis* infections in nonhuman primates. *Am. J. Trop. Med. Hyg.* 1988;38:574–581.

31. Perdue MH, Ramage JK, Burget D, Marshall J, Masson S. Intestinal mucosal injury is associated with mast cell activation and leukotriene generation during Nippostrongylus-induced inflammation in the rat. *Dig. Dis. Sci.* 1989;34:724–731.

32. Swieter M, Ghali WA, Rimmer C, Befus D. Interferon-alpha/beta inhibits IgE-dependent histamine release from rat mast cells. *Immunology* 1989;66:606–610.

33. Miller HR. Mucosal mast cells and the allergic response against nematode parasites. *Vet. Immunol. Immunopathol.* 1996;54:331–336.

34. Newlands GF, Miller HR, MacKellar A, Galli SJ. Stem cell factor contributes to intestinal mucosal mast cell hyperplasia in rats infected with *Nippostrongylus brasiliensis* or *Trichinella spiralis,* but anti-stem cell factor treatment decreases parasite egg production during *N. brasiliensis* infection. *Blood* 1995;86:1968–1976.

35. Miller HR, Newlands GF, McKellar A, Inglis L, Coulson PS, Wilson RA. Hepatic recruitment of mast cells occurs in rats but not mice infected with *Schistosoma mansoni. Parasite Immunol.* 1994;16:145–155.

36. Bidri M, Vouldoukis I, Mossalayi MD, Debre P, Guillosson JJ, Mazier D, Arock M. Evidence for direct interaction between mast cells and *Leishmania* parasites. *Parasite Immunol.* 1997;19:475–483.

37. Von Stebut, E. Immunology of cutaneous leishmaniasis: the role of mast cells, phagocytes and dendritic cells for protective immunity. *Eur. J. Dermatol.* 2007;17:115–122.

38. Lantz CS, Boesiger J, Song CH, Mach N, Kobayashi T, Mulligan RC, Nawa Y, Dranoff G, Galli SJ. Role for interleukin-3 in mast-cell and basophil development and in immunity to parasites. *Nature* 1998;392:90–93.

39. McLauchlan PE, Roberts HC, Loxton NJ, Wastling JM, Newlands GF, Chappell LH. Mucosal mast cell responses and release of mast cell protease-I in infections of mice with *Hymenolepis diminuta* and *H. microstoma*: modulation by cyclosporin A. *Parasite Immunol.* 1999;21:151–161.

40. Koyama K, Ito Y. Mucosal mast cell responses are not required for protection against infection with the murine nematode parasite *Trichuris muris. Parasite Immunol.* 2000;22:13–20.

41. Onah DN, Uchiyama F, Nagakui Y, Ono M, Takai T, Nawa Y. Mucosal defense against gastrointestinal nematodes: responses of mucosal mast cells and mouse mast cell protease 1 during primary *Strongyloides venezuelensis* infection in FcRgamma-knockout mice. *Infect. Immun.* 2000;68:4968–4971.

42. Urban JF, Jr., Schopf L, Morris SC, Orekhova T, Madden KB, Betts CJ, Gamble HR, Byrd C, Donaldson D, Else K, Finkelman FD. Stat6 signaling promotes protective immunity against *Trichinella spiralis* through a mast cell- and T cell-dependent mechanism. *J. Immunol.* 2000;164:2046–2052.

43. Sasaki Y, Yoshimoto T, Maruyama H, Tegoshi T, Ohta N, Arizono N, Nakanishi K. IL-18 with IL-2 protects against *Strongyloides venezuelensis* infection by activating mucosal mast cell-dependent type 2 innate immunity. *J. Exp. Med.* 2005;202:607–616.

44. Wiener Z, Pocza P, Racz M, Nagy G, Tolgyesi G, Molnar V, Jaeger J, Buzas E, Gorbe E, Papp Z, Rigo J, Falus A. IL-18 induces a marked gene expression profile change and increased Ccl1 (I-309) production in mouse mucosal mast cell homologs. *Int. Immunol.* 2008;20:1565–1573.

45. Issekutz TB, Palecanda A, Kadela-Stolarz U, Marshall JS. Blockade of either alpha-4 or beta-7 integrins selectively inhibits intestinal mast cell hyperplasia and worm expulsion in response to *Nippostrongylus brasiliensis* infection. *Eur. J. Immunol.* 2001;31:860–868.

46. McDermott JR, Bartram RE, Knight P A, Miller HR, Garrod DR, Grencis RK. Mast cells disrupt epithelial barrier function during enteric nematode infection. *Proc. Natl. Acad. Sci. USA* 2003;100:7761–7766.

47. Gurish MF, Bryce PJ, Tao H, Kisselgof AB, Thornton EM, Miller HR, Friend DS, Oettgen HC. IgE enhances parasite clearance and regulates mast cell responses in mice infected with *Trichinella spiralis. J. Immunol.* 2004;172:1139–1145.

48. Li E, Zhou P, Petrin Z, Singer SM. Mast cell-dependent control of *Giardia lamblia* infections in mice. *Infect. Immun.* 2004;72:6642–6649.

49. Onah DN, Nawa Y. Mucosal mast cell-derived chondroitin sulphate levels in and worm expulsion from FcRgamma-knockout mice following oral challenge with *Strongyloides venezuelensis. J. Vet. Sci.* 2004;5:221–226.

50. Pennock JL, Grencis RK. *In vivo* exit of c-kit + /CD49d(hi)/beta7+ mucosal mast cell precursors from the bone marrow following infection with the intestinal nematode *Trichinella spiralis. Blood* 2004;103:2655–2660.

51. Li E, Zhao A, Shea-Donohue T, Singer SM. Mast cell-mediated changes in smooth muscle contractility during mouse giardiasis. *Infect. Immun.* 2007;75:4514–4518.

52. Ierna MX, Scales HE, Saunders KL, Lawrence CE. Mast cell production of IL-4 and TNF may be required for protective and pathological responses in gastrointestinal helminth infection. *Mucosal. Immunol.* 2008;1:147–155.

53. Villasenor-Cardoso MI, Salaiza N, Delgado J, Gutierrez-Kobeh L, Perez-Torres A, Becker I. Mast cells are activated by *Leishmania mexicana* LPG and regulate the disease outcome depending on the genetic background of the host. *Parasite Immunol.* 2008;30(8):425–434.

54. Romao PR, Da Costa Santiago H, Ramos CD, De Oliveira CF, Monteiro MC, De Queiroz Cunha F, Vieira LQ. Mast cell degranulation contributes to susceptibility to *Leishmania major. Parasite Immunol.* 2009;31:140–146.

55. Blum LK, Thrasher SM, Gagliardo LF, Fabre V, Appleton JA. Expulsion of secondary *Trichinella spiralis* infection in rats occurs independently of mucosal mast cell release of mast cell protease II. *J. Immunol.* 2009;183:5816–5822.

56. Pennock JL, Grencis RK. The mast cell and gut nematodes: damage and defence. *Chem. Immunol. Allergy* 2006;90:128–140.

57. Erb KJ, Holloway JW, Le Gros G. Mast cells in the front line: innate immunity. *Curr. Biol.* 1996;6:941–942.

58. Malaviya R, Abraham SN. Mast cell modulation of immune responses to bacteria. *Immunol. Rev.* 2001;179:16–24.

59. Abraham SN, Arock M. Mast cells and basophils in innate immunity. *Semin. Immunol.* 1998;10:373–381.

60. Malaviya R, Abraham SN. Clinical implications of mast cell-bacteria interaction. *J. Mol. Med.* 1998;76:617–623.

61. Sher A, Hein A, Moser G, Caulfield JP. Complement receptors promote the phagocytosis of bacteria by rat peritoneal mast cells. *Lab Invest.* 1979;41:490–499.

62. Prodeus AP, Zhou X, Maurer M, Galli SJ, Carroll MC. Impaired mast cell-dependent natural immunity in complement C3-deficient mice. *Nature* 1997;390:172–175.

63. Tavarela Veloso F, Vaz Saleiro J. Mast cells in Whipple's disease. *J. Submicrosc. Cytol.* 1982;14:515–520.

64. Church MK, Norn S, Pao GJ, Holgate ST. Non-IgE-dependent bacteria-induced histamine release from human lung and tonsillar mast cells. *Clin. Allergy* 1987;17:341–353.

65. Brzezinska-Blaszczyk E, Gaik A, Czuwaj M, Kuna P. Histamine release from human pulmonary mast cells induced by bacterial antigens. *Allergol. Immunopathol. (Madr)* 1988;16:375–378.

66. Wize J, Wojtecka-Lukasik E, Maslinski S. Collagen-derived peptides release mast cell histamine. *Agents Actions* 1986;18:262–265.

67. Konig B, Konig W, Scheffer J, Hacker J, Goebel W. Role of *Escherichia coli* alpha-hemolysin and bacterial adherence in infection: requirement for release of inflammatory mediators from granulocytes and mast cells. *Infect. Immun.* 1986;54:886–892.

68. Scheffer J, Vosbeck K, Konig W. Induction of inflammatory mediators from human polymorphonuclear granulocytes and rat mast cells by haemolysin-positive and -negative *E. coli* strains with different adhesins. *Immunology* 1986;59:541–548.

69. Gross-Weege W, Konig W, Scheffer J, Nimmich W. Induction of histamine release from rat mast cells and human.basophilic granulocytes by clinical *Escherichia coli* isolates and relation to hemolysin production and adhesin expression. *J. Clin. Microbiol.* 1988;26:1831–1837.

70. Barbuti G, Moschioni M, Censini S, Covacci A, Montecucco C, Montemurro P. *Streptococcus pneumoniae* induces mast cell degranulation. *Int. J. Med. Microbiol.* 2006;296:325–329.

71. Kramer S, Sellge G, Lorentz A, Krueger D, Schemann M, Feilhauer K, Gunzer F, Bischoff SC. Selective activation of human intestinal mast cells by *Escherichia coli* hemolysin. *J. Immunol.* 2008;181:1438–1445.

72. Magerl M, Lammel V, Siebenhaar F, Zuberbier T, Metz M, Maurer M. Non-pathogenic commensal *Escherichia coli* bacteria can inhibit degranulation of mast cells. *Exp. Dermatol.* 2008;17:427–435.

73. Lutton DA, Bamford KB, O'Loughlin B, Ennis M. Modulatory action of *Helicobacter pylori* on histamine release from mast cells and basophils *in vitro*. *J. Med. Microbiol.* 1995;42:386–393.

74. Nakajima S, Bamba N, Hattori T. Histological aspects and role of mast cells in *Helicobacter pylori*-infected gastritis. *Aliment Pharmacol. Ther.* 2004;20(Suppl. 1):165–170.

75. Ebmeyer J, Furukawa M, Pak K, Ebmeyer U, Sudhoff H, Broide D, Ryan AF, Wasserman S. Role of mast cells in otitis media. *J. Allergy Clin. Immunol.* 2005;116:1129–1135.

76. Chatterjea D, Burns-Guydish SM, Sciuto TE, Dvorak A, Contag CH, Galli SJ. Adoptive transfer of mast cells does not enhance the impaired survival of Kit(W)/Kit(W-v) mice in a model of low dose intra-peritoneal infection with bioluminescent *Salmonella typhimurium*. *Immunol. Lett.* 2005;99:122–129.

77. Wei OL, Hilliard A, Kalman D, Sherman M. Mast cells limit systemic bacterial dissemination but not colitis in response to *Citrobacter rodentium*. *Infect. Immun.* 2005;73:1978–1985.

78. Gekara NO, Weiss S. Mast cells initiate early anti-Listeria host defences. *Cell. Microbiol.* 2008;10:225–236.

79. Xu X, Zhang D, Lyubynska N, Wolters PJ, Killeen NP, Baluk P, McDonald DM, Hawgood S, Caughey GH. Mast cells protect mice from *Mycoplasma pneumonia*. *Am. J. Respir. Crit. Care Med.* 2006;173:219–225.

80. Carvalho M, Benjamim C, Santos F, Ferreira S, Cunha F. Effect of mast cells depletion on the failure of neutrophil migration during sepsis. *Eur. J. Pharmacol.* 2005;525:161–169.

81. Malaviya R, Ikeda T, Ross EA, Jakschik BA, Abraham SN. Bacteria—mast cell interactions in inflammatory disease. *Am. J. Ther.* 1995;2:787–792.

82. Malaviya R, Abraham SN. Interaction of bacteria with mast cells. *Methods Enzymol.* 1995;253:27–43.

83. Malaviya R, Ross E, Jakschik BA, Abraham SN. Mast cell degranulation induced by type 1 fimbriated *Escherichia coli* in mice. *J. Clin. Invest.* 1994;93:1645–1653.

84. Malaviya R, Ross EA, MacGregor JI, Ikeda T, Little JR, Jakschik BA, Abraham SN. Mast cell phagocytosis of FimH-expressing enterobacteria. *J. Immunol.* 1994;152:1907–1914.

85. Malaviya R, Ikeda T, Ross E, Abraham SN. Mast cell modulation of neutrophil influx and bacterial clearance at sites of infection through TNF-alpha. *Nature* 1996;381:77–80.

86. Dreskin SC, Abraham SN. Production of TNF-alpha by murine bone marrow derived mast cells activated by the bacterial fimbrial protein, FimH. *Clin. Immunol.* 1999;90:420–424.

87. Lin, TJ, Gao Z, Arock Z, Abraham SN. Internalization of FimH+ *Escherichia coli* by the human mast cell line (HMC-1 5C6) involves protein kinase C. *J. Leukoc. Biol.* 1999;66:1031–1038.

88. Malaviya R, Gao Z, Thankavel K, van der Merwe PA, Abraham SN. The mast cell tumor necrosis factor alpha response to FimH-expressing *Escherichia coli* is mediated by the glycosylphosphatidylinositol-anchored molecule CD48. *Proc. Natl. Acad. Sci. USA* 1999;96:8110–8115.

89. Shin JS, Gao Z, Abraham SN. Involvement of cellular caveolae in bacterial entry into mast cells. *Science* 2000;289:785–788.

90. Malaviya R, Ikeda T, Abraham SN. Contribution of mast cells to bacterial clearance and their proliferation during experimental cystitis induced by type 1 fimbriated *E. coli*. *Immunol. Lett.* 2004;91:103–111.

91. von Kockritz-Blickwede M, Goldmann O, Thulin P, Heinemann K, Norrby-Teglund A, Rohde M, Medina E. Phagocytosis-independent antimicrobial activity of mast cells by means of extracellular trap formation. *Blood* 2008;111:3070–3080.

92. Rocha-de-Souza CM, Berent-Maoz B, Mankuta D, Moses AE, Levi-Schaffer F. Human mast cell activation by *Staphylococcus aureus*: interleukin-8 and tumor necrosis factor alpha release and the role of Toll-like receptor 2 and CD48 molecules. *Infect. Immun.* 2008;76:4489–4497.

93. Okayama Y. Mast cell-derived cytokine expression induced via Fc receptors and Toll-like receptors. *Chem. Immunol. Allergy* 2005;87:101–110.

94. Lorentz A, Schwengberg S, Sellge G, Manns MP, Bischoff SC. Human intestinal mast cells are capable of producing different cytokine profiles: role of IgE receptor cross-linking and IL-4. *J. Immunol.* 2000;164:43–48.

95. Lorentz A, Bischoff SC. Regulation of human intestinal mast cells by stem cell factor and IL-4. *Immunol. Rev.* 2001;179:57–60.
96. Bischoff, SC, Sellge G, Manns MP, Lorentz A. Interleukin-4 induces a switch of human intestinal mast cells from proinflammatory cells to Th2-type cells. *Int. Arch. Allergy Immunol.* 2001;124:151–154.
97. Bischoff SC, Lorentz A, Schwengberg S, Weier G, Raab R, Manns MP. Mast cells are an important cellular source of tumour necrosis factor alpha in human intestinal tissue. *Gut* 1999;44:643–652.
98. Arock M, Ross E, Lai-Kuen R, Averlant G, Gao Z, Abraham SN. Phagocytic and tumor necrosis factor alpha response of human mast cells following exposure to Gram-negative and Gram-positive bacteria. *Infect. Immun.* 1998;66:6030–6034.
99. Sun G, Liu F, Lin TJ. Identification of *Pseudomonas aeruginosa*-induced genes in human mast cells using suppression subtractive hybridization: up-regulation of IL-8 and CCL4 production. *Clin. Exp. Immunol.* 2005;142:199–205.
100. Malaviya R, Abraham SN. Role of mast cell leukotrienes in neutrophil recruitment and bacterial clearance in infectious peritonitis. *J. Leukoc. Biol.* 2000;67:841–846.
101. Brzezinska-Blaszczyk E, Rdzany RS. Lipoteichoic acids selectively stimulate rat mast cells to cysteinyl leukotriene generation and affect mast cell migration after tumor necrosis factor (TNF)-priming. *Immunol. Lett.* 2007;109:138–144.
102. Imajo N, Kuriharav, Fukuishi N, Inukai A, Matsushita S, Noda S, Toyoda M, Yoshioka M, Teruya H, Nishii Y, Matsui N, Akagi M. Lipoteichoic acid improves the capability of mast cells in the host defense system against bacteria. *Inflamm. Res.* 2009;58:797–807.
103. Supajatura V, Ushio H, Wada A, Yahiro K, Okumura K, Ogawa H, Hirayama T, Ra C. Cutting edge: VacA, a vacuolating cytotoxin of *Helicobacter pylori*, directly activates mast cells for migration and production of proinflammatory cytokines. *J. Immunol.* 2002;168:2603–2607.
104. Krishnaswamy G, Martin R, Walker E, Li C, Hossler F, Hall K, Chi DS. *Moraxella catarrhalis* induces mast cell activation and nuclear factor kappa B-dependent cytokine synthesis. *Front. Biosci.* 2003;8:a40–a47.
105. Sutherland RE, Olsen JS, McKinstry A, Villalta SA, Wolters PJ. Mast cell IL-6 improves survival from Klebsiella pneumonia and sepsis by enhancing neutrophil killing. *J. Immunol.* 2008;181:5598–5605.
106. Orinska Z, Maurer M, Mirghomizadeh F, Bulanova E, Metz M, Nashkevich N, Schiemann F, Schulmistrat J, Budagian V, Giron-Michel J, Brandt E, Paus R, Bulfone-Paus S. IL-15 constrains mast cell-dependent antibacterial defenses by suppressing chymase activities. *Nat. Med.* 2007;13:927–934.
107. Malaviya R, Twesten NJ, Ross EA, Abraham SN, Pfeifer JD. Mast cells process bacterial Ags through a phagocytic route for class I MHC presentation to T cells. *J. Immunol.* 1996;156:1490–1496.
108. Marietta EV, Weis JJ, Weis JH. CD28 expression by mouse mast cells is modulated by lipopolysaccharide and outer surface protein A lipoprotein from *Borrelia burgdorferi*. *J. Immunol.* 1997;159:2840–2848.
109. Mielcarek N, Hornquist EH, Johansson BR, Locht C, Abraham SN, Holmgren J. Interaction of *Bordetella pertussis* with mast cells, modulation of cytokine secretion by pertussis toxin. *Cell. Microbiol.* 2001;3:181–188.
110. Trivedi NN, Caughey GH. Mast cell peptidases: chameleons of innate immunity and host defense. *Am. J. Respir. Cell. Mol. Biol.* 2009;42(3):257–267.
111. Huang C, De Sanctis GT, O'Brien PJ, Mizgerd JP, Friend DS, Drazen JM, Brass LF, Stevens RL. Evaluation of the substrate specificity of human mast cell tryptase beta I and demonstration of its importance in bacterial infections of the lung. *J. Biol. Chem.* 2001;276:26276–26284.
112. Thakurdas, SM, Melicoff E, Sansores-Garcia L, Moreira DC, Petrova Y, Stevens RL, Adachi R. The mast cell-restricted tryptase mMCP-6 has a critical immunoprotective role in bacterial infections. *J. Biol. Chem.* 2007;282:20809–20815.
113. Malaviya R, Navara C, Uckun FM. Role of Janus kinase 3 in mast cell-mediated innate immunity against Gram-negative bacteria. *Immunity* 2001;15:313–321.
114. Kanamaru Y, Sumiyoshi K, Ushio H, Ogawa H, Okumura K, Nakao A. Smad3 deficiency in mast cells provides efficient host protection against acute septic peritonitis. *J. Immunol.* 2005;174:4193–4197.

115. Akira S, Uematsu S, Takeuchi O. Pathogen recognition and innate immunity. *Cell* 2006;124:783–801.
116. Kumar H, Kawai T, Akira S. Toll-like receptors and innate immunity. *Biochem. Biophys. Res. Commun.* 2009;388:621–625.
117. Dabbagh K, Lewis DB. Toll-like receptors and T-helper-1/T-helper-2 responses. *Curr. Opin. Infect. Dis.* 2003;16:199–204.
118. Marshall JS, McCurdy JD, Olynych T. Toll-like receptor-mediated activation of mast cells: implications for allergic disease? *Int. Arch. Allergy Immunol.* 2003;132:87–97.
119. Kulka M, Alexopoulou L, Flavell RA, Metcalfe DD. Activation of mast cells by double-stranded RNA: evidence for activation through Toll-like receptor 3. *J. Allergy Clin. Immunol.* 2004;114:174–182.
120. Triantafilou K, Vakakis E, Orthopoulos G, Ahmed MA, Schumann C, Lepper PM, Triantafilou M. TLR8 and TLR7 are involved in the host's immune response to human parechovirus 1. *Eur. J. Immunol.* 2005;35:2416–2423.
121. Ronnberg E, Guss B, Pejler G. Infection of mast cells with live streptococci causes a Toll-Like receptor 2- and cell–cell contact-dependent cytokine and chemokine response. *Infect. Immun.* 2009. doi: 10.1128/IAI.01004-09.
122. Supajatura V, Ushio H, Nakao A, Okumura K, Ra C, Ogawa H. Protective roles of mast cells against enterobacterial infection are mediated by Toll-like receptor 4. *J. Immunol.* 2001;167:2250–2256.
123. Supajatura V, Ushio H, Nakao A, Akira S, Okumura K, Ra C, Ogawa H. Differential responses of mast cell Toll-like receptors 2 and 4 in allergy and innate immunity. *J. Clin. Invest.* 2002;109:1351–1359.
124. Ikeda T, Funaba M. Altered function of murine mast cells in response to lipopolysaccharide and peptidoglycan. *Immunol. Lett.* 2003;88:21–26.
125. Jawdat DM, Rowden G, Marshall JS. Mast cells have a pivotal role in TNF-independent lymph node hypertrophy and the mobilization of Langerhans cells in response to bacterial peptidoglycan. *J. Immunol.* 2006;177:1755–1762.
126. Mallen-St Clair J, Pham CT, Villalta SA, Caughey GH, Wolters PJ. Mast cell dipeptidyl peptidase I mediates survival from sepsis. *J. Clin. Invest.* 2004;113:628–634.
127. Liu PT, Stenger S, Li H, Wenzel L, Tan BH, Krutzik SR, Ochoa MT, Schauber J, Wu K, Meinken C, Kamen DL, Wagner M, Bals R, Steinmeyer A, Zugel U, Gallo RL, Eisenberg D, Hewison M, Hollis BW, Adams JS, Bloom BR, Modlin RL. Toll-like receptor triggering of a vitamin D-mediated human antimicrobial response. *Science* 2006;311:1770–1773.
128. Nizet V, Ohtake T, Lauth X, Trowbridge J, Rudisill J, Dorschner RA, Pestonjamasp V, Piraino J, Huttner K, Gallo RL. Innate antimicrobial peptide protects the skin from invasive bacterial infection. *Nature* 2001;414:454–457.
129. Niyonsaba F, Iwabuchi K, Someya A, Hirata M, Matsuda H, Ogawa H, Nagaoka I. A cathelicidin family of human antibacterial peptide LL-37 induces mast cell chemotaxis. *Immunology* 2002;106:20–26.
130. Yoshioka M, Fukuishi N, Kubo Y, Yamanobe H, Ohsaki K, Kawasoe Y, Murata M, Ishizumi A, Nishii Y, Matsui N, Akagi M. Human cathelicidin CAP18/LL-37 changes mast cell function toward innate immunity. *Biol. Pharm. Bull.* 2008;31:212–216.
131. Di Nardo A, Vitiello A, Gallo RL. Cutting edge: mast cell antimicrobial activity is mediated by expression of cathelicidin antimicrobial peptide. *J. Immunol.* 2003;170:2274–2278.
132. Di Nardo A, Yamasaki K, Dorschner RA, Lai Y, Gallo RL. Mast cell cathelicidin antimicrobial peptide prevents invasive group A *Streptococcus* infection of the skin. *J. Immunol.* 2008;180:7565–7573.
133. Mekori YA, Metcalfe DD. Mast cells in innate immunity. *Immunol. Rev.* 2000;173:131–140.
134. Bischoff SC. Physiological and pathophysiological functions of intestinal mast cells. *Semin. Immunopathol.* 2009;31:185–205.
135. Bischoff SC, Kramer S. Human mast cells, bacteria, and intestinal immunity. *Immunol. Rev.* 2007;217:329–337.
136. Karkowska-Kuleta J, Rapala-Kozik M, Kozik A. Fungi pathogenic to humans: molecular bases of virulence of *Candida albicans, Cryptococcus neoformans* and *Aspergillus fumigatus*. *Acta Biochim. Pol.* 2009;56:211–224.

137. Sheldon WH, Bauer H. Tissue mast cells and acute inflammation in experimental cutaneous mucormycosis of normal, 48/80-treated, and diabetic rats. *J. Exp. Med.* 1960;112:1069–1084.
138. Niide O, Suzuki Y, Yoshimaru T, Inoue T, Takayama T, Ra C. Fungal metabolite gliotoxin blocks mast cell activation by a calcium- and superoxide-dependent mechanism: implications for immuno-suppressive activities. *Clin. Immunol.* 2006;118:108–116.
139. Olynych TJ, Jakeman DL, Marshall JS. Fungal zymosan induces leukotriene production by human mast cells through a dectin-1-dependent mechanism. *J. Allergy Clin. Immunol.* 2006;118:837–843.
140. Castleman WL, Owens SB, Brundage-Anguish LJ. Acute and persistent alterations in pulmonary inflammatory cells and airway mast cells induced by Sendai virus infection in neonatal rats. *Vet. Pathol.* 1989;26:18–25.
141. Opengart K, Eyre P, Domermuth CH. Increased numbers of duodenal mucosal mast cells in turkeys inoculated with hemorrhagic enteritis virus. *Am. J. Vet. Res.* 1992;53:814–819.
142. Sorden SD, Castleman WL. Virus-induced increases in bronchiolar mast cells in brown Norway rats are associated with both local mast cell proliferation and increases in blood mast cell precursors. *Lab Invest.* 1995;73:197–204.
143. Sorden SD, Castleman WL. Virus-induced increases in airway mast cells in brown Norway rats are associated with enhanced pulmonary viral replication and persisting lymphocytic infiltration. *Exp. Lung Res.* 1995;21:197–213.
144. Sun Q, Wang D, She R, Li W, Liu S, Han D, Wang Y, Ding Y. Increased mast cell density during the infection with velogenic Newcastle disease virus in chickens. *Avian Pathol.* 2008;37:579–585.
145. Kimman TG, Terpstra GK, Daha MR, Westenbrink F. Pathogenesis of naturally acquired bovine respiratory syncytial virus infection in calves: evidence for the involvement of complement and mast cell mediators. *Am. J. Vet. Res.* 1989;50:694–700.
146. Sugiyama K. Histamine release from rat mast cells induced by Sendai virus. *Nature* 1977;270:614–615.
147. Gomperts BD, Baldwin JM, Micklem KJ. Rat mast cells permeabilized with Sendai virus secrete histamine in response to Ca^{2+} buffered in the micromolar range. *Biochem. J.* 1983;210:737–745.
148. Mokhtarian F, Griffin DE. The role of mast cells in virus-induced inflammation in the murine central nervous system. *Cell Immunol.* 1984;86:491–500.
149. Ogunbiyi PO, Black WD, Eyre P. Parainfluenza-3 virus-induced enhancement of histamine release from calf lung mast cells: effect of levamisole. *J. Vet. Pharmacol. Ther.* 1988;11:338–344.
150. Franceschini B, Russo C, Dioguardi N, Grizzi F. Increased liver mast cell recruitment in patients with chronic C virus-related hepatitis and histologically documented steatosis. *J. Viral Hepat.* 2007;14:549–555.
151. Shirato K, Taguchi F. Mast cell degranulation is induced by A549 airway epithelial cell infected with respiratory syncytial virus. *Virology* 2009;386:88–93.
152. Morimoto M, Yamada M, Arizono N, Hayashi T. Lactic dehydrogenase virus infection enhances parasite egg production and inhibits eosinophil and mast cell responses in mice infected with the nematode *Nippostrongylus brasiliensis. Immunology* 1998;93:540–545.
153. Sanchez LF, Hotta H, Hotta S, Homma M. Degranulation and histamine release from murine mast cells sensitized with dengue virus-immune sera. *Microbiol. Immunol.* 1986;30:753–759.
154. King CA, Marshall JS, Alshurafa H, Anderson R. Release of vasoactive cytokines by antibody-enhanced dengue virus infection of a human mast cell/basophil line. *J. Virol.* 2000;74:7146–7150.
155. King CA, Anderson R, Marshall JS. Dengue virus selectively induces human mast cell chemokine production. *J. Virol.* 2002;76:8408–8419.
156. Brown MG, Huang YY, Marshall JS, King CA, Hoskin DW, Anderson R. Dramatic caspase-dependent apoptosis in antibody-enhanced dengue virus infection of human mast cells. *J. Leukoc. Biol.* 2009;85:71–80.
157. Brown MG, King CA, Sherren C, Marshall JS, Anderson R. A dominant role for FcgammaRII in antibody-enhanced dengue virus infection of human mast cells and associated CCL5 release. *J. Leukoc. Biol.* 2006;80:1242–1250.
158. Bannert N, Farzan M, Friend DS, Ochi H, Price KS, Sodroski J, Boyce JA. Human mast cell progenitors can be infected by macrophagetropic human immunodeficiency virus type 1 and retain virus with maturation *in vitro. J. Virol.* 2001;75:10808–10814.

159. Li Y, Li L, Wadley R, Reddel SW, Qi JC, Archis C, Collins A, Clark E, Cooley M, Kouts S, Naif HM, Alali M, Cunningham A, Wong GW, Stevens RL, Krilis SA. Mast cells/basophils in the peripheral blood of allergic individuals who are HIV-1 susceptible due to their surface expression of CD4 and the chemokine receptors CCR3, CCR5, and CXCR4. *Blood* 2001;97:3484–3490.

160. Marone G, de Paulis A, Florio G, Petraroli A, Rossi FW, Triggiani M. Are mast cells MASTers in HIV-1 infection? *Int. Arch. Allergy Immunol.* 2001;125:89–95.

161. Marone G, Florio G, Petraroli A, Triggiani M, de Paulis A. Human mast cells and basophils in HIV-1 infection. *Trends Immunol.* 2001;22:229–232.

162. Sundstrom JB, Ellis JE, Hair GA, Kirshenbaum AS, Metcalfe DD, Yi H, Cardona AC, Lindsay MK, Ansari AA. Human tissue mast cells are an inducible reservoir of persistent HIV infection. *Blood* 2007;109:5293–5300.

163. Sundstrom JB, Hair GA, Ansari AA, Secor WE, Gilfillan AM, Metcalfe DD, Kirshenbaum AS. IgE-FcepsilonRI interactions determine HIV coreceptor usage and susceptibility to infection during ontogeny of mast cells. *J. Immunol.* 2009;182:6401–6409.

164. Qi JC, Stevens RL, Wadley R, Collins A, Cooley M, Naif HM, Nasr N, Cunningham A, Katsoulotos G, Wanigasek Y, Roufogalis B, Krilis SA. IL-16 regulation of human mast cells/basophils and their susceptibility to HIV-1. *J. Immunol.* 2002;168:4127–4134.

165. Sundstrom JB, Little DM, Villinger F, Ellis JE, Ansari AA. Signaling through Toll-like receptors triggers HIV-1 replication in latently infected mast cells. *J. Immunol.* 2004;172:4391–4401.

166. Nelson AM, Auerbach A, Man YG. Failure to detect active virus replication in mast cells at various tissue sites of HIV patients by immunohistochemistry. *Int. J. Biol. Sci.* 2009;5:603–610.

167. Feger F, Varadaradjalou S, Gao Z, Abraham SN, Arock M. The role of mast cells in host defense and their subversion by bacterial pathogens. *Trends Immunol.* 2002;23:151–158.

168. Burke SM, Issekutz TB, Mohan K, Lee PW, Shmulevitz M, Marshall JS. Human mast cell activation with virus-associated stimuli leads to the selective chemotaxis of natural killer cells by a CXCL8-dependent mechanism. *Blood* 2008;111:5467–5476.

169. Wang Z, Lai Y, McLeod DT, Cogen AL, DiNardo A. TLR2-activation turn mast cells in skin sentinels against viruses. *J. Invest. Dermatol.* 2010;130:S124.

CHAPTER 10

CELLULAR IMMUNITY OF THE SKIN: LANGERHANS CELLS AND DENDRITIC CELLS

Karen E. Burke[1] and Niroshana Anandasabapathy[2]

[1]Department of Dermatology, Mt. Sinai Medical Center, New York, NY
[2]Laboratory of Cellular Physiology and Immunology,
The Rockefeller University, New York, NY

10.1 INTRODUCTION

The skin is not only the body's largest organ but also the most exposed to the surrounding environment. Thus, the skin must provide a physical barrier and the first line of immune surveillance against biologic pathogens and chemical irritants. This is accomplished by a network of sophisticated and specialized antigen-presenting cells: Langerhans cells (LCs) in the epidermis and several distinct types of interstitial dendritic cells (DCs) in the dermis. LCs and DCs are the sentinels that recognize not only foreign environmental antigens such as irritating chemicals (thereby inducing contact hypersensitivity) and microorganisms (thus protecting through antimicrobial immunity) but also tumors (providing antitumor immunity) and allogens (causing skin graph rejection). The extended dendrites of these unique cells form a network within the epidermis and in the dermis, to create an immunologic barrier primed to recognize, capture, and process pathogens and foreign antigens for presentation to naïve and memory T lymphocytes, thereby initiating and then modulating the subsequent immune response. Furthermore, LCs and DCs play a significant role in inducing peripheral immunologic tolerance to innocuous environmental proteins and to self-antigens, thus helping to prevent autoimmune disease. Understanding how to modulate these functions may lead to therapeutic strategies to inhibit cancers and to abrogate metastases (particularly skin cancers such as melanoma) and to fight serious viral infections such as HIV.

Innate Immune System of Skin and Oral Mucosa: Properties and Impact in Pharmaceutics, Cosmetics, and Personal Care Products, First Edition. Nava Dayan and Philip W. Wertz.
© 2011 John Wiley & Sons, Inc. Published 2011 by John Wiley & Sons, Inc.

10.2 HISTORIC PERSPECTIVES

Langerhans cells were first described in 1868 by Paul Langerhans when he was still a medical student in Berlin [1]. Because of their long dendrites, Langerhans mistakenly thought these were of neural origin and functioned as "intra-epidermal receptors for extracutaneous signals of the nervous system." About 100 years after the discovery of LCs, Birbeck et al. [2] noted using electron microscopy that the numerous "clear cells" (LCs) in vitiligo lesions had a distinctive intracytoplasmic organelle that now carries his name. These cells were indeed LCs with their unique "Birbeck granule." LCs were later also found to make up most of the cellular infiltrate of histiocytosis X [3].

In the early 1970s, Steinman and Cohn [4] discovered a distinct dendritic cell (DC) subpopulation in the mouse spleen. Morphology, endocytic activity, and adherence properties distinguished these cells from macrophages. These DCs lacked both surface immunoglobulins and T-lymphocyte markers and did not proliferate with mitogen stimulation; therefore, they could not be considered lymphocytes. Epidermal LCs were similar to the newly observed splenic DCs; however, they were still postulated to be part of the peripheral nervous system or of neural crest origin (related to melanocytes) or of ectodermal origin. The presence of LCs in vitiligo, a disease diagnosed by an absence of epidermal melanocytes, provided some evidence against neural crest lineage. When Silverberg et al. [5] observed the accumulation of LCs in the dermis with close apposition of these LCs to lymphocytes in response to contact sensitizers, they postulated that LCs did play a role in antigen transport and induction of contact allergic reactions. This concept was strengthened after the expression of Fc- and complement receptors [6,7] and of mixed histocompatibility antigens type II (MHC-II, also called "Ia antigens") [8,9] on the surface of LCs was demonstrated.

Breakthrough bone marrow chimera experiments in 1979 proved that LCs are of macrophage–monocyte lineage derived from the bone marrow hematopoietic system: By reconstituting lethally irradiated recipient mice with donor allogeneic or semi-allogeneic hematopoietic progenitor cells, the resultant LCs were shown to be partially of donor origin after transplantation [10,11]. Also, LCs were observed to express other markers that are selectively expressed in hematopoietic cells, such as CD45 (LCA, leukocyte common antigen) [12] and cutaneous lymphocyte-associated antigen (CLA, primarily expressed on skin-homing T cells) [13]. Extensive experiments in tissue culture further clarified the hematopoietic ontogeny of LCs. The marker CD34 + selectively identifies only myeloid precursors and myeloid cells: CD34 + precursor cells were shown to develop into LCs or into a monocyte/macrophage phenotype, which ultimately differentiates into non-LC DCs [14,15]. This differentiation pathway is critically dependent on the sequential presence of specific cytokines.

The antigen-presenting function of LCs was confirmed in humans shortly thereafter [16,17]. In 1985, at a meeting at the Rockefeller University, Schuler and Steinman concluded that LCs are indeed part of the "DC family" [18]. LCs became "the model" to study DCs. In LCs, granulocyte-macrophage colony-stimulating factor (GM-CSF) was shown to be necessary for survival and growth [19]. Reorganization of the cell surface during activation and maturation was observed [18,20]. DC capacities including translocation of MHC-II molecules to the surface [21], T-cell stimulation [18], and downregulation of antigen presentation to induce tolerance [22] were first demonstrated in LCs.

Now we realize that LCs have unique features that distinguish them from other types of DCs [23]. Also, research within the past 8 years has demonstrated that the skin has several types of DCs in addition to LCs: at least four other dendritic cell subclasses have been identified in the dermis. The characterization of these DCs is quite complex because DCs can arise from several types of progenitor cells, and different functional phenotypes of DCs can be generated from the same precursor cell. Furthermore, as the LCs and DCs encounter a foreign antigen and migrate, they mature and both their surface markers and their functional interactions change.

10.3 LANGERHANS CELLS

10.3.1 Distribution

LCs are the epidermal resident dendritic cell population. LCs make up about 3–5% of the suprabasal, stratum spinosum layer of the epidermis [24] including the mucosal epithelia lining the ocular oral and vaginal surfaces [25]. They are scattered without desmosomal connections between keratinocytes. In light microscopic sections, LCs cannot be detected by routine histologic staining, but only either by staining with gold chloride or by staining of membrane-bound adenosine triphosphatase (ATPase) or adenosine diphosphatase (ADPase) for human and murine LCs, respectively [26].

As summarized in Tables 10.1 and 10.2 [26–33], LCs can also be visualized with antibodies to surface molecules, including specific "cluster of differentiation" (CD) surface markers. As summarized in Table 10.1, human LCs express CD45

TABLE 10.1 Surface Markers and Characteristics of Human LCs [26–32]

Surface marker	Epidermal LC
Panhematopoietic (CD45[a])	+
Specific for LCs and some DCs (CD207 = langerin)	+
Mixed histocompatibility complex (MHC-II, HLA-DR)	+
Thymocyte, brain/astrocyte marker (CD1a[b])	+
Calcium-bound protein on melanomas (S-100 protein)	+
Monocyte, macrophage, neutrophil, B cells (CD14[c])	+
Integrin (CD11c)	+
Distinguishing features	
Radioresistant [31]	+
Require TGF-β for growth [32]	+

[a] CD indicates "cluster of differentiation," the designation of cell membrane molecules used to classify leukocytes as defined by numbered references to monoclonal antibodies to which they bind.
[b] CD1a is the most useful marker for detecting human LCs since it is exclusively expressed in LCs in both normal and inflamed tissues.
[c] CD14 is also found on monocytes, macrophages, neutrophils, some B cells, and some leukemias (B cell CLL, acute nonlymphacytic leukemia); CD14 functions as a signal transducer leading to oxidative bursts and/or secretion of TNF-α.

(a panhematopoietic marker), mixed histocompatibility complexes-II (MHC-II and HLA-DR), CD1a (also found on thymocytes and brain astrocytes), S-100 protein (a calcium-bound protein seen in melanomas), CD14 (also found on monocytes, macrophages, neutrophils, and B cells), CD11c (integrin), and CD207 or langerin (a lectin unique to LCs and some dermal DCs, as described below). As shown in Table 10.2, murine LCs are identified as CD207+ (langerin+), MHC-II+, CD11b+, CD103−, and CD11c+ (integrin+). CD11b and CD103 are the markers that most clearly distinguish between langerin+ epidermal LCs (CD11b+, CD103−) and one subset of langerin+ dermal DCs (CD11b low, CD103+). Also, epidermal cell adhesion molecule (gp40) (EpCAM or CD326) is high in epidermal LCs and low in langerin+ dermal DCs [29,31].

The most useful of these markers for detecting human LCs is CD1a since this is exclusively expressed in LCs in both normal and inflamed tissue [26]. CD1a is not present in murine skin, so MHC-II is the most frequently used marker for noninflamed

TABLE 10.2 Surface Markers and Characteristics of Murine LCs and DCs [26–33]

Surface marker	Epidermal		Dermal[a]			
	Resident LC	Migrating LC	Resident DC	Resident DC	Resident DC	Resident DC
Specific for LCs and some DCs (CD207 = langerin)	+	+	+	+	−	−
Mixed histocompatibility complex (MHC-II[b])	+	+	+	+	+	+
Integrin αM (CD11b[c])	High	High	Low	Low	Low	High
Integrin α$_{IEL}$ chain (CD103[d])	−	−	+	−	−	−
Integrin (CD11c[c])	High	High	High	High	High	High
Epidermal cellular adhesion molecule (gp40) (CD326 = EpCAM)	+	+	Low	−	−	−
Distinguishing features						
Radioresistant [31]	+	+	−	−	−	−
Require TGF-β for growth [32]	+	+	−	−	−	−
Cellular lifespan [31]	Long life		Short life			
Time in lymph node poststimulation (days) [33]	3–4		2			
Repopulate after depletion [33]	Slowly[e]		Quickly[e]			
Are required for CD8 response	No	No	Yes			

[a] Blanks indicate that these markers were not measured or published.

[b] Since CD1a is not present in murine skin, MHC-II is the most frequently used marker for noninflamed murine skin.

[c] CD11b is also found on monocytes, macrophages, some B cells, natural killer cells, some leukemias (B-cell CLL, hairy cell, acute nonlymphocytic).

[d] CD103 is also found on interstitial, intraepithelial lymphocytes, some circulating leukocytes, some T cells, and some leukemias (B-cell CLL, hairy cell).

[e] Epidermal LC repopulate slowly after depletion—only partially after 2–4 weeks (in patches); at 8 weeks, LCs are still depleted in "patchy" areas. In contrast, dermal LCs repopulate quickly and are present in the skin within 4 days after depletion, with about 50% repopulation after 2 weeks.

murine skin [26]. Subset populations of epidermal and dermal DCs will be discussed in the following section [27].

LC density depends on age, sex, anatomic location, and steady-state versus active inflammation [26]. Their density decreases with age and with exposure to UV. In humans, LC numbers are decreased on the cornea, palms and soles, genitalia, and buccal mucosa—all places where there is constant contact with environmental allergens and irritants, most of which are benign. The greatest density is on the eyelids, thus protecting the eye without obscuring vision (as would occur if the cornea had a high density of LCs). LC density increases after contact with environmental allergens, irritants, and infections (particularly viruses). Inflammatory cytokines released in inflammation further stimulate an increase in number and activity of LCs.

In the absence of inflammation, the turnover of LCs is relatively slow ($t\frac{1}{2}$ = 53–78 days) [33,34]. Ablation with langerin-DTR (diphtheria toxin receptor) showed that reconstitution requires several weeks [34]. (This is relatively slow compared to only a few days for reconstitution of splenic or lymph node DCs [35].) LCs are largely radioresistant [31] and are capable of repopulating the skin from the host, independent of donor circulating precursor cells, while the other DCs are more similar to lymphoid organ DCs that are eliminated following lethal irradiation and are replaced by donor precursor cells [36–38]. LCs are thought to be replenished from the hair follicle since after a first degree UVB burn, which abolishes epidermal LCs but not the dermal hair follicle, LCs are restored [39]. Indeed, the bulge of the hair follicle has been shown to be the site of not only LCs but also keratinocyte, melanocyte, and mast cell progenitors [40].

LCs are unique from other DC subsets, as shown in Tables 10.1 and 10.2. In addition to being radioresistant, they produce and depend upon transforming growth factor-β1 (TGF-β1) for their growth [32]. Their development is also unique. In mice, a wave of LC precursors is recruited to the epidermis on about embryonic day 18. After birth, LCs acquire a DC morphology, express major histocompatibility class II (MHC-II) molecules, CD207 (langerin), and CD11c (integrin). These LC precursors proliferate between postnatal days 2 and 7 [41]. After this early proliferative burst, fully differentiated and radioresistant LCs divide slowly but can maintain their numbers without further input from the bone marrow [42]. These immature steady-state LCs reside in the epidermis. Upon stimulation by encountering foreign antigens or inflammation, surface markers change, so new "subpopulations" evolve [28–30,43] (as will be explained in more detail in the next sections).

10.3.2 Morphology

The morphology of dendritic cells is shown in Figure 10.1. Figure A shows murine epidermal LCs stained with antibodies by immunohistochemistry (a) for Langerin and (b) for murine MHC-II; these are stellate with extensive dendritic fibers extending in all directions, forming a network within the stratum spinosum layer. Panel (c) shows the LC nuclei labeled with DAPI (4'6-diamidino-2-phenylindole·2HCl stain) and (d) is a composite photograph of all of these three stains. With low-powered scanning electron microscopy, these processes are thin, long, and spiny or sheet-like as seen in Figure 10.1. B. When viewed alive by phase contrast microscopy, the DCs extend delicate, flower-like processes that bend, retract, and re-extend in nonpolarized movements for

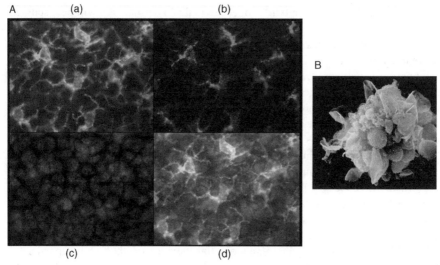

Figure 10.1   A. Appearance of murine dendritic cells. LCs in a sheet of epidermis, stained by immunohistachemistry with antibodies against (a) Langerin and (b) murine MHC-II, and (c) with nuclei labeled with DAPI; (d) is an overlay of all three stains. (*See the color version of this figure in Color Plate section* with (a) Langerin stained green, (b) MHC-II stained red, and (c) nuclei stained blue.) B. Scanning electron micrograph of a cluster of DCs with nested T cells. A (a-d). Courtesy of R. Steinman and J. Idoyaga [44], Laboratory of Cellular Physiology and Immunology, the Rockefeller University, New York; B. Courtesy of Gilla Kaplan, Laboratory Mycobacterial Immunity and Pathogenesis, University of Medicine and Dentistry, New Jersey).

one to several days. As pointed out by Banchereau and Steinman [44], this shape and motility enable them to accomplish their function of capturing antigens and of selecting and processing the antigens for specific T cells.

By high-powered electron microscopy, LCs have a folded nucleus and are identified by their distinctive, intracytoplasmic *Birbeck granules* that (when mature) are rod shaped with a vacuole at one end, resembling a tennis racquet (Figure 10.2). Only recently has the function of these Birbeck granules begun to be elucidated. Antigen capture seems to be a consequence of binding to langerin, a calcium-dependent lectin that specifically binds mannose and other sugars and is found only in LCs and some dermal DCs [45]. This binding actually induces formation of Birbeck granules and then routes the antigen into the Birbeck granules for further processing [45].

10.4   DISTINCT SUBSETS OF DERMAL DENDRITIC CELLS

The dendritic cell system is quite complex [28–30,42]. As more surface makers are discovered, as new models are studied, and as different biologic pathogens are investigated, this complexity increases. Our understanding is enhanced almost every month, though many details remain to be clarified and many questions are as yet unanswered. The complexity arises since (1) DCs arise from several different types

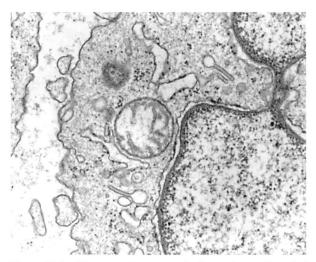

Figure 10.2   Electron microscopy of a Langerhans cell with the Birbeck granules, tennis racquet-shaped organelles specific for Langerhans cells. (Courtesy of N. Romani, Department of Dermatology and Venereology, Innsbruck Medical University.)

of progenitor cells [46]; (2) different functional phenotypes of DCs can be generated from the same precursor cell [46] (as determined by the function required, generating a sequential encounter with specific cytokines); (3) when the LC or DC encounters a foreign antigen, different states of maturation ensue, changing the surface markers, the functions, and the activities [43]. Thus the steady-state population is different from the inflammatory response population, and it is difficult to distinguish actual subpopulations from temporal variances. Also, DC subsets in the mouse are not exactly like those in humans: murine and human CD surface markers are different, and in laboratory research, DCs studied in the mouse are derived from bone marrow or spleen, while those in adult humans are almost exclusively generated from peripheral blood [28,30,46]. Furthermore, *in vitro* models are limited because they often cannot fully reflect true biologic complexity, and LC cultures in standard conditions (for even a few days) usually differ significantly from LC freshly isolated from skin [47].

Although the entire epidermal resident dendritic cell population consists of LCs, a small population of migrating LCs is found in the dermis as they travel en route to the skin-draining lymph nodes. In humans, these migrating LCs are CD207 + (langerin +) and CD14 +; in mice, they are identified as CD207 +, CD11b +, EpCAM + (as shown in Table 10.2) [30]. In addition to these migrating LCs, the dermis of the mouse was found to contain two other resident populations of CD207 + (langerin-expressing) cells [48]. This observation led to considerable confusion in the field until these DCs were found to be quite different from LCs despite their shared expression of CD207. In humans, the langerin + dermal DCs, unlike epidermal LCs, are radiosensitive and derive from precursors in the blood [49]. In mice some are CD103 + while others are CD103−. Langerin + dermal dendritic cells, unlike LCs, are EpCAM− (or EpCAM-low) and radiosensitive; these are derived from and repopulate from precursors in the blood after radiation injury [48–50] and develop independent of TGF-β [51], but depend on the DC hematopoietin Flt3L [52]. Two other populations of CD207$-$ DCs are also present in the dermis, distinguished from each other by low and high expression of CD11b [42].

As shown in murine skin, in addition to LCs these other distinctive subsets of dermal DCs migrate to skin-draining lymph nodes where they are likely to present antigens to T cells [42]. The precise functions of each subset are being investigated. The CD103$+$, CD207$+$ dermal DC is believed to "cross present" skin-derived antigens to CD8 T cells [53]. Some data also support a role of CD103$+$ cells in priming CD8$+$ responses against HSV infection [54]. Henri et al. published an excellent detailed review of the experiments to date examining and clarifying dermal DC subsets and functions [42].

The study of human dermal resident DC subsets in the steady state (without inflammation) has been hindered by the paucity of cells that can be isolated from skin by conventional techniques. Nevertheless, by addition of growth factors hematopoietins and cytokines (GM-CSF, Flt3L, and TNF-alpha) to *in vitro* skin sheet cultures of skin explants, several groups have studied dermal DC populations. Banchereau et al. [55] demonstrated that several skin subsets can be derived from CD34$+$ precursors. In addition to CD1a^{high}, CD14$-$, HLA$-$, DR$+$, CD207$+$ LCs, they identified two human dermal DC populations: one population derived from dermal cultures was CD1a$-$, CD14$+$, HLA$-$, DR$+$ (dermal CD14$+$ cells) and another was CD1a^{dim}, CD14$-$, HLA$-$, DR$+$ (CD1a dermal DCs). In this particular model, LCs were observed to efficiently prime suppressor CD8 naive T cells and to induce differentiation of CD4 T cells into T-helper 2 cells. The CD14$+$ dermal DC population instead primes helper CD4 T cells to induce naive B cell maturation into plasma cells, a process characterized by immunoglobulin isotype switching. The CD1a^{high} population was observed to prime CD8 T cell responses less efficiently than LCs, but with greater efficiency than CD14$+$ dermal DCs [55].

Because *in vitro* culture methods may induce changes in maturation and cell surface phenotype markers of dendritic cells that do not naturally occur *in vivo*, other classification methods of dermal DCs have also been performed *in situ* followed by *ex vivo* functional testing. In both mouse and humans, the integrin CD11c is considered a general marker of dendritic cells. Blood-derived circulating antigen-1 (BCDA-1, also called CD1c), BDCA-2 (CD303), BDCA-3 (CD141), and BCDA-4 (CD304/neuropilin-1) further label DC subsets in human peripheral blood and tissue [56]. Zaba et al. [56] used these markers to identify BDCA-1 (CD1c$+$), CD14$-$, CD1a$+$ dermal DCs in normal skin. These DCs were found to be mainly immature or to lack the cell surface proteins needed for further differentiation and antigen presentation [56]. A population of BDCA-3 cells (distinct from BDCA-1 cells), comprising about 10% of the total CD11c$+$ population, was also observed. Functional analysis of these subsets is pending. In contrast to the CD34$+$ culture system described above, these researchers did not observe many CD14$+$ cells in normal skin.

The environmental milieu of human skin changes quite dramatically with inflammation, stimulating changes in DC subsets. For example, the inducible dermal

DC subsets called "TIP-DCs" (which are CD11c +, BDCA-1−) observed in psoriasis produce intracellular nitric oxide synthase and tumor necrosis factor (TNF) [57]. The review by Zaba et al. [43] describes and classifies the various DC resident populations in normal and inflamed human skin.

10.5 T CELLS IN THE SKIN

T cells have very diversified antigen receptors, allowing them to respond to many different antigens. *Naive T cells* (i.e., those that have not yet encountered antigen) circulate through the blood and lymph nodes. DCs bring antigens from peripheral tissues into the lymph nodes. Upon encountering antigens presented by the DCs, the T cell differentiates further and becomes specialized as an *effector cell*, competent to produce cytokines that can stimulate B cells and other T cells or mediate cell killing. While early in an immune response T cells are effectors, later in the response *memory T cells* persist to maintain further surveillance against continued or recurrent antigen challenge. Because T cells can maintain a memory, the immune system can be educated and vaccines can be made to create these types of memory to specific antigens.

T cells are present both in normal human skin and in inflamed skin where they have been implicated in the pathogenesis of psoriasis [57,58]. In 2006, one study estimated twice as many T cells in normal human skin compared to the numbers of T cells in circulation [59]. Of the 20 billion T cells estimated in human skin, most are memory T cells (marked by CD45RO) and with a diverse repertoire of T cell receptors, suggesting an ability to recall and respond to a variety of antigens. *T regulatory cells*, which protect against autoimmunity and dampen immune responses, have also been detected in the skin.

The importance of intact cutaneous immunosurveillance by T cells is remarkable. Transplant recipients on immunosuppressive medications that target T cells have 65–250-fold higher incidence of squamous cell cancers [60], proving that these resident T cells are effective in detecting abnormal mutations of their own skin cells. Though T cell memory responses in the skin have been implicated in the etiology of many dermatologic diseases such as fixed drug, lymphomatoid papulosis, and contact hypersensitivity, psoriasis is perhaps the most studied model system for T-cell-mediated cutaneous inflammation. In 2004, it was demonstrated that grafts of nonpsoriatic skin from psoriasis patients, but not those from healthy donors, could transfer psoriatic disease into immunodeficient mice in a manner dependent on the grafted T cells [61]. This finding demonstrated that cutaneous T cells, even from nonlesional skin, were sufficient to mediate disease without additional contributions from the blood.

Dermatologists observe malignant T cell responses as well both in Sezary syndrome and in CTCL. Recent studies have begun to trace the origin of malignant Sezary syndrome T cells to central memory T cells, while CTCL T cell clones were observed to derive from skin resident effector memory T cells [62]. Clark has published an excellent, detailed review of the role of T cells in the skin [63].

10.6 ANTIGEN PRESENTATION

10.6.1 Toll-Like Receptors

In addition to the many cell surface markers described above, both steady-state and migrating LCs and DCs express a recently identified group of pattern recognition receptors known as *Toll-like receptors* (*TLRs*) [64]. These are transmembrane, leucine-rich glycoproteins with a cytoplasmic tail domain homologous to the interleukin 1 (IL-1) receptor [65–67]. TLRs detect and bind components of microorganisms, thereby initiating various intracellular signaling cascades [65–67] such as nuclear factor-κB (NF-κB). This in turn promotes expression of genes involved in immune responses such as cytokines, chemokines, costimulatory molecules, and adhesion molecules [65–67]. TLRs are also found on keratinocytes, monocytes, macrophages, T and B lymphocytes, dermal mast cells, endothelial cells of the skin's microvasculature, and stromal cells such as fibroblasts and adipocytes [64,68].

Ten TLRs have been identified in humans [26,64]; undoubtedly many more will be discovered. The pathogen and specific ligand(s) of each are listed in Table 10.3. TLR2 is essential for the recognition of bacterial lipoproteins and peptidoglycans. TLR4 recognizes bacterial lipopolysaccharide and TLR5 recognizes flagellin, a component of bacterial flagella. TLR6 participates in the discrimination of lipoproteins, and TLR9 recognizes bacterial CpG DNA sequences. TLRs may also be involved in the recognition of viral components. TLR2 can form a heterodimer with either TLR1 or TLR6 to recognize tri- or diacyl lipopeptides of bacteria [64–67]. TLR2/6 with CD36 recognizes lipoteichoic acid of Gram-positive bacteria [64–67].

TABLE 10.3 Toll-Like Receptors [64–67]

TLR	Cellular location[a]	Pathogen	Specific ligand
TLR1/2 heterodimer	CM	Bacteria	Triacyl lipopeptides
TLR2/6 heterodimer	CM	Bacteria	Diacyl lipopeptides
TLR2/6 heterodimer with CD 36	CM	Bacteria, Gram-positive	Lipoteichoic acid
TLR2	CM	Bacteria fungi	Pepidoglycans, various components
TLR3	IOM	Virus	dsRNA of replication cycle
TLR4 (with CD14)	CM	Bacteria, Gram-negative	Lipopolysaccharide
TLR5	CM	Bacteria	Flagellin
TLR6	CM	Bacteria	Lipoproteins
TLR7	IOM	Viruses imidazoquinoline:	ssRNA compounds
TLR8	IOM	Viruses imidazoquinoline:	ssRNA compounds
TLR9	IOM	Bacteria dsDNA virus: herpes simplex	CpG in dsDNA (pG) dsDNA
TLR10		Unknown	Unknown

[a] CM: cell membrane; IOM: intracellular organelle membrane (e.g., endosomal or lysosomal membrane).

TLRs can also be classified into two groups based upon cellular location [64–67]. TLRs 1, 2, 4, 5, and 6 are found on the cell membranes and can be activated by extracellular pathogen-associated molecular patterns (PAMPs). In contrast, TLRs 3, 7, 8, and 9 are found in membranes of intracellular organelle compartments, such as endosomes and lysosomes [64–67]. The intracellular location of TLRs 3, 7, 8, and 9 enables them to detect nucleic acids (DNA or RNA) that have been released from viruses or bacteria and degraded within endosomes and lysosomes inside the cell [64–67].

Our understanding of the specificity and mechanisms of action of TLRs [69] can lead to important potential therapeutic uses. Indeed, imiquimod (Aldara (5%), Zyclara (3.75%)) is the first TLR ligand approved by the FDA for treatment of human disease [70,71]. Dermatologists use topical imiquimod to treat genital warts, actinic keratoses, and superficial basal cell carcinomas [70,71]. Indeed, topical imiquimod is possibly the most effective topical medication for treatment of actinic keratosis and UV-damaged skin since the UV-induced mutations in the p53 and p16 genes (mutations noted to be very high percentages in actinic keratoses and even higher in skin cancers) are reversed after 1–4 months of topical application (Eggert Stockpleth, private communication).

As described above, LCs do not only express TLRs but may also participate in mediating TLR responses [72–74]. LC-like DCs derived from human cord blood express mRNA for TLRs 1–10 [75]. LC-like DCs are most responsive to TLR2 and TLR7/8 ligands, indicating that in response to TLR recognition, both antibacterial and antiviral action is initiated. In fact, loss of TLRs 2, 4, and 5 on LCs abolishes bacterial recognition [74]. Also, activation of LC-like DCs by TLR3 produces type I interferon (IFNα/β), indicating that these cells may be involved in antiviral immunity [75,76]. Freshly isolated LCs purified from human skin were found to express only TLRs 1, 2, 3, 5, 6, and 10 and to respond to ligands of TLR2 and 3 by producing TNF-α but not interleukin 12 (IL-12) or IFNα/β [76]. Furthermore, in response to peptidoglycans, these LCs produced IL-10, suggesting that they play a role in tolerance against commensal Gram-positive bacteria [76].

10.6.2 Langerin

The importance of langerin as a recognition receptor for carbohydrates on the surfaces of pathogens has recently been studied [77]. Both langerin and CD1a are required for presentation of nonpeptide antigens from *Mycobacterium leprae* by LCs to T cells [78]. Using ovalbumin fused to a langerin-specific monoclonal antibody to target antigens to langerin leads to loading antigen on both MHC-I and MHC-II molecules with subsequent presentation of the antigenic peptides to effector and regulatory T cells [79].

Thus, langerin routes antigens to different cellular compartments involved in antigen presentation to promote recognition by different specific T cells. This understanding of the role of langerin in modulating infections is extremely important and may lead to therapeutic breakthroughs for the treatment of serious viral diseases such as acquired immunodeficiency syndrome (AIDS).

10.6.3   Maturation and Migration of LCs and DCs

As presented above, LCs and DCs perform the two distinct functions: (1) capturing antigen and (2) initiating the immune response by presentation to specific T lymphocytes. These distinct functions are executed by LCs and DCs in different stages of development. The subpopulations are identified by the surface markers previously described and by the cytokines secreted—both of which vary (a) by state of LC or DC maturity, (b) by position in either "peripheral" tissues (skin, mucosa, and blood) or "central" (lymphatic vessels and lymph node), and (c) by type of antigen encountered (contact allergen, infectious pathogen, autoantigen, or tumor antigen).

Immature, "steady-state" LCs and DCs capture the antigen and process it by forming MHC–peptide complexes, thus preparing for antigen presentation. As these LCs and DCs migrate to the specific T cell areas of the lymph nodes, they further differentiate and mature. With maturation, the LCs and DCs express new surface membrane molecules that bind and activate regulator or effector T cells [80,81], and they synthesize cytokines that modulate regulator or effector T-cell proliferation and differentiation [82,83]. The maturing, evolving LCs and DCs also alter production of chemokines and chemokine receptors that act to intensify their own movement into lymphatics [84,85].

10.6.4   Tolerance

As important as it is to recognize foreign antigens, it is equally necessary to avoid reactions to innocuous environmental antigens and to self. Seasonal allergies and contact allergies to benign common substances (such as nickel in jewelry, coins, and utensils) are the result of an unnecessary excessive immune response, and systemic diseases such as juvenile diabetes, multiple sclerosis, systemic lupus erythematosis, psoriasis, and rheumatoid arthritis are all examples of autoimmunity. Paul Ehrlich stated, "The formation of tissue autotoxins would . . . constitute a danger threatening the organism more frequently and much more severely than all exogenous injuries [86]."

Steinman and Nussenzweig [87] have proposed that LCs and DCs not only induce immunity but also play a critical role in establishing antigen-specific tolerance. The induction of tolerance can be beneficial even with acute infection, in order to prevent reaction to self-antigens released from dying, infected cells. Also, because nonpathogenic environmental antigens (such as commensal organisms in our airways and gastrointestinal tract) may cross-react with lymphocyte receptors for pathological antigens [88], an effective mechanism for peripheral tolerance is required [89,90]. Immature LCs and DCs are ideally poised to execute this tolerizing function. In the steady state (i.e., in the absence of acute infection or inflammation), LCs and DCs are immature cells that capture both innocuous environmental antigens and self-antigens. They then mature as they move to the lymph nodes where they can either (1) activate effector T cells to *induce immunity* or (2) *induce tolerance* either by (a) inhibiting or deleting effector T cells or (b) by expanding regulatory T cells.

Steinman and Nussenzweig [87] provide evidence that proteins captured and processed by LCs and DCs in the steady state are tolerogenic. Thus, "when the same proteins are presented during infection, the immune response is able to focus on the pathogen, not on self or environmental antigens that are presented along with pathogens. Reciprocally, chronic inflammatory diseases against otherwise nonpathogenic antigens would be directed primarily to proteins that are not presented by DCs in the steady state" [87].

In the steady state, immature LCs and DCs capture the antigen to form MHC–peptide complexes, then migrate from epithelial surfaces (and deeper tissues) via afferent lymphatic vessels to lymph nodes where they go to the T-cell area and die, as evident by the fact that few DCs are found in efferent lymphatic vessels [91]. (In mice, the lifespan of most DCs in lymphoid tissues is <2 days [92].) LCs in skin draining lymph nodes are found to contain melanin granules captured from keratinocytes, melanocytes, and extracellular matrix [93] and apoptotic intestinal epithelial cells are captured by DCs before entering mesenteric lymphatics [94]. Thus, self-antigens are constantly processed and presented as MHC–peptide complexes to resting T cells [95]. Then, via the newly recognized lectin receptors on their surfaces, the migratory DCs bind to intercellular adhesion molecule-3 on resting T cells [96]. Elegant experiments demonstrated that the mechanisms of inducing peripheral tolerance by immature DCs involve both *deletion of specific effector T cells* [97] and *induction of regulatory T cells* (i.e., those T cells that usually inhibit the response of helper and killer lymphocytes by producing regulatory cytokines, including IL-10). This evidence has been well summarized by Steinman and Nussenzweig [87].

On the other hand, when immature DCs that could possibly induce tolerance are exposed to a stimulus for maturation (such as a TLR agonist), the outcome instead of tolerance is immunity. Then, the migrating cells would mature, thereby expressing different cellular receptors and secreting different cytokines, thus inducing an immune response instead of tolerance.

10.7 THERAPEUTIC IMPLICATIONS

10.7.1 Viral Infection

The fact that LCs and DCs have specific TLRs that recognize viral antigens suggests that they play a role in the pathogenesis of viral infections. Both *in vitro* and in patients, dengue virus has been shown to infect human LCs [98]. After tick bites, encephalitis virus can be found within LCs [99].

Infection by herpes simplex might also be directly regulated by LCs and DCs. Interestingly, herpes simplex virus often recurs at sites of previous infection after sun exposure. This might be explained by the fact that UVB exposure is known to alter LC behavior: (1) LCs lose their antigen-presenting capacity; (2) they lose their ability to activate the Th1 subset of CD4 + T cells, thereby inducing clonal anergy instead of CD4 + -cell-mediated immunity; (3) they continue to activate the Th2 subset that augments humoral responses and can additionally inhibit cell-mediated activity. Furthermore, UVB-irradiated LCs are known to produce antigen-specific immunologic tolerance in mice after intravenous infusion [47]. Because CD103 + dermal resident dendritic cells migrating to the skin draining LNs were demonstrated recently to be central to the immune response to HSV, their role alongside LCs should be considered as well in the setting of UVB and HSV recrudescence [30].

These UVB-induced impairments of the LCs' antigen-presenting functions were studied *in vitro* by Takashima [47]. In these studies, to ensure the tissue culture model reflected biologic reality, the LCs were carefully evaluated for cell surface markers and cytokine profiles that demonstrated no contamination by other cell types and normal LC function—particularly the ability to activate naïve and primed T cells. Even after long-term culture, these *in vitro* LCs were indistinguishable from LC freshly isolated from murine skin [47].

By investigating the UVB-induced impairment of LCs' antigen-presenting abilities, Takashima [47] found that although high fluences of UVB are cytotoxic, a single exposure at low, nontoxic fluences ($25-100 \text{ J/m}^2$) significantly inhibits LC antigen-presenting capabilities through increased production of hydrogen peroxide. Normally, the migrating, maturing LC activates the T cell, which in turn induces terminal maturation of the LC. However, the UVB-sensitized LCs were found to undergo apoptosis when they next interacted with antigen-specific T cells in the antigen's presence. And these LCs were susceptible to this T-cell-mediated apoptosis even 16 h after UVB irradiation. Thus, UVB induces antigen-specific immunosuppression by premature cell death of LCs.

Other recent research has concentrated on the interaction of LCs with the HIV-1 virus. Since LCs are found within the epithelium of the foreskin, vagina, and anus (although less dense than in other anatomic locations), these are prime targets for HIV-1 infection [100,101]. Indeed, immature LCs were found to bind efficiently and specifically to the HIV-1 envelope glycoprotein gp120 through langerin [102] leading to the assumption that binding led to infection of LCs and subsequent transinfection of T cells. However, by coculturing LCs and T cells, langerin was found to promote a natural barrier to HIV-1 transmission by LCs: instead of promoting infection, binding of langerin to gp120 prevents T-cell infection [103]. Blocking langerin with a monoclonal antibody to langerin or by saturation of langerin binding with high concentrations of virus abolishes this protective effect, resulting in HIV-1 infection of LCs and subsequent transmission of the virus to T cells [103].

Thus, langerin-mediated capture of HIV-1 with internalization is essential for protection by LCs against T-cell infection [103]. If LCs are treated with lipopolysaccharide or tumor necrosis factor, they express less langerin and fail to prevent T-cell infection by HIV-1 [104]. Thus, with absent or diminished langerin, the normally HIV-1 protective LCs promote T-cell infection by the virus.

The role of dermal DCs in HIV-1 infection has not been fully clarified. Earlier tissue culture experiments showed that DCs can drive the replication of virus within T cells [105,106]. DCs can either replicate HIV, which then infects T cells in large numbers, or simply capture and transmit HIV to permissive T cells [87]. During chronic infection, when patients are largely asymptomatic, the immature, steady-state

DCs may take up sizable quantities of virus and support viral replication [107,108]. The virus may then induce tolerance by stimulating regulatory T cells and/or deleting HIV-reactive cells [87]. Possibly modulating langerin expression or LC-T cell interactions could lead to prevention of HIV-1 infection and transmission.

Hopefully, our understanding of the interactions of the HIV-1 virus with epidermal LCs and with various subsets of dermal DCs will lead to therapeutic interventions that could inhibit or prevent infection and transmission.

10.7.2 Cancer Metastases

Possibly our understanding of LC and DC biology will also lead to advances in developing therapies for cancers, particularly those of epithelial origin such as melanoma and squamous cell carcinomas of the head and neck, as well as T-cell lymphomas. Although treatments by surgical excision followed by chemotherapy and/or radiation successfully eliminate the majority of tumor cells, abolishing the few persistent cells that later metastasize is an unsolved problem. Using the specificity of the LC and DC antigen presentation with subsequent T-cell differentiation to specific cytotoxic populations might well overcome the cancer-generated immune suppression that facilitates metastases.

Kalinski et al. [109] are studying the interactions of DCs with T cells by manipulating cytokine activation. They found that maturation of DCs leads to an interleukin 12 (IL-12)-secreting population of DCs. This IL-12 in turn stimulates naïve T cells to differentiate into a subpopulation of CD4$+$ helper cells called Th1 cells that activate cellular immunity to protect against intracellular infections and cancer. Exposing these DC cells to prostaglandin E_2 (PGE$_2$, an immunosuppressive factor) stopped the DC-induced Th1 differentiation. Treatment with glucocorticoids induces an antagonist population of CD4$+$ helper T cells called Th2 cells, which suppress Th1 activity and initiate the humoral immune response. The Th2 cells secrete the immune-suppressive cytokine IL-10. Exposure to IL-10 stops the DCs from maturing into IL-12-producing DC cells. Kalinski unexpectedly found that he could actually transform Th2 cells into Th1 cells by interaction with primed mature DC cells. Thus, primed DCs and cytokines can alter T-cell differentiation and response.

The therapeutic concept is to culture the patient's immature DCs and instruct them by exposure to tumor antigen and specific, sequential cytokine stimulation *ex vivo*. Hopefully, when reinjected, these mature DCs will migrate into the lymph nodes to turn on specific Th1 cells. This approach was successful in a B16 melanoma mouse model. The B16 melanoma is a particularly aggressive tumor because these cells downregulate MHC-I molecules and antigen-processing functions, produce a vascular growth factor that inhibits DC function and T-cell immunity, and produces galectin-1, a negative regulator of T-cell activation and survival. Indeed the *ex vivo* engineered DCs induced Th1 tumor-specific cells, achieving significant reduction in tumor growth. Human trials have begun with 70 melanoma patients and 23 colorectal cancer patients. Hopefully, this DC therapy will achieve greater efficacy than the first generation of melanoma vaccines that focused only on melanoma antigens.

10.8 CONCLUSIONS

The LC and DC system of immune surveillance, which begins with identification and capture of antigens and is followed by presentation to specific effector or regulator T lymphocytes, is incredibly elegant and exact.

Our understanding is ever-evolving as researchers delve into the complexity of the distinct subsets of immature, steady-state LCs and DCs followed by temporal changes as these cells mature in executing their functions: Surface markers change; cytokines released vary with maturation and degrees of inflammation; migration and maturation of LCs and DCs are self-regulated and are modulated by other cell types (particularly by effector and/or regulator T cells). Laboratory studies are particularly difficult because murine and human surface markers are not the same and because tissue culture models do not always reflect biologic reality, especially since the *in vivo* microenvironment changes with time and situation (such as exposure to microbes and microbial products, cytokines, foreign and self-antigens, and host tumors and donor tissue grafts). The beauty of the LC–DC system is that the functions of both immunity and tolerance can be accomplished. Understanding the precise mechanisms of these LCs and DCs may lead to innovative therapies not only in fighting bacterial and viral infections as well as cancer, but also in abrogating autoimmune disease and tissue transplant rejection.

REFERENCES

1. Langerhans P. Über die verven der menschlichen haut. *Virchows Arch. Pathol. (Pathol. Anat.)* 1868; 44:325–332.
2. Birbeck MS, et al. An electron microscopic study of basal melanocytes and high-level clear cell (Langerhans cell) in vitiligo. *J. Invest. Dermatol.* 1961;37:51–58.
3. Basset F, Turiaf J. Identification par la microscopic electronique de particules de nature probablement virale dans les lesions granulomateuses d'une histiocytose "X" pulmonaire. *C. R. Acad. Sci. (Paris)* 1965;261:3701–3714.
4. Steinman RM, Cohn ZA. Identification of a novel cell type in peripheral lymphoid organs of mice. I. Morphology, quantitation, tissue distribution. *J. Exp. Med.* 1973;137:1142–1150.
5. Silberberg I, Baer RL, et al. The role of Langerhans cells in allergic contact hypersensitivity: a review of findings in man and guinea pigs. *J. Invest. Dermatol.* 1976;66:210–217.
6. Stingl G, Wolff-Schreiner EC, et al. Epidermal Langerhans cells bear Fc and C3 receptors. *Nature* 1977;268:245–246.
7. Burke KE, Gigli I. Receptors for complement of Langerhans cells. *J. Invest. Dermatol.* 1980;75:46–50.
8. Klareskog L, Malmnas-Tjernlund U, et al. Epidermal Langerhans cells express Ia antigens. *Nature* 1977;268:248–250.
9. Rowden G, Lewis MG, et al. Ia antigen expression on human epidermal Langerhans cells. *Nature* 1977;268:247–248.
10. Katz S, Tamaki K, et al. Epidermal Langerhans cells are derived from cells originating in bone marrow. *Nature* 1979;282:324–325.
11. Frelinger JG, Hood L, et al. Mouse epidermal Ia molecules have a bone marrow origin. *Nature* 1979;282:321–323.
12. Caux C, Dezutter-Dambuyant C, Schmitt D, et al. GM-CSF and TNF-alpha cooperate in the generation of dendritic Langerhans cells. *Nature* 1992;360:258–261.

13. Roszik F, Strunk D, Simonetsch I, et al. Expression of monoclonal antibody HECA-452-defined selectin ligands on Langerhans cells in normal and diseased skin. *J. Invest. Dermatol.* 1994;102:773–780.

14. Caux C, Vanbervliet B, Massacrier C, et al. CD34- hematopoietic progenitors from human cord blood differentiate along two independent dendritic cell pathways in response to GM-CSF + TNF alpha. *J. Exp. Med.* 1996;184:695–706.

15. Caux C, Vanbervliet B, Massacrier C, et al. Interleukin-3 cooperates with tumor neuro-factor alpha for the development of human dendritic Langerhans cells from cord blood CD34 + hematopoietic progenitor cells. *Blood* 1996;87:2376–2385.

16. Braathen LR, Thorsby E. Studies on human epidermal Langerhans cells. I. Allo-activating and antigen-presenting capacity. *Scand. J. Immunol.* 1980;11:401–408.

17. Bjercke S, Elgo J, et al. Enriched epidermal Langerhans cells are potent antigen-presenting cells for T cells. *J. Invest. Dermatol.* 1984;83:286–289.

18. Schuler G, Steinman RM. Murine epidermal Langerhans cells mature into potent immunostimulatory dendritic cells *in vitro*. *J. Exp. Med.* 1985;161:526–546.

19. Witmer-Pack MD, Olivier W, et al. Granulocyte/macrophage colony-stimulating factor is essential for the viability and function of cultured murine epidermal Langerhans cells. *J. Exp. Med.* 1987;166:1484–1498.

20. Romani N, Lenz A, et al. Cultured human Langerhans cells resemble lymphoid dendritic cells in phenotype and function. *J. Invest. Dermatol.* 1989;93:600–609.

21. Pierre P, Turley SJ, et al. Developmental regulation of MHC class II transport in mouse dendritic cells. *Nature* 1997;388:787–792.

22. Romani N, Koide S, et al. Presentation of exogenous protein antigens by dendritic cells to T cell clones: intact protein is presented best by immature epidermal Langerhans cells. *J. Exp. Med.* 1989;169:1169–1178.

23. Romani N, Clausen BE, Stoitzner P. Langerhans Cells & More: Langerin-expressing dendritic cell subsets in the skin. *Immunol Rev*, 2010;234:120–141.

24. James WD. The skin: basic structure and function. In: Odom RB, James WD, Berger TG, editors. *Andrews' Diseases of the Skin: Clinical Dermatology*, 9th edition. New York: WD Saunders Company, 2000. pp. 2–3.

25. Iwasaki A. Mucosal dendritic cells. *Annu. Rev. Immunol.* 2007;25:381–418.

26. Schwartz T.Chapter 5. Immunology. In: Bolognia JL, Jorizzo JL, Rapini RP, et al., editors. *Dermatology*. New York: Mosby, 2003. pp. 66–81.

27. Stingl G, Maurer D, et al., The epidermis: an immunologic microenvironment. In: Freedberg BI, Eizen RZ, Wolff K, et al., editors. *Fitzpatrick's Dermatology in General Medicine*. New York: McGraw Hill, 1999. pp. 343–376.

28. Merad M, Ginhoux F, et al. Origin, homeostasis and function of Langerhans cells and other langerin-expressing dendritic cells. *Nat. Rev. Immunol.* 2008;8:935–947.

29. Igyarto BZ, Kaplan DH. The evolving function of Langerhans cells in adaptive skin immunity. *Immunol. Cell Biol.* 2010;88:361–365.

30. Heath WR, Carbone FR. Dendritic cell subsets in primary and secondary T cell responses at body surfaces. *Nat. Immunol.* 2009;10:1237–1243.

31. Bursch LS, Wang L, Igyart B, et al. Identification of a novel population of Langerin + dendritic cells. *J. Exp. Med.* 2007;204:3147–3156.

32. Kaplan DH. TGF-beta1 is required for the development of epidermal Langerhans cells. *J. Exp. Med.* 2007;204:2545–2552.

33. Shlokovskaya E, Roediger B, Fazekas de St Groth B. Epidermal and dermal dendritic cells display differential activation and migratory behavior while sharing the ability to stimulate CD4 + T cell proliferation *in vivo*. *J. Immunol.* 2008;181:418–430.

34. Vishwanath M, et al. Development of intravital intermittent confocal imaging system for studying Langerhans cell turnover. *J. Invest. Dermatol.* 2006;126:2452–2457.

35. Kissenpfennig A, et al. Dynamics and function of Langerhans cells *in vivo*: dermal dendritic cells colonize lymph node areas distinct from slower migrating Langerhans cells. *Immunity* 2005;22:643–654.

36. Jung S, et al. *In vivo* depletion of CD11c + dendritic cells abrogates priming of CD8 + T cells by exogenous cell-associated antigens. *Immunity* 2002;17:211–220.

37. Merad M, et al. Depletion of host Langerhans cells before transplantation of donor alloreactive T cells prevents skin graft versus host disease. *Nat. Med.* 2004;10:510–517.

38. Liu K, et al. Origin of dendritic cells in peripheral lymphoid organs of mice. *Nat. Immunol.* 2007;8:578–583.

39. Gilliam AC, et al. The human hair follicle: a reservoir of CD40 + B7-deficient Langerhans cells that repopulate epidermis after UVB exposure. *J. Invest. Dermatol.* 1998;110:422–427.

40. Blanbain C, Fuchs E. Epidermal stem cells of the skin. *Annu. Rev. Cell Dev. Biol.* 2006;22:339–373.

41. Chorro L, et al. Langerhans cell (LC) proliferation mediates neonatal development, homeostasis, and inflammation-associated expansion of the epidermal LC network. *J. Exp. Med.* 2009;206:3089–3100.

42. Henri S, Guilliams M, Poulin LF, et al. Disentangling the complexity of the skin dendritic cell network. *Immunol. Cell. Biol.* 2010;88(4):366–375.

43. Zaba LC, Krueger JG, Lowes MA. Resident and "inflammatory" dendritic cells in human skin. *J. Invest. Dermatol.* 2009;129(2):302–308.

44. Banchereau J, Steinman RM. Dendritic cells and the control of immunity. *Nature* 1998;392:245–252.

45. Valladeau J, Kane O, et al. Langerin, a novel C-type lectin specific to Langerhans cells, is an endocytic receptor that induces the formation of Birbeck granules. *Immunity* 2000;12:71–81.

46. Ardavín C, Martinez del Hoyo G, et al. Origin and differentiation of dendritic cells. *Trends Immunol.* 2001;22:691–700.

47. Takashima A. Long-lived epidermal dendritic cells: breakthrough methodology opens big doors. *Dermatol. Focus* 1999;18:1–12.

48. Bursch LS, et al. Identification of a novel population of langerin + dendritic cells. *J. Exp. Med.* 2007;204:3147–3156.

49. Ginhoux F, et al. Blood-derived dermal langerin + dendritic cells survey the skin in the steady state. *J. Exp. Med.* 2007;204:3133–3146.

50. Poulin LF, Henri S, de Bovis B. The dermis contains langerin + dendritic cells that develop and function independently of epidermal Langerhans cells. *J. Exp. Med.* 2007;204:3119–3131.

51. Nagao K, et al. Murine epidermal Langerhans cells and langerin-expressing dermal dendritic cells are unrelated and exhibit distinct functions. *Proc. Natl. Acad. Sci. USA* 2009;106:3312–3317.

52. Merad M, Manz MG. Dendritic cell homeostasis. *Blood* 2009;113:3418–3427.

53. Henri S, et al. CD207 + CD103 + dermal dendritic cells cross-present keratinocyte-derived antigens irrespective of the presence of Langerhans cells. *J. Exp. Med.* 2010;207:189–206.

54. Bedoui S, et al. Cross-presentation of viral and self antigens by skin derived CD103 + dendritic cells. *Nat. Immunol.* 2009;10:488–495.

55. Klechevsky E, Banchereau J, et al. Functional specializations of human epidermal Langerhans cells and CD14 + dermal dendritic cells. *Immunity* 2008;29(3):497–510.

56. Zaba LC, et al. Normal human dermis contains distinct populations of CD11c BDCA-1 + dendritic cells and CD163FXIIIA + macrophages. *J. Clin. Invest.* 2007;117:2517–2525.

57. Lowes MA, et al. Increase in TNF-alpha and inducible nitric oxide synthase-expressing dendritic cells in psoriasis and reduction with efalizumab (anti-CD11a). *Proc. Natl. Acad. Sci. USA* 2005;102:19057–19062.

58. Boyman, O, Hefti H, Conrad C, et al. Spontaneous development of psoriasis in a new animal model shows an essential role for resident T cells and tumor necrosis factor-alpha. *J. Exp. Med.* 2004;199:731–736.

59. Clark RA, Chong B, Mirchandani N, et al. The vast majority of CLA + T cells are resident in normal skin. *J. Immunol.* 2006;176:4431–4439.

60. Berg D, Otley, CC. Skin cancer in organ transplant recipients: epidemiology, pathogenesis, and management. *J. Am. Acad. Dermatol.* 2002;47:1–17.

61. Boyman O, Hefti HP, Conrad C, Nickoloff BJ, Suter M, Nestle FO. Spontaneous development of psoriasis in a new animal model shows an essential role for resident T cells and tumor necrosis factor-alpha. *J. Exp. Med.* 2004;199(5):731–736.

62. Campbell JJ, Clark RA, Watanbe R, et al. Sezary syndrome and MF arise from distinct T cell subsets: a biological rationale for their distinct behaviors. *Blood* 2010;116(5):767–771.

63. Clark RA. Skin resident T cells: the ups and downs of on-site immunity. *J. Invest. Dermatol.* 2010;130:362–370.
64. Miller, LS. Toll-like receptors in skin. *Adv. Dermatol.* 2008;24:71–87.
65. Iwasaki A, Medzhitov R. Toll-like receptor control of the adaptive immune responses. *Nat. Immunol.* 2004;5:987–995.
66. Kawai T, Akira S. TLR signaling. *Semin. Immunol.* 2007;19:24–32.
67. Trinchieri G, Sher A. Cooperation of Toll-like receptor signals in innate immune defense. *Nat. Rev. Immunol.* 2007;7:179–190.
68. Miller LS, Modlin RL. Toll-like receptors in the skin. *Semin. Immunoptathol.* 2007;29:15–26.
69. Kang SS, Kaula LS, et al. Toll-like receptors: applications to dermatologic disease. *J. Am. Acad. Dermatol.* 2006;54:951–983.
70. Schiller M, Metze D, et al. Immune response modifiers: mode of action. *Exp. Dermatol.* 2006;15:331–41.
71. Gupta AK, Cherman AM, et al. Viral and nonviral uses of imiquimod: a review. *J. Cutan. Med. Surg.* 2004;8:338–352.
72. Fujita H, Asahina A, et al. Langerhans cells exhibit low responsiveness to double-stranded RNA. *Biochem. Biophys. Res. Commun.* 2004;319:832–839.
73. Burns RP, Jr., Ferbel B, et al. The imidazoquinolines, imiquimod and R-848, induce functional, but not phenotypic, maturation of human epidermal Langerhans cells. *Clin. Immunol.* 2000;94:13–23.
74. van der Aar AM, Sylva-Steenland RM, et al. Loss of TLR2, TLR4 and TLR 5 on Langerhans cells abolishes bacterial recognition. *J. Immunol.* 2007;178:1986–1990.
75. Renn CN, Sanchez DJ, et al. TLR activation of Langerhans cell-like dendritic cells triggers an antiviral immune response. *J. Immunol.* 2006;177:298–305.
76. Flacher V, Bouschbacher M, et al. Human Langerhans cells express a specific TLR profile and differentially respond to viruses and Gram-positive bacteria. *J. Immunol.* 2006;177:7959–7967.
77. Figdor CG, van Kooyk Y, Adema GJ. C-type lectin receptors on dendritic cells and Langerhans cells. *Nat. Rev. Immunol.* 2002;2:77–84.
78. Hunger RE, et al. Langerhans cells utilize CD1a and langerin to efficiently present nonpeptide antigens to T cells. *J. Clin. Invest.* 2004;113:701–708.
79. Idoyaga J, et al. Cutting edge: langerin/CD207 receptor on dendritic cells mediates efficient antigen presentation on MHC I and II products *in vivo. J. Immunol.* 2008;180:3647–3650.
80. Caux C, Vanbervliet B, Massacrier C, et al. B70/B7-2 is identical to CD86 and is the major functional ligand for CD28 expressed on human dendritic cells. *J Exp Med.* 1994;180:1841–1847.
81. Tseng S-Y, Otsuii M, Gorski K, et al. B7-DC, a new dendritic cell molecule with potent costimulatory properties for T cells. *J. Exp. Med.* 2001;193:839–846.
82. Lanzavecchia A, Messi, M, Lanzavecchio A, et al. Kinetics of dendritic cell activation: impact on priming of TH1, TH2 and nonpolarized T cells. *Nat. Immunol.* 2000;1:311–316.
83. Elbner S, Ratzinger G, Krosbacher B, et al. Production of IL-12 by human monocyte-derived dendritic cells is optimal when the stimulus is given at the onset of maturation, and is further enhanced by IL-4. *J. Immunol.* 2001;166:633–641.
84. Sallusto F, Schaerli P, Loetscher P, et al. Rapid and coordinated switch in chemokine receptor expression during dendritic cell maturation. *Eur. J. Immunol.* 1998;28:2760–2769.
85. Sozzani S, Allavena P, Vecchi A, et al. Rapid and coordinated switch in chemokine receptor expression during dendritic cell maturation. *J. Leukoc. Biol.* 1999;66:1–9.
86. Himmelweit F. *Collected Papers of Paul Ehrlich.* London: Pergamon, (1956–1960). p. 253.
87. Steinman RM, Nussenzweig MC. Avoiding horror autotoxicus: the importance of dendritic cells in peripheral T cell tolerance. *PNAS* 2002;99:351–358.
88. Mason D. Antigen cross-reactivity: essential in the function of TCRs. *Immunologist* 1998;6:220–222.
89. Kamradt T, Mitchison NA. Tolerance and autoimmunity. *N. Engl. J. Med.* 2001;344:655–664.
90. Maloy KJ, Powrie F. Regulatory T cells in the control of immune pathology. *Nat. Immunol.* 2001;2:816–822.
91. Matsuno K, Kudo S, Ezaki T, et al. Isolation of dendritic cells in the rat liver lymph. *Transplantation* 1995;60:765–768.

92. Steinman RM. The dendritic cell system and its role in immunogenicity. *Annu. Rev. Immunol.* 1991;9:271–296.
93. Hemmi H, Yosino M, Yamazuki H, et al. Skin antigens in the steady state are trafficked to regional lymph nodes by transforming growth factor-beta1-dependent cells. *Int. Immunol.* 2001;13:695–704.
94. Huang F-P, Platt N, Wykes M, et al. A discrete subpopulation of dendritic cells transports apoptotic intestinal epithelial cells to T cell areas of mesenteric lymph nodes. *J. Exp. Med.* 2000;191:435–442.
95. Steinman RM, Turley S, Mellman I, et al. The induction of tolerance by dendritic cells that have captured apoptotic cells. *J. Exp. Med.* 2000;191:411–416.
96. Geijtenbeek TBH, Torenson R, van Vliet SJ, et al. DC-SIGN, a dendritic cell-specific HIV-1-binding protein that enhances trans-infection of T cells. *Cell* 2000;100:575–585.
97. Hawiger D, Inaba K, Dorsett Y, et al. Dendritic cells induce peripheral T cell unresponsiveness under steady state conditions *in vivo*. *J. Exp. Med.* 2001;194:769–780.
98. Wu SJL, Grouard-Vogel G, Sun W, et al. Human skin Langerhans cells are targets of dengue virus infection. *Nat. Med.* 2000;6:816–820.
99. Labuda M, Austyn JM, Zuffova E, et al. Importance of localized skin infection in tick-borne encephalitis virus transmission. *Virology* 1996;219:357–366.
100. Hladik F, McElrath MJ. Setting the stage: host invasion by HIV. *Nat. Rev. Immunol.* 2008;8:447–457.
101. Piguet V, Steinman RM. The interaction of HIV with dendritic cells: outcomes and pathways. *Trends Immunol.* 2007;28:503–510.
102. Turville SG, et al. Diversity of receptors binding HIV on dendritic cell subsets. *Nat. Immunol.* 2002;3:975–983.
103. de Witte L, et al. Langerin is a natural barrier to HIV-1 transmission by Langerhans cells. *Nat. Med.* 2007;13:367–371.
104. Fahrbach KM, et al. Activated CD34-derived Langerhans cells mediate transinfection with human immunodeficiency virus. *J. Virol.* 2007;81:6858–6868.
105. Cameron PU, Freudenthal PS, Barker JM, et al. Dendritic cells exposed to human immunodeficiency virus type-1 transmit a vigorous cytopathic infection to CD4$^+$ T cells. *Science* 1992;257:383–387.
106. Pope M, Betjes MG, Romani N, et al. Conjugates of dendritic cells and memory T lymphocytes from skin facilitate productive infection with HIV-1. *Cell* 1994;78:389–398.
107. Zaitseva M, Blauvelt A, Lee S, et al. Expression and function of CCR5 and CXCR4 on human Langerhans cells and macrophages: implications for HIV primary infection. *Nat. Med.* 1997;3:1369–1375.
108. Granelli-Piperno A, Delgado E, Finkel V, et al. Immature dendritic cells selectively replicate macrophagetropic (M-tropic) human immunodeficiency virus type 1, while mature cells efficiently transmit both M- and T-tropic virus to T cells. *J. Virol.* 1998;72:2733–2737.
109. Kalinski P. Dendritic cells with the right staff: the third generation anti-melanoma vaccine. *Dermatol. Focus* 2006;24:1–10.

PART IV

INNATE IMMUNITY RESPONSE TO STRESS AND AGING

CHAPTER *11*

CHANGES IN SKIN IMMUNITY WITH AGE AND DISEASE

Barbara Geusens[1], Ilse Mollet[1], Chris D. Anderson[2], Sarah Terras[1], Michael S. Roberts[3,4], and Jo Lambert[1]

[1]*Department of Dermatology, Ghent University Hospital, Ghent, Belgium*
[2]*Department of Dermatology, Linköping University, Linkoping, Sweden*
[3]*Therapeutics Research Centre, Department of Medicine, Southern Clinical Division, Princess Alexandra Hospital, University of Queensland, Woolloongabba, Australia*
[4]*School of Pharmacy & Medical Sciences, University of South Australia, North Terrace, Adelaide, Australia*

11.1 INTRODUCTION

The skin is one of our key defenses to invasion from outside the body as well as in maintaining the homeostasis within. This defense consists of both a physical barrier and an active response system to physical, chemical, microorganisms, and allergens. Nondermatologists and nonimmunologists may misinterpret the skin as a tissue simply defined by its structural characteristics and cells (e.g., collagen/elastin and fibroblast-rich dermis, and its continually proliferating keratinocyte (KC)-rich epidermis). Current understanding of cutaneous immune defense mechanisms has recognized that the human immune system is comprised of two coordinated mechanisms by which our body defends against infection and disease: innate and adaptive immunity. Although both the innate and the adaptive immune systems protect against invading organisms, they differ in a number of ways (Table 11.1). Innate immunity is an evolutionarily ancient part of our defense system that is common among plants and animals, vertebrates and invertebrates, and consists of mechanisms that exist before infection. It elicits a rapid response and involves a collection of preexisting, nonspecific anatomical, secretory, and cellular mechanisms to combat infection. Innate immunity provides the first line of defense against infection, works with a limited repertoire of recognition molecules, and typically acts as a broad-spectrum and rapid defense mechanism to clear pathogens or reduce their spread. Adaptive immunity, on the other hand, exists only in vertebrates. It develops more slowly and reacts following education by a specific immune stimulus (antigen). It is highly

Innate Immune System of Skin and Oral Mucosa: Properties and Impact in Pharmaceutics, Cosmetics, and Personal Care Products, First Edition. Nava Dayan and Philip W. Wertz.

TABLE 11.1 Comparison of Innate and Adaptive Immune Responses

Innate	Adaptive
non-specific	specific
response is antigen-independent	response is antigen-dependent
immediate maximal response	lag time between exposure and maximal response
no immunologic memory	immunologic memory

adaptive and provides specific recognition of foreign antigens, leading to immunological memory.

Only if innate immunity is unable to control the potential pathogen will the adaptive immune system be fully activated. The innate immune system first initiates and influences the nature of the adaptive response and in a next step a recognized bidirectional effect, whereby the adaptive immune response may focus and amplify innate responses to relevant sites of specific antigen, is established [1]. Because activation of the adaptive immune system can require several days, the innate immune system effectively buys the body time until the slower effector molecules of both the innate and the adaptive systems appear to fight. It is clear that although each system has distinct responsibilities, neither is effective alone and each is influenced by the other.

11.2 INNATE IMMUNITY

Innate immunity involves naive immune mechanisms (i.e., without previous "education") that are used by the host to immediately defend itself. As the first line of defense against pathogen attack, the innate immune system recognizes possible invading pathogens and distinguishes pathogenic microorganisms from nonpathogens. Innate immunity consists of three major components: (1) the physical/anatomical barriers, (2) the cellular components, and (3) the chemical/secretory molecules (Figure 11.1). A coordinated physiological response in the relevant organ results in the recognition and destruction of pathogens.

11.2.1 The Anatomical and Physical Barriers of Innate Immunity

The anatomical barrier of an epidermal surface is the first physical structure of the innate immune system that prevents most pathogens and environmental toxins from harming the host. The skin plays a vital role in protecting the individual from the external environment by producing sweat and sebum and forming a stratum corneum (SC) that guards our inner environment. It impedes the penetration of microbial organisms, chemical irritants, and toxins; absorbs and blocks solar and ionized radiation; inhibits water loss; and yet permits and possibly encourages microbial colonization of nonpathogens [2]. The stratum corneum is the outermost layer of the epidermis that results from the terminal differentiation of the keratinocytes and forms the primary layer of protection. It is composed of large, polyhedral, plate-like

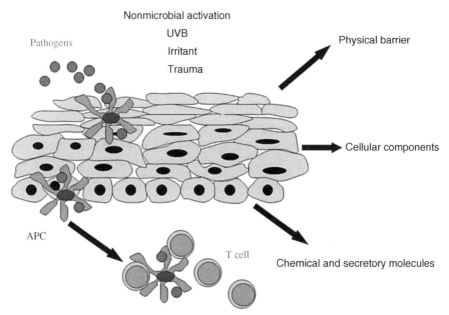

Figure 11.1 The innate immune response in skin as the first line of defense against pathogen attacks consists of three major sets of elements: the physical/anatomical barriers, the cellular components, and the chemical/secretory molecules. In response to microbial or nonmicrobial provocation, innate immunity (i) releases antimicrobial agents, (ii) induces inflammatory mediators including cytokines and chemokines, and (iii) influences the adaptive immune response (adapted and modified from *Fitzpatrick's Dermatology in General Medicine*, Chapter 22).

envelopes with extracellular lipid lamellae consisting of ceramides, free fatty acids, and cholesterol in a tightly packed and usually orthorhombic conformation. In addition, the SC is often covered by sebum exuded from the sebaceous glands, adjacent to hair follicles. The sebum and skin lipids create an acidic environment at the outer surface of the stratum corneum, providing further protection, that inhibits colonization by certain bacteria such as *Staphylococcus aureus*. Also, glycosaminoglycans (GAGs) are structural elements that contribute actively to the immune defense system of the skin. In general, GAGs influence cytokine/chemokine production, leukocyte recruitment, and inflammatory cell maturation [3,4]. Among them, hyaluronan (HA) is best known in clinical applications for its role in triggering an inflammatory response [5–7].

A similar phenomenon occurs with mucosal membranes that cover the surface of gastrointestinal (GI), urogenital, and respiratory tracts. In the mouth and the upper gastrointestinal tract, digestive enzymes and secretions such as saliva, tears, and mucus are produced that inhibit microbial growth. In addition, nonpathogenic microbes colonize the epithelium of the gut and prevent invasion by pathogenic microbes. Specialized physical elements such as cilia of bronchopulmonary tree prevent the inhaled foreign particles from entering the alveolar space. Thus, when considered together, the anatomical, physical barrier is the first innate immune defensive shield. Given these vital functions of this physical barrier, it is not surprising that a break in the barrier, as often occurs in patients with severe burn or large wounds, results in high morbidity and mortality. Less dramatic, defects in the barrier, for instance, in filaggrin production can also result in impaired immune response.

11.2.2 The Cells of the Innate Immunity

The cellular compartment of the innate immune system consists of phagocytes, mast cells, natural killer (NK) cells, and natural killer T (NKT-$\gamma\delta$) cells. All these cells rapidly differentiate into short-lived effector cells whose main role is to rid the body of infecting organisms.

11.2.2.1 Phagocytes Phagocytes are immune cells that engulf, that is, phagocytose, pathogens, or particles. They generally patrol the body searching for pathogens, but are also able to react to cytokines. The phagocytic cells of the immune system include macrophages, neutrophils, and dendritic cells (DCs).

Macrophages Macrophages are large phagocytic leukocytes that are able to move outside the vascular system by moving across the cell membrane of capillary vessels and entering the areas between cells in pursuit of invading pathogens. In tissues, organ-specific macrophages are differentiated from phagocytic cells present in the blood called monocytes. Monocytes originate from hematopoietic cells in the bone marrow in response to growth factors, such as macrophage colony-stimulating factor (M-CSF), granulocyte–macrophage colony-stimulating factor (GM-CSF), and interleukin (IL)-3 [8]. After entering the blood from the bone marrow, monocytes continue to differentiate into macrophages as they migrate into tissues. Macrophages are the most efficient phagocytes, and can phagocytose substantial numbers of bacteria or other cells or microbes [9]. The binding of bacterial molecules to receptors on the surface of a macrophage triggers it to engulf and destroy the bacteria through the generation of a "respiratory burst," causing the release of reactive oxygen species. Pathogens also stimulate the macrophage to produce cytokines, which summons other cells to the site of infection [9]. A number of important cytokines are secreted by macrophages in response to microbes, including IL-1, IL-6, TNF-α, IL-8, IL-12, and IL-10. IL-1, IL-6, and TNF-α play a critical role in inducing the acute-phase response in the liver and in inducing fever for effective host defense. TNF-α induces a potent inflammatory response to contain infection. IL-8 is important as a mediator of polymorphonuclear cells (PMNs) chemotaxis to the site of infection. The production of IL-12 by macrophages on pathogen recognition activates T cells and NK cells and is critical for the outcome of infection. Finally, IL-10 is produced by several types of cells, including T helper 1 (Th1) cells, monocytes/macrophages, and keratinocytes, and is known to suppress cytokine synthesis and downregulate major histocompatibility complex (MHC) class II expression and inhibit release of reactive oxygen intermediates [10].

Granulocytes Neutrophils along with two other cell types, eosinophils and basophils, are known as granulocytes due to the presence of granules in their cytoplasm or as polymorphonuclear cells due to their distinctive lobed nuclei. They have classically been known as the most important cells in combating bacterial and fungal infections. This activity requires specific functions driven by specific receptors, including formyl methionyl leucyl peptide (FMLP), GM-CSF, and IL-8 receptors [11]. Also, pattern recognition receptors (PRRs) including at least 10 Toll-like receptors (TLRs), recognizing conserved molecular structures related mostly to pathogens, were described and extensively studied [12]. The cytoplasmic granules (lysosomes) contain many secretory components, including lysozymes (e.g., myeloperoxidase), proteases (elastase, cathepsin G, etc.), cationic proteins, and human neutrophil defensins. These secretory elements play an integral part in defending our bodies against pathogens and lead to direct killing of the microbial organisms [13]. Lysozyme, for example, attacks bacterial peptidoglycan cell walls [14]. Neutrophils have the capacity to migrate to the site of infection, detect the pathogen using their receptors, phagocytose, and induce several important effector mechanisms such as triggering the production of cytokines.

Dendritic Cells Dendritic cells are phagocytic cells present in tissues that are in contact with the external environment, mainly the skin—where they are often called Langerhans cells in the epidermis and dermal dendritic cells (DDCs) in the dermis—and the inner mucosal lining of the nose, lungs, stomach, and intestines. They are named for their resemblance to neuronal dendrites, but dendritic cells are not connected to the nervous system. They are heterogeneous, professional antigen-presenting cells (APCs) that are uniquely equipped with molecules and strategically placed between internal and external environments, which enable them to link the innate and adaptive immune systems (Figure 11.2) [15]. Hematopoietic

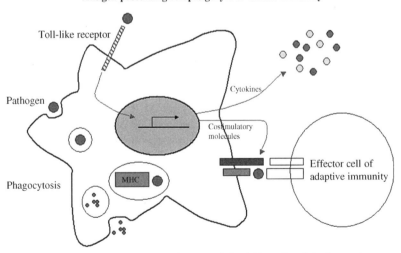

Antigen-presenting cell/phagocyte of innate immunity

Toll-like receptor

Pathogen

Cytokines

Costimulatory molecules

Phagocytosis

MHC

Effector cell of adaptive immunity

Figure 11.2   APCs such as macrophages and dendritic cells of the innate immune system survey the environment and recognize pathogens through receptors such as TLRs. Activation of APCs by pathogens leads to phagocytosis and expression of cytokines and costimulatory molecules. On the other hand, APCs present pathogenic antigens (through MHC molecules) and costimulatory molecules to effector cells of the adaptive immune system to direct their response (adapted and modified from Ref. 15).

precursor stem cells differentiate into immature dendritic cells (iDCs) that are recruited to the periphery where they continuously sample antigens and process them in an endosomal–MHC II complex-dependent pathway. These iDCs then migrate to the regional lymph nodes where they phenotypically mature and express a number of cell surface molecules and secrete a number of cytokines, which are important in their migration to and interactions with T cells, B cells, and NK cells to elicit their specific responses and differentiate into functionally mature DCs.

11.2.2.2   Mast Cells   Mast cells are widely viewed in the context of immediate-type immune reactions. This is surprising as mast cells store not only histamines, prostaglandins, and leukotrienes but also a large array of cytokines, chemokines, including immediate-type cytokines, such as IL-4 that modulates antigen-presenting cell functions, or tumor necrosis factor (TNF). In consequence, mast cells also affect more complex immune responses including T cell or B cell-mediated immunity. More important, mast cells affect the priming during both the innate and the effector phase during adaptive immune responses [16]. Mast cells are a type of innate immune cells that reside in the connective tissue and in the mucous membranes and are intimately associated not only with defense against pathogens and wound healing but also with allergy and anaphylaxis [17]. When activated, mast cells rapidly release characteristic granules, rich in histamine and heparin, along with various hormonal mediators and chemokines or chemotactic cytokines into the environment. Histamine dilates blood vessels, causing the characteristic signs of inflammation, and recruits neutrophils and macrophages.

11.2.2.3   Natural Killer Cells   Natural killer cells are our major defense against viral infections and malignancies before the adaptive immune responses have had a chance to launch. Simply put, NK cells are large granular lymphoid cells without a specific antigenic receptor that T cells and B cells express. NK cells do not rearrange immunoglobulin (Ig) or T cell receptor (TCR) genes and therefore neither Ig nor the TCR/CD3 complex is expressed at the cell surface, except for the zeta chain. Their function is to survey the body looking for altered cells, be they transformed or infected with viruses. Normal, healthy, nucleated cells express MHC class I molecules. NK cells have "killer inhibitory receptors" that recognize these self-MCH class I molecules, which results in a negative signal to the NK cells. After malignant transformation or virus infection, the nucleated cells lose expression of their MHC class I molecules. The NK cells encounter it, become activated, and kill the malignant cells. In addition, NK cells become activated in response to interferons (IFNs) or macrophage-derived cytokines [18]. Target cell lysis takes place by a secretory mechanism via exocytosis of cytoplasmic granules containing perforins that damage membrane and granzyme that damages DNA or by a nonsecretory mechanism via Fas–Fas ligand interaction [19,20]. In addition, there are data suggesting that the binding of NK ligands to the target cell's death receptors such as TRAIL-R [21] induces cell death. Regardless of mechanism of induction, apoptosis is a very effective way to protect the body against viral and malignant spread. In contrast to cell lysis that may lead to the release of pathogens, apoptosis leads to destroying the virus inside the cell.

11.2.2.4 NKT Cells Unlike NK cells, NKT cells are innate lymphocytes that express an αβ T cell receptor that recognizes glycolipid antigens presented in the context of CD1d molecules expressed on professional antigen-presenting cells [22]. NKT cells are found throughout the lymphoid compartment, in the circulation, and comprise the majority of hepatic lymphocytes. They are rare cells, constituting only about 1% or less of the total lymphocyte pool. Classified as innate lymphocytes (because they express a highly invariant TCR that recognizes lipids instead of peptides), NKT cells are known for their critical importance in the clearance of viral and bacterial infections as well as facilitating antitumor immunity and regulating immune tolerance and autoimmunity [22,23].

11.2.2.5 Keratinocytes Keratinocytes that form 95% of all epidermal cells were believed to function purely in maintaining the structure of the epidermis via their production of cytokeratins and in maintaining the physical barrier to a variety of exogenous microorganisms. In the last decade, after observations that keratinocytes express Toll-like receptors, are potent source of cytokines, chemokines, and antimicrobial peptides (AMPs), and are able to express the class II MHC antigens, it has become clear that keratinocytes may not only actively participate in epidermal immune responses but may also play key initiating roles [24]. For a complete overview of the role of keratinocytes in innate immunity, we refer to Pivarcsi et al. [25].

11.2.3 The Components of the Innate Immunity for Recognition and Response

11.2.3.1 Chemical Components The soluble/secretory/chemical group of the innate immune system includes the chemical components that are constitutively produced by a number of cells that prevent pathogen colonization and growth at the interface. Examples of specialized chemical innate barriers include lactic and fatty acids in skin secretions that provide a low pH (5.6–6.4) and the degradation product of sebum-derived triglycerides that contribute to making a hostile environment for pathogen growth. Similarly, the low pH of the stomach and the vagina inhibit microbial growth. Hydrolytic enzymes present in the stomach, such as pepsin, are capable of cleaving proteins.

11.2.3.2 Pattern Recognition Receptors Pathogen recognition by the innate immune system happens through a limited number of germline-encoded receptors. These receptors are special in that they recognize not one specific but many similar molecules; they are less stringent and more promiscuous receptors than their adaptive counterparts. They are referred to as pattern recognition receptors. PRRs have evolved to recognize patterns that are common among pathogens but not present in the host called pathogen-associated molecular patterns (PAMP). LPS is a cell wall component of Gram-negative bacteria, and is recognized by PRRs present on antigen-presenting cells and other cells. Macrophages and dendritic cells of the innate immune system continually survey the environment and recognize PAMPs [26]. This is in contrast to the cells of adaptive immune system that can create a large repertoire of specificity by combination of genetic material.

PRRs of the innate immune system are not confined to the cell membrane. They are also present in intracellular compartments, circulating plasma, and tissues. Once activated, these receptors participate in phagocytosis, opsonization, activation of complement and coagulation cascades, activation of proinflammatory signaling pathways, and induction of apoptosis. Examples of receptors are macrophage scavenger receptor (MSR), macrophage mannose receptor (MMR), protein kinase receptor (PKR), and soluble Mannan binding lectin and ficolins. Expression of a mannose binding receptor on the cell surface of keratinocytes mediates killing of *Candida albicans*. The keratinocyte mannose binding receptor (KcMR) resembles the macrophage mannose receptor but does not internalize mannose efficiently [27].

Among the most well-known of all PRRs are the Toll-like receptors. These transmembrane proteins have ligand binding domains composed of leucine-rich repeats. TLRs are located on the cell surface or in the intracellular compartments and play an important role as primary sensors of invading pathogens and initiators of inflammatory and immune responses [26]. They recognize a diverse set of PAMPs, bind certain antigenic ligands of infectious agents, and activate distinct signaling pathways resulting in a similar but not identical pattern of antimicrobial mediators. TLR1–TLR6 are expressed on the cell surface and recognize bacterial components; TLR2 associates with TLR1 or TLR6 to recognize lipopeptides from bacteria, peptidoglycan, and lipoteichoic acid; TLR4/CD14 is activated by LPS derived from Gram-negative bacteria; TLR5 recognizes flagellin. On the other hand, the intracellular TLRs bind viral and bacterial components in the cytoplasm; TLR3 recognizes dsRNA that is produced during virus replication, TLR7 and TLR8 recognize (G + U)-rich-ss RNA, and, finally, TLR9 recognizes unmethylated CpG DNA primarily found in bacteria [28]. In the past several years, compelling studies have demonstrated that epidermal keratinocytes express at least seven members (TLR1–TLR6 and TLR9) of the human TLR family, suggesting an important role for keratinocytes in cutaneous host defense [29–32].

The mechanisms of downstream signaling and responses of TLR activation are not fully understood. Commonly, TLRs couple with adaptor molecules and initiate signals. At least four different adaptor molecules are known: myeloid differentiation factor 88 (MyD88), TIR domain-containing adaptor, TIR domain-containing adaptor protein inducing IFN-β (TRIF), and TRIF-related adaptor molecule. Most TLRs activate adaptor molecule MyD88 that in turn activates MAPK kinases and the transcription factor NF-KB. This leads to expression of several proinflammatory and regulatory cytokines and chemokines, including IL-1-β, TNF-α, IL-6, and IL-12 [28]. Microbial stimulation of TLRs also leads to the activation of signaling pathways that result in production of antimicrobials, triggering of dendritic cell maturation, induction of costimulatory molecules, and increased antigen-presenting capacity. All these activities help to initiate and direct adaptive immune responses. In this way, TLRs have been recognized as the link between innate and adaptive immunity.

11.2.3.3 Complement Following invasion of the epithelial barrier, one of the first innate defense mechanisms that awaits pathogens is the alternative pathway of complement. The complement system is best known for induction of phagocytosis (opsonization) and bacterial lysis. Unlike the classic complement pathway that requires antibody triggering, the lectin-dependent pathway and the alternative pathway of complement activation can be spontaneously activated by microbial surfaces in the absence of specific antibodies. Upon activation, the circulating proteins of the complement system participate in enzymatic cascades resulting in the destruction of pathogenic organisms. In addition, the complement system is involved in modulating other parts of the immune system such as mast cell activation, neutrophil recruitment, and inflammation [33].

11.2.3.4 Antimicrobial Compounds

Antimicrobial Peptides Antimicrobial peptides refer to a group of small peptides containing less than 100 amino acids, which have an inherent ability to kill a broad range of pathogens, including Gram-negative and Gram-positive bacteria, fungi, and viruses. They are an important evolutionary conserved innate host defense mechanism in many organisms. AMPs are produced by epithelial cells, keratinocytes, and circulating cells. Of peptides discovered in humans with the ability to kill pathogens, cathelicidins (LL-37) and defensins (BD-1–BD-3) are the two main groups that are the most thoroughly studied [13]. Human β-defensins (HBDs) are produced, constitutively or as result of inflammatory stimuli, by keratinocytes and by epithelia of mucous membranes. Cathelicidin, or LL-37, produced in epithelia and by neutrophils, inhibits the growth of many bacteria and some protozoan parasites, as well as the replication of lentivirus [34]. Their function, once considered to be only antimicrobial—membrane insertion and pore formation—has now been understood to involve many more immunological activities [35]. They act as important communicators and regulators by driving cytokine expression in keratinocytes. Some defensins have been shown to stimulate immature dendritic cells and subsets of T cells [36] and play a chemoattractant role for neutrophils, mast cells, and other immune cells [37,38]. Cathelicidins are also chemoattractants for neutrophils, monocytes, and T lymphocytes [39]. AMPs are produced in part not only by the epithelial surfaces as a first-line defense system but also by PMNs, macrophages, platelets, lymphocytes, dendritic cells, and mast cells. AMP production increases with inflammation and injury, and they also have important roles in host repair and adaptive immune response.

iNOS Activation of TLRs appears to be directly involved in the induction of antimicrobial activities of keratinocytes. Historically, keratinocytes were known to possess antimicrobial activities long before the description of the first mammalian TLR. In these early reports, antimicrobial activity of keratinocytes was attributed to phagocytosis and nitric oxide (NO) production. NO is a free radical and it has a pronounced antimicrobial activity against viruses, mycobacteria, protozoans, bacteria, and fungi. Indeed, iNOS-deficient mice show increased susceptibility to *Leishmania major*, *Porphyromonas gingivalis*, *Toxoplasma gondii,* and *Mycobacterium tuberculosis* infection, suggesting a protective effect of iNOS-derived NO against these microorganisms [40].

11.2.3.5 Chemokines, Cytokines, and Other Mediators
Other circulating components important to innate immunity were first described in the setting of their activity on cells participating in adaptive responses. This diverse group of regulators,

generally referred to as cytokines, includes the growing list of interleukins, IFNs, chemokines, the tumor necrosis factor family, and growth factors. Also, neuropeptides, including neurotransmitters and neurohormones, eicosanoids—an ensemble of lipid mediators regulating inflammatory and immunological reactions, and reactive oxygen species are produced by keratinocytes and other epidermal cells.

Keratinocytes express numerous cytokines in response to microbial products, which are involved in the induction of immune response, and act as cytoprotective factors for the keratinocytes themselves. *S. aureus* and *C. albicans* induce the expression of TNF-α, IL-1β, and IL-6 in cultured keratinocytes [41–43]. TNF-α not only enhances the bactericidal properties of neutrophils but also promotes adhesion of neutrophils to endothelial cells, partially by inducing the expression of E-selectin and adhesion molecules on endothelial cells. In addition, TNF-α, IL-1β, and IL-6 are also implicated in the induction of antimicrobial peptide expression in keratinocytes.

Migration of leukocytes from peripheral blood vessels into inflamed skin involves a tightly controlled sequence of events involving the activation of vessel endothelium, transendothelial migration, and chemotaxis. Chemokines, a superfamily of small cytokine-like chemotactic proteins, have been shown to critically regulate leukocyte trafficking into the skin [44]. Skin pathogenic microorganisms such as *S. aureus*, *Borrelia burgdorferi*, and *C. albicans* and several PAMPs induce abundant expression of IL-8/*CXCL8*, in keratinocytes in a TLR-NF-κB-pathway-dependent manner. IL-8, a chemokine now referred to as CXC chemokine ligand 8 (CXCL8), is one of the most potent neutrophil chemoattractants and it is also required for the transendothelial migration of neutrophils [45]. In addition to IL-8, pathogens and microbial products stimulate the expression of other chemokines in keratinocytes such as RANTES (regulated on activation, normal T expressed and secreted)/*CCL5* and MCP-1 (monocyte chemoattractant protein-1)/*CCL2* that regulate the recruitment of various classes of phagocytic cells, T cells, and eosinophils into the site of infection and regulate their functions [41].

The diversity of cytokines and the complexity of their interactions make it impossible for us to address this part of the immune system in detail. Therefore, we refer to other handbooks.

11.3 ADAPTIVE IMMUNITY

As cutaneous adaptive immunity is somewhat peripheral to the main focus on innate immunity here and is discussed in more detail elsewhere [46–49], our discussion will be as a brief overview only.

Adaptive immunity is triggered in vertebrates when a pathogen evades the innate immune system and generates a threshold level of antigen.

Following are the major functions of the adaptive immune system:

- The recognition of specific "nonself" antigens in the presence of "self" during the process of antigen presentation.
- The generation of responses that are tailored to maximally eliminate specific pathogens or pathogen-infected cells.

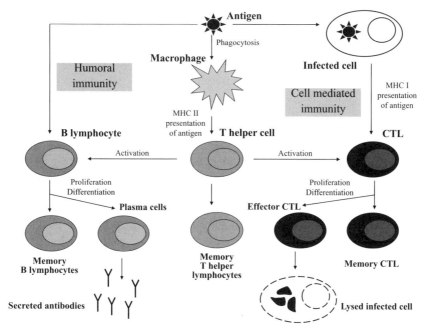

Figure 11.3   Basic model of human adaptive immunity. MHC, major histocompatibility complex; CTL, cytotoxic T lymphocytes.

- The development of immunological memory in which each pathogen is "remembered" by a signature antibody. These memory cells can be called upon to quickly eliminate a pathogen should subsequent infections occur.

B and T lymphocytes mediate the effector functions that define the adaptive immune response (Figure 11.3). They are derived from the same pluripotential hematopoietic stem cells, and are indistinguishable from one another until they are activated. B cells are principally found in the spleen and lymph nodes where they can differentiate after activation into Golgi-rich "cellular factories" for the production and secretion of immunoglobulin. T cells may demonstrate incredible potential recirculating migratory pattern through the blood vessels, lymph nodes, and most tissues of the body. B cells play a large role in the humoral immune response, whereas T cells are intimately involved in cell-mediated immune responses. The peripheral blood contains 20–50% of circulating lymphocytes; the rest move within the lymphatic system or are in the peripheral tissues.

11.3.1   Antigen Presentation

The host's cells express "self" antigens. These antigens are different from those on the surface of bacteria ("nonself" antigens) or on the surface of virally infected host cells ("missing-self"). The adaptive response is triggered by recognizing nonself and missing-self antigens. With the exception of nonnucleated cells, all cells are capable of presenting antigen and of activating the adaptive response. Some cells are specially equipped to present antigen and prime naive T cells. Dendritic cells, B cells, and—to a lesser extent—macrophages are equipped with special immunostimulatory receptors that allow enhanced activation of T cells and are termed professional antigen-presenting cells. Several T cell subgroups can be activated by professional APCs, and each type of T cell is specially equipped to deal with each unique toxin or bacterial and viral pathogen. The type of T cell activated and the type of response generated depend, in part, on the context in which the APC first encountered the antigen.

Antigen presentation stimulates T cells to become either "cytotoxic" $CD8^+$ cells or "helper" $CD4^+$ cells. Dendritic cells engulf exogenous pathogens, such as bacteria, parasites, or toxins in the tissues and then migrate, via chemotactic signals, to the T cell-enriched lymph nodes. During migration, dendritic cells undergo a process of maturation in which they lose most of their ability to engulf other pathogens and develop an ability to communicate with T cells. In the lymph node, the dendritic cell will display the "nonself" antigens on its surface by coupling them to a "self"-receptor called the major histocompatibility complex (also known in humans as human leukocyte antigen (HLA)). This MHC–antigen complex is recognized by T cells passing through the lymph node. Exogenous antigens are usually displayed on MHC class II molecules, which activate $CD4^+$ helper T cells.

Endogenous antigens are produced by viruses replicating within a host cell. The host cell displays virally associated proteins on its surface to T cells by coupling them to MHC. Endogenous antigens are typically displayed on MHC class I molecules and activate $CD8^+$ cytotoxic T cells (CTLs). With the exception of nonnucleated cells (including erythrocytes), MHC class I is expressed by all host cells.

11.3.2   T Lymphocytes

Several different subsets of T cells have been discovered, each with a distinct function. These include helper, cytotoxic, memory, regulatory, natural killer, and γδ T cells. Only helper and cytotoxic T cells are briefly discussed here (Figure 11.3).

T cells that express the CD4 protein on their surface are called T helper cells because they assist other leukocytes (e.g., macrophages, B cells, and cytotoxic T cells) in immunological processes. Helper T cells are presented peptide antigens associated with MHC class II on the surface of APCs. Once activated, they divide rapidly and secrete cytokines that regulate and assist in the immune response. These cells can differentiate into one of several subtypes, including Th1–Th3, Th17, T_{FH}, and others, which secrete different cytokines to facilitate a different type of immune response. The mechanism by which T cells are directed into a particular subtype is poorly understood, though signaling patterns from the APC are thought to play an important role.

Cytotoxic T cells destroy virally infected cells and tumor cells, and are also implicated in transplant rejection. These cells are also known as $CD8^+$ T cells, since they express the CD8 glycoprotein at their surface. Naive cytotoxic T cells are activated when their T cell receptor strongly interacts with a peptide-bound MHC class I molecule. Once activated, the CTL undergoes clonal expansion in which it gains functionality, and divides rapidly, to produce an army of "armed" effector cells. Activated CTL will then travel throughout the body in search of cells bearing that unique MHC class I peptide. When exposed to these infected or dysfunctional somatic cells, effector CTL releases perforin and granulysin: cytotoxins that form pores in the target cell's plasma membrane, allowing ions and water to flow into the infected cell and causing it to burst or lyse.

11.3.3 B Lymphocytes

B cells are the major cells involved in the creation of antibodies that circulate in blood plasma and lymph, known as humoral immunity. Antibodies (or immunoglobulin) are large Y-shaped proteins used by the immune system to identify and neutralize foreign objects. In mammals, there are five types of antibodies: IgA, IgD, IgE, IgG, and IgM, differing in biological properties and each having evolved to handle different kinds of antigens. Upon activation, B cells produce antibodies, each of which recognizes a unique antigen and neutralize specific pathogens.

Like the T cell receptor, B cells express a unique B cell receptor (BCR), in this case, an immobilized antibody molecule. The BCR recognizes and binds to only one particular antigen (Figure 11.3). A critical difference between B cells and T cells is how each cell "sees" an antigen. T cells recognize their cognate antigen in a processed form—as a peptide in the context of an MHC molecule, while B cells recognize antigens in their native form. Once a B cell encounters its cognate (or specific) antigen (and receives additional signals from a helper T cell (predominately Th2 type)), it further differentiates into an effector cell, known as a plasma cell.

The plasma secrete antibodies that bind to antigens, making them easier targets for phagocytes, and trigger the complement cascade. About 10% of plasma cells will survive to become long-lived antigen-specific memory B cells. Already primed to produce specific antibodies, these cells can be called upon to respond quickly if the same pathogen reinfects the host, while the host experiences few, if any, symptoms.

11.4 CHANGES IN SKIN IMMUNITY WITH AGE

Aging is a process of progressive decreases in the maximal functioning and reserve capacity of all organs in the body, including the skin. The naturally occurring functional decline in the skin is often compounded and accelerated by chronic environmental insults, such as ultraviolet (UV) radiation. Aging occurs at the cellular level and reflects both a genetic program and cumulative environmentally imposed damage. Aging mechanisms are attributed to the shortening of telomeres—the terminal portions of eukaryotic chromosomes, decreased DNA repair capacity, and decline in the immune system [50]. Evidence indicates that the immune system deteriorates with age, and is referred to as "immunosenescence." Some reports attribute immunosenescence to adaptive immunity dysfunction [51], while others indicate the contrary, demonstrating that innate cells are also affected in advanced age [52,53].

11.4.1 Aging of the Innate Immune System

Innate immunity represents the first line of host defense and provides the basis for an adequate response to pathogens. However, innate immunity generally declines with age [54]. Aging is frequently associated with a decreased function of epithelial barriers of the skin, lung, or gastrointestinal tract, which enables pathogenic organisms to invade mucosal tissues, resulting in an increased challenge for the aged innate immune system [55].

Besides phagocytic cells (neutrophils, monocytes, macrophages, and DCs) and NKs, soluble mediators such as cytokines, chemokines, hormones, and oxygen-free radicals are also of importance within the innate immune system. Elevated plasma concentrations of IL-6, IL-1β, TNF-α, prostaglandin E2, and anti-inflammatory mediators, such as IL-1 receptor antagonist, soluble TNF receptor, and acute phase proteins, have been described in elderly populations and were postulated as predictive markers of functional disability, frailty, and mortality [56]. Evidence from healthy subjects reveals that such factors are associated with an hyperinflammatory state, referred to as "inflammaging," in advanced aged persons [57]. Chronic inflammation supports the development and progression of age-related diseases, such as osteoporosis, neurodegeneration, and atherosclerosis. In renal failure, particularly in patients treated with hemodialysis, the skin is prematurely aged [58]. Subclinical inflammation may be caused by the chronic stimulation of the innate immune system by degradation products and by the partial inability of the aged immune system to eliminate certain pathogens. The age-related changes that occur in the innate immune response are summarized in Table 11.2.

11.4.1.1 Neutrophils Neutrophils are short-lived cells that play an important role in host defense to both bacterial and fungal infections and during acute inflammation. They are normally found in circulating blood, where they constitute the predominant phagocytic cell type but readily migrate to sites of infection. Neutrophil numbers in the blood and neutrophil precursors in the bone marrow are well preserved in healthy elderly persons [59]. Neutrophils are recruited from the periphery along a gradient of chemotactic factors produced at the site of infection. This includes adhesion to vascular endothelial cells and migration into the affected tissue. Neither the adhesive nor adhesion capacities seem to be affected during aging [60,61]. The results concerning neutrophil chemotaxis with aging are somewhat contradictory [53]. It should be noted, however, that there are several limitations associated with the use of phagocytes from elderly subjects. For example, various clinical conditions and the frequent use of drugs by elderly individuals are likely to be confounding factors in interpreting intrinsic effects of aging on innate immune cells, and thus more valid results are obtained if the cells are isolated from "healthy elderly subjects" [62]. As a consequence, this may cause variation among different studies. Age-dependent functional defects are seen in the phagocytic ability of neutrophils of the elderly population [63]. This is especially the case for opsonized bacteria like *Escherichia coli* and *S. aureus*. The reduced response of neutrophils to *S. aureus* is of particular clinical importance bearing in mind the increased susceptibility to this pathogen in elderly persons. A hypothesis is stated that alterations in the signal transduction pathways of the various receptors involved—as a result of aging—may lead to changes in membrane fluidity, which in turn affects neutrophil functions such as phagocytosis, chemotaxis, and superoxide anion production [64,65]. Interestingly, phagocytosis of unopsonized bacterial targets occurs at the same level in young and old subjects [66]. This suggests that receptors for innate recognition of bacterial components (e.g., the LPS receptor CD14) are not affected by aging. In contrast, the expression of the Fcγ receptor CD16 is significantly reduced in neutrophils from elderly donors [60]. In addition, it has been shown that Fc receptor-mediated superoxide production is significantly reduced in elderly persons [53]. Thus, both Fc receptor-mediated superoxide generation and phagocytosis are decreased in elderly persons, suggesting that a decline in Fc receptor-triggered effector

TABLE 11.2   Age-related Changes in the Innate Immune System

Cell type	Status quo	Age-related increase	Age-related decrease	Ref.
Neutrophils	No change in number of cells	TLR4 expression	TLR2 expression	[53]
	No change in fMPL receptor levels	Membrane fluidity	Chemotaxis	
	No change in cholesterol content	Phospholipid content	Free radical production	
			Phagocytic capacity	
			Bactericidal activity	
Macrophages	No change in number of cells	Prostaglandin E$_2$ production	Chemotaxis	[67,68]
			Wound healing	
			MHC class II expression	
			TRL4 expression	
			P38 and ERK MAPK signalling	
			JAK/STAT signaling	
			Oxidative burst	
			Phagocytic capacity	
NK cells		Total number of cells	Proliferative response to IL-2	[88,89]
			Cytotoxicity	
			Production of IFN-γ	
			Production of chemokines	
NKT cells		Total number of cells IL-10 and IL-4	Production of IFN-γ	[90–92]
			Cytotoxicity	
			Production of chemokines	
Dendritic cells			Capacity to stimulate antigen specific T cells	[83]

responses is of particular importance in age-related neutrophil dysfunction. It could thus be envisioned that the above-described age-associated alterations could result in a continuous influx of impotent neutrophils that fail to contain an infection and, quite probably, contribute to host tissue damage from eventual release of toxic substances.

11.4.1.2 Macrophages   Macrophages are affected by advanced age in many of their biological functions [67]. The number of blood monocytes in elderly persons appears to be similar compared to that in young subjects. However, a significant decrease in macrophage precursors and macrophages in the bone marrow of elderly persons has been described [68]. Macrophages can destroy microbes via products of the respiratory burst induced by IFN-γ. Studies on rats have demonstrated a 75% decrease in the ability of macrophages from aged animals to produce superoxide anion following incubation with IFN-γ. As a consequence of decreased respiratory burst in elderly individuals, the intercellular killing of bacteria is hindered and thus may cause the elderly to have infections of longer duration [52]. Aging human and rodent macrophage populations appear to have reduced levels of MHC class II molecules [68,69], which may contribute to poor CD4$^+$ T cell responses. Upon stimulation with saturating amounts of IFN-γ, macrophages from aged mice expressed half of the MHC class II molecules at the cell surface than macrophages from young mice [70]. As a consequence, antigen-pulsed macrophages from old mice stimulated lower levels of T cell proliferation than macrophages from young mice [70,71]. The reduced capacity in antigen presentation is one of the dysfunctions of macrophages that may lead to increased susceptibility to microbial infection in elderly. Other functions of macrophages that are affected by age are phagocytosis and clearance of infectious organisms [72,73]. This may be due to the inability of aged macrophages to recognize invading pathogens, as aging macrophages demonstrate decreased expression of TLRs [74]. Alternatively, aging macrophages may not be able to migrate to the site of infections, as macrophage chemotactic response to complement-derived factors is impaired in the elderly.

Macrophages may also actively contribute to dysregulated immune function by their secretion of immunosuppressive substances, particularly prostaglandins (PGE). Macrophages from old mice have higher PGE$_2$ production than those from young mice [75]. This can affect multiple cells of the immune system. PGE$_2$ can inhibit the function of DCs, the primary professional antigen-presenting cell. Also, PGE$_2$ directly inhibits T cells, and T cells from the elderly may be more susceptible to such inhibition than T cells from the young [76]. PGE$_2$ also suppresses IL-12 secretion, decreases surface expression of MHC class II molecules on APCs, and enhances IL-10 secretion, resulting in downregulation of T cell function.

Although the overall results reveal a decreased cellular function with aging, controversies exist as a result of differences in the activation state of the macrophages, their source, or particular experimental conditions (*in vitro* versus *in vivo*) [50,52]. Reactive nitrogen intermediates offer conflicting results with regard to aging. Both decreased and increased levels of iNOS mRNA in mice were observed and the opposite results are likely the result of differences in experimental protocols. The same is true for properties like chemotaxis and phagocytosis. While some reports have shown decreased chemotaxis and phagocytosis in macrophages from aged humans and mice, other studies using aged rats found completely opposite results of even no age-related defects (reviewed in Ref. 50).

Skin is also affected with advanced age, and these changes have implication for its function as a protective barrier, including its ability to heal wounds [77]. Macrophages play an important role during the inflammatory phase of wound healing, as they keep the wound bed free from infection and promote angiogenesis [78]. Studies performed in mice have demonstrated defective wound healing [79,80] associated with decreased percentage of phagocytic macrophages [80], as well as impaired macrophage function [79,80].

11.4.1.3 Dendritic Cells   Dendritic cells play a critical role in linking the innate and the adaptive immune systems. They capture and process antigens, interact with T cells, B cells, and NK cells—functioning as antigen-presenting cells, and secrete a variety of cytokines. The role of DCs in immunosenescence and in chronic inflammatory state in aging is poorly understood. *In vitro* generated DCs, originating from peripheral blood monocytes (monocyte-derived dendritic cells (MODCs) from elderly persons, are phenotypically and functionally similar to those from younger persons [81,82]. However, MODCs migration, micro-pinocytosis, and receptor-dependent and receptor-independent phagocytosis are impaired in aging [83]. The reduced uptake of antigen may also affect antigen processing and presentation, and thus effective T cell responses in aging. As phagocytosis of apoptotic cells results in an anti-inflammatory response [84], this decreased ability to phagocytose may contribute to the proinflammatory background observed in elderly individuals. *In vivo* data from mice suggest that aged dendritic cells have an impaired capacity to stimulate antigen-specific T cells and that DC *in vivo* trafficking to drain lymph nodes is affected by aging, as a result of an impaired expression of the lymph node homing marker CCR7 [85]. MODCs from aged persons also display impaired migration. However, in humans, the cell surface receptors are comparable between young and aged, thus the defect appears to be in downstream signaling pathways [83]. Phosphoinositide 3 kinase (PI3K) positively regulates both phagocytosis and migration of DCs [86]. A decreased activation of PI3K—and the PI3-AKT pathway, as evidenced by impaired phosphorylation of AKT shown in MODCs of aged subjects, therefore leads to impaired phagocytosis and migration of MODCs [83].

These age-related defects in micropinocytosis, phagocytosis, and migration could contribute to impairments in immunity in old age. They could specifically have implications on the use of DC-based immunotherapy against cancer in elderly persons.

11.4.1.4 Natural Killer Cells   The cytotoxic capacity of NK cells has been extensively analyzed in elderly people and has been associated with controversy. With the introduction of strict criteria to select only the very healthy elderly to analyze the effect of senescence on the immune system, it was found that NK cell cytotoxicity is not significantly affected by aging [87]. On the contrary, other groups have demonstrated a decreased or defective NK cell cytotoxicity function as a consequence of aging [88,89]. Unlike T cells and B cells, the absolute number of NK cells is increased in aged individuals. NK cells are able to directly kill cells by releasing perforin and granzymes. These enzymes activate caspases and induce apoptosis of the target cell. NK cell proliferation, expression of CD69, and killing of NK-resistant cell lines in response to IL-2 are also decreased with aging, whereas other NK cell functions such as TNF-α production or perforin synthesis are not significantly altered. Taken together, these results indicate that senescence is associated with a defective functional capacity of NK cells that is partially compensated by an increased number of mature NK cells [90].

11.4.1.5 NKT Cells   Only a limited number of studies have examined the effects of aging on NKT cell number and function, although studies do exist both in mice and humans. In general, it is accepted that as age advances, the absolute number of NKT cells within the lymphoid compartment increases [91–93]. It is not clear, however, whether the increase results from a longer life span of NKT cells (versus conventional lymphocytes) [94], active expansion of the population within the aged immune microenvironment, or perhaps an age-related alteration in recruitment from the peripheral circulation to the lymphoid compartment. Interestingly, several reports have shown an age-related decrease of CD1d-restricted NKT cells in the peripheral circulation and decreased proliferative capacity [95–97], which might support the notion that aging causes differential trafficking of the NKT cell population. Although NKT cells are known for their capacity to influence both antigen-presenting cell and T cell function, only a few studies have examined the contribution of NKT cells to immunosenescence. Systemic inhibition of NKT cell activation significantly prevented the age-associated decline of both *in vitro* T cell proliferative responses and *in vivo* delayed-type hypersensitivity responses [92]. In these studies, it was further reported that NKT cells contributed to the age-associated increase in the immunosuppressive cytokine, IL-10 [92]. Additional reports demonstrated that NKT cells contribute to the age-associated increase in IL-4, a cytokine that is known to directly inhibit various aspects of T cell immunity and antigen-presenting cell function [98,99], while other work demonstrated an age-related decrease in IFN-γ [100]. Finally, it has also been shown that age negatively affects NKT cell-mediated cytotoxic activity in mice [101,102]. Although NKT cells have been shown to play a significant role in shaping the overall immune response and advanced age appears to alter NKT cell number and function, more research is required in both experimental animal models and humans to fully appreciate the impact of aging on NKT cell biology and further understand the mechanisms by which NKT cells might contribute to immunosenescence.

11.5 CHANGES IN INNATE SKIN IMMUNITY WITH DISEASE

11.5.1 Immunity in Psoriasis

Psoriasis vulgaris is a common chronic inflammatory skin disorder affecting 2–3% of the worldwide population [103]. The disease is characterized by epidermal hyperproliferation and aberrant differentiation and maturation of keratinocytes, resulting in the formation of raised, well-demarcated, erythematous oval plaques with adherent silvery scales (Figure 11.4) [104–106]. Several comorbidities are seen with psoriasis, such as rheumatoid arthritis, with psoriatic arthritis bridging the two, diabetes mellitus, Crohn's disease, ulcerative colitis, nail disease, alcoholism, and depression. The metabolic syndrome and cardiovascular diseases may develop in direct correlation with the duration and severity of psoriasis. These disorders aggravate psoriasis morbidity and, by increasing cardiovascular mortality, reduce life expectancy by 3–4 years [107–109].

11.5.1.1 Pathogenesis Although the exact etiology of psoriasis is still unclear, the disorder is now considered to be an organ-specific T cell-driven autoimmune disease, evolving over time during a complex interplay between genetic and

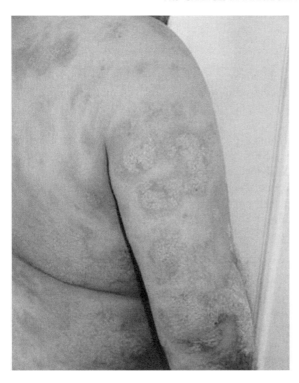

Figure 11.4 Psoriasis vulgaris involving the back and right arm of a man. (*See the color version of this figure in Color Plate section.*)

environmental factors [110]. Both innate immunity, with cellular and molecular components, and adaptive immunity contribute to the pathophysiology of psoriasis [101,110,111].

The Cells Major cellular components of the skin's innate immune system implicated in the pathogenesis of psoriasis are keratinocytes, neutrophils, mast cells, macrophage subsets, natural killer cells, NKT cells, and dendritic cell subsets [112].

Keratinocytes Psoriatic keratinocytes have an extended capacity to resist induction of apoptosis, in contrast to keratinocytes derived from normal skin [113]. They are a rich source of antimicrobial peptides such as LL-37 (cathelicidin), human β-defensins, and S100A7 (psoriasin) [106]. The activation and hyperproliferation of KCs result from the action of cytokines produced by Th17 cells such as IL-17A, IL-17F, and IL-22 on KCs. Activated KCs might produce IL-23, probably resulting in a cross talk between KCs and Th17 cells, in concordance with IL-23 produced by dermal dendritic cells [114]. KCs also have a potential accessory role in skin immune responses. KCs are responsive to key DC-derived and T cell-derived cytokines, such as IFN, TNF-α, IL-17, and IL-20 family of cytokines. In turn, KCs will produce proinflammatory cytokines, such as IL-1, IL-6, and TNF-α, and chemokines, such as CXCL8, CXCL10, and CXCL20 [106].

Neutrophils The primary abnormality in a developing psoriatic lesion is the epidermal perivascular accumulation of neutrophils, resulting in microscopically detectable microabscesses, referred to as Munro abscesses. As these microabscesses may enlarge, they become clinically visible as sterile 2–3 mm pustules [112].

NKT Cells   Natural killer T cells are a heterogeneous subpopulation of innate memory T cells that coexpress T cell receptors and NK cell receptors, such as CD94 and CD161 [32,110,112]. NKT cells play an important role in the earliest phase of an infection, because of their capacity to perform direct cytotoxicity and produce cytokines, such as IFN-γ, affecting the subsequent development of adaptive immunity [32,112]. Activated NKT cells, producing IFN-γ, may therefore represent an important link between innate and adaptive immunity in psoriasis [32]. NKT cell numbers are significantly increased in psoriatic plaques, compared to the number of this cell population in nonlesional psoriatic skin or in normal human skin [115]. In contrast, circulating NKT cell numbers in patients with psoriasis are decreased, tending to be related to disease activity [116].

Dendritic Cell Subsets   Dendritic cells are professional antigen-presenting cells, which can take up antigen in the tissue they reside in and then migrate to the draining lymph nodes in order to activate naive T cells and generate specific T cell responses [112]. Myeloid dendritic cells (mDCs), such as dermal dendritic cells, and plasmacytoid dendritic cells (pDCs) are major subsets of DC that accumulate and are activated in psoriatic skin lesions [101]. Myeloid DC induce autoproliferation of T cells and production of Th1 cytokines, such as IFN-γ, and TNF-α. Plasmacytoid DC produces the innate cytokine IFN-α. Clinical observations point to an important role of IFN-α as an inducer of psoriasis [101,106].

Dendritic cells are major sentinels of the immune system, linking innate and adaptive immunity [106]. They promote the activation and maturation of T cells within psoriatic skin. DC- and T cell-derived cytokines then promote the inflammatory epidermal hyperplasia by producing a typical pattern of cytokines that is dominated by TNF-α, IL-17, IFN-γ, and IL-22 [117,118]. DCs secrete IL-23, inducing production of proinflammatory cytokines by Th17 cells, such as IL-17A, IL-17F, and IL-22. These cytokines will act on KCs, resulting in their activation and hyperproliferation [114].

The Soluble Components of Skin Innate Immune System   Key molecular components of the innate part of the skin immune system, involved in the pathogenesis of psoriasis, include antimicrobial peptides, Toll-like receptors, heat shock proteins (HSPs), complement system, and a wide array of cytokines and chemokines [112].

AMPs   AMPs are small proteins produced by epithelial cells. They provide frontline protection against skin pathogens [119]. Higher concentrations of antimicrobial peptides HBD-2 and HBD-3, and human cathelicidin peptide (hCAP) LL-37 are present in the epidermis of psoriatic skin lesions, compared to the levels of these AMPs in normal human skin and in uninvolved psoriatic skin [120,121]. LL-37 is stored in the granules of neutrophils, which are typically present in clusters in the stratum corneum of lesional psoriatic skin. Bacterial skin infections are rare in psoriatic skin lesions, although there is skin barrier disruption. This is probably due to the increased expression of AMPs in psoriatic lesional skin [120,121].

TLRs   Toll-like receptors belong to the group of pattern recognition receptors that recognize molecular structures shared by many pathogens, so-called pathogen-associated molecular patterns [103,112]. TLR1, TLR2, and TLR5 are constitutively expressed by healthy epidermal KCs, but their expression levels are highest in the cytoplasm of proliferating basal KCs. TLR1, TLR2, and TLR5 are expressed throughout the epidermis of normal human skin. In contrast, in lesional psoriatic skin, TLR1 and TLR2 are highly expressed in nonproliferating KCs of the upper epidermis, close to the keratin layer, but not in the basal KC layer. TLR5 is downregulated by basal KCs of lesional psoriatic skin, compared to nonlesional psoriatic skin. The role of TLRs in the pathogenesis of psoriasis is not fully understood. A possible role for TLRs in innate immunity activation in psoriasis needs further investigation [32,101,103,112].

HSPs   In psoriatic skin, an elevated expression of heat shock proteins, such as HSP27, HSP60, and HSP70 and their receptors are present [122]. HSPs can act as danger signals leading to the destruction of endocytosed pathogens, the activation of phagocytes and DCs and of NF-κB in fibroblasts, and the resultant initiation of adaptive immune responses [1,112,123].

Complement System   Activation of complement proteins may be involved in the psoriatic process [124]. Complement protein activation products, such as C5a des Arg, have been isolated from psoriatic scales. When the skin disease becomes chronic, it has been hypothesized that stratum corneum autoantibody-mediated complement activation induced the immigration of neutrophils that damaged the epidermis. This could lead to epidermal hyperplasia and to secondary immune activation such as lymphocytic infiltration [112].

Cytokines and Chemokines   Cytokines and chemokines are critical for cell–cell interactions, activation and migration of effector cells, and the generation of an effective immune response [101]. A cytokine networking theory for the cause of psoriasis was hypothesized almost 20 years ago. This theory postulates that cytokines orchestrate the multicellular plotting among immunocytes, such as DCs and T cells, and the cross talk between activated dermal immunocytes and epidermal KCs, resulting in the formation of a psoriatic plaque [24,125]. The psoriatic plaque is characterized by the presence of elevated levels of Th1-type cytokines, including IFN-γ, TNF-α, and IL-2, but not Th2-type cytokines, such as IL-4, IL-5, or IL-10 [126]. These observations led to the definition of psoriasis as a Th1-type disease [127].

Recent interest has put the spotlight on a new subset of T helper cells, Th17 cells, which secrete IL-17. This cell type is specialized in immunosurveillance of epithelium; it secretes IL-22, a key cytokine linking adaptive immune effectors and epithelial dysregulation in psoriasis [106]. Increasing evidence suggests that Th17 cells are also key players in the pathogenesis of psoriasis. DCs and KCs in lesional psoriatic skin produce high levels of IL-23, a cytokine that supports the development and proliferation of Th17 cells [128,129]. No statistically significant differences in peripheral levels of IL-17A have been found in psoriatic patients compared to the levels of this cytokine in controls. This suggests that lesional skin infiltrated by Th17 cells is the major site of production of IL-17A in psoriasis [130].

Some of the cellular and humoral elements of the innate part of the skin immune system in psoriasis are upregulated or increased in uninvolved psoriatic skin, and practically all are upregulated or increased in lesional psoriatic skin [112]. An increased presence of $CD4^+$ and $CD8^+$ T lymphocytes in peripheral blood and lesional skin of psoriasis patients points to an involvement of the adaptive immune system in the pathogenesis of this immune-mediated disease [111]. The major populations of T cells that play a role in psoriasis are $CD4^+$ Th1 and Th17 T cells, $CD8^+$ T cells, NKT cells, and regulatory T cells (Tregs). These cells are all mature, skin-homing, activated memory cells. Both $CD4^+$ and $CD8^+$ T cells respond to processed polypeptides presented by mature APCs [101]. It has been demonstrated that Treg cell activity is deficient in the peripheral blood and lesional skin of patients with psoriasis. Although the absolute number of circulating Tregs in patients with psoriasis is normal compared to healthy controls, circulating Tregs have defective suppressor cell activity. Increased numbers of Tregs are present in psoriatic plaques, compared to healthy skin, but they are defective in their ability to suppress effector $CD4^+$ T cell proliferative responses in skin lesions [131].

11.5.1.2 Treatment As psoriasis is a lifelong relapsing disease, conventional systemic therapies such as methotrexate, acitretin, and cyclosporine A are of limited value as their long-term use is associated with cumulative organ toxic effects, which may limit their therapeutic use. Recent advances in the understanding of immunopathogenesis of psoriasis have led to the development of highly effective biological therapies, characterized by highly selective mechanisms of action and designed to target the molecular mechanisms of the disease. The biological agents can be classified into three major therapeutic classes, according to their mechanisms of action: T cell antagonists, TNF-α antagonists, and an IL-12/IL-23 p40 agonist have been demonstrated to relieve symptoms of psoriasis and arrest disease progression. There are two variants of T cell antagonists, namely, efalizumab (Raptiva®), a chimeric monoclonal anti-CD11 antibody, which has been withdrawn from the market due to safety concerns, and alefacept (Amevive®), the lymphocyte function antigen (LFA)-3-imunoglobulin G-Fc fusion protein. They both interfere with T cell recruitment, T cell activation, and T cell expansion and have validated the concept of a role of T cells in psoriasis [132,133].

TNF-α antagonists include the chimeric monoclonal antibody infliximab (Remicade®), the human monoclonal antibody adalimumab (Humira®), and the genetically engineered Fc fusion protein etanercept (Enbrel®). TNF-α antagonists bind to TNF-α, making it functionally inactive and blocking its proinflammatory effects [134,135]. The IL-12/IL-23 p40 agonist ustekinumab (Stelara®) is a human monoclonal antibody that binds to the shared p40 protein subunit of IL-12 and IL-23, which are two cytokines with fundamental roles in inflammation and immunity [136].

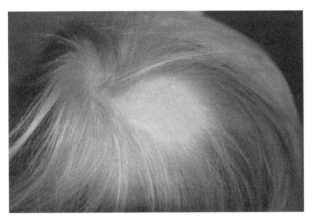

Figure 11.5   Alopecia areata lesion on the scalp of a child.

Targeting both IL-12 and IL-23 is a highly effective therapeutic approach in chronic plaque psoriasis [114]. Current biological therapies are well tolerated, and some are more effective than conventional systemic therapies [137]. To date, limited safety data are available regarding ustekinumab. Another anti-p40 antibody, ABT 874, is currently being tested in clinical trials [114].

11.5.2 Immunity in Alopecia Areata

Hair loss or alopecia is a very common problem among adults and children, both in men and women. It can be caused by a large amount of conditions and has great impact on the quality of life. One type of immune-mediated hair loss is alopecia areata (AA).

Alopecia areata occurs in 0.1–0.2% of the population, equally affecting men and women [138]. Clinically, a sudden onset of nonscarring, unifocal, patchy hair loss on the scalp occurs. Exclamation point hairs, which are broken-off stubby hairs, are diagnostic features of this disorder (Figure 11.5). The patches of hair loss may evolve to complete loss of scalp hair, a phenomenon called alopecia totalis, or to complete loss of all body hairs, a phenomenon called alopecia universalis [139]. Alopecia areata has a very unpredictable course and often resolves spontaneously without treatment within a year in 34–50% of patients [140].

11.5.2.1 Pathogenesis   The exact pathogenesis of alopecia areata is still undetermined, but it is thought to be a tissue-specific, T cell-mediated autoimmune disease of the hair follicle, with possible involvement of genetic and environmental factors. To date, the major hypothesis involves a T cell-mediated attack of anagen hair follicles, which have lost their immune privilege [141].

The hair follicle in the anagen phase and the nail epithelium are two sites of immune privilege in the skin [12,142]. This immune privilege is mainly established by low or absent expression of major histocompatibility complex class I and II [120,143,144]. It is supported by the local production of potent immunosuppressants such as transforming growth factor (TGF)-β1, insulin growth factor (IGF)-1, and α-melanocyte-stimulating hormone (α-MSH) [12]. Also, a reduction in the number and functional activity of Langerhans cells is present [120].

Normally, MHC class I is expressed on all nucleated cells [145]. Cells that have low or altered expression of MHC class I molecules are attacked by natural killer cells. This would mean that normal hair follicles would be attacked by NK cells. However, in normal skin, very few perifollicular NK cells are present around human anagen hair follicles [12,120]. In addition, almost no CD4$^+$ or CD8$^+$ T cells are found in the anagen hair bulb. Langerhans cells are also rare [120]. In AA on the contrary, more perifollicular NK cells were found, compared to normal skin. So, it is suggested that in normal skin, an active NK cell suppression would be present to maintain the immune privilege [12]. It was shown that in normal skin, a strong expression of macrophage migration inhibitory factor (MIF), which is a potent NK cell inhibitor, is present on the epithelium of the hair follicle. In AA on the contrary, a decreased expression of MIF was seen. Apart from this, the skin in alopecia areata has a strong extra- and intrafollicular MHC class I chain-related A (MICA) expression, unlike an almost complete absent expression of MICA in normal anagen hair follicles. Also, the circulating NK cells and CD8$^+$ cells in the blood of alopecia areata patients were more sensitive to MHC class I chain-related A stimulation. This taken all together points to an important role of NK cells, which are excessively stimulated and activated, in the pathogenesis of alopecia areata [12].

In alopecia areata hair follicles, augmented expression of MHC class I and, to a lesser extent, MHC class II was found, which was thought to be indicative of a breakdown of the immune privilege. During treatment, a downregulation of this expression was measured, indicating a restoration of the immune privilege [144]. As IFN-γ induces ectopic MHC class I expression, it is most likely to be also responsible for initiating the collapse of the hair follicle IP [12]. In normal cells, IFN-γ also leads to upregulation of NKG2D, which is an activating receptor on NK cells, so the theory of an IFN-γ-induced collapse of hair follicle immune privilege, that simultaneously facilitates an attack of NK2GD + NK cells on hair follicles becomes attractive [12].

Gilhar et al. [146] demonstrated that alopecia areata is mediated by T cells that recognize a follicular autoantigen. Autoreactive T cells were found in scalp biopsies from alopecia areata patients [147]. They most favorably attack melanocyte-associated antigens, since hair follicles are attacked only in the anagen/growth phase of the hair cycle, characterized by active melanogenesis [142]. This would also explain why recovering hair follicles in alopecia areata are often nonpigmented [12]. Melanocyte-associated antigens are also targeted in other immune diseases such as vitiligo [148].

11.5.2.2 Treatment: Restoration of Hair Follicle Immune Privilege Alopecia areata has an unpredictable course: limited patches can regrow spontaneously without treatment, though relapse and gradual progression may also be seen. Strong evidence-based studies proving the efficacy of any treatment of alopecia areata are still lacking [149].

Topical corticosteroids are often the preferred therapy. They are thought to suppress the inflammatory reaction seen in alopecia areata. Intralesional corticoids can be used for treating alopecia areata manifestation in eyebrows or for other small spots of alopecia areata [139,141]. The use of systemic corticoids is limited due to side effects, although initial satisfactory results were seen especially in moderate disease. Unfortunately, relapse is frequent [150]. On the contrary, contact immunotherapy with diphenylcyclopropenone (DPCP), squaric acid dibutyl ester (SADBE), and dinitrochlorobenzene (DCNB) has a low side effect profile and can be used when more conservative treatments fail [141]. Topical immunotherapy is effective in 30–60% of the cases [151,152]. Treatment with psoralen and ultraviolet A (PUVA), which most likely has an immunomodulatory effect, has poor or mixed results and is limited by the potential long-term side effects [153].

The abnormal expression of MHC class I in human hair follicles can be downregulated by treatment with α-MSH, IGF-1, or TGF-β1 *in situ* and by FK506 (tacrolimus), suggesting that these immunomodulators are possible candidates for the restoration of the immune privilege [12]. Recently, a number of case reports were published of successful treatment of AA with efalizumab [48,154]. A larger, placebo-controlled study, however, showed no effectiveness of 3 and 6 months treatment with efalizumab in patients with moderate-to-severe alopecia areata [155]. Efaluzimab was recently withdrawn from the market for safety concerns.

An open-label study with etanercept, a TNF-α inhibitor, showed that etanercept is ineffective in treating alopecia areata [156]. This is consistent with the finding that patients receiving treatment with etanercept, infliximab, and adalimumab are reported to have development or recurrence of alopecia areata [157,158]. This suggests that TNF-α may not play an essential role in the inflammatory pathway of alopecia areata [141].

11.6 INNATE IMMUNITY IN SKIN REACTIVITY

11.6.1 Response at a Tissue Level

The three elements in innate immunity (the barrier, the cells, and the secretory components) gain their effectiveness by orchestration of a response in a tissue. In this response, neurological, physiological, and tissue biological components operate in a spectrum that includes subliminal, subtle, obvious, or very obvious manifestations. The skin is eminently available for observation of the spectrum of changes relevant for a discussion of innate immunity. The physiological preparation for the arrival of potential pathogens begins long before the actual appearance of the pathogens—a "danger" situation is anticipated by the tissue. The reactivity of the skin to external stimuli is a homeostatic mechanism that includes innate preparedness for possible bacterial invasion after tissue trauma—possibly because phylogenetically, injury has always been associated with risk for microbial invasion.

11.6.2 Skin Puncture Scenario

A sharp trauma can be sensed by the skin innervation and communicated centrally. A more intense sharp (or other noxious) trauma is not only communicated centrally but also induces a reaction locally, not only at the actual point of the stimulation but also around it, the classical triple response of Lewis [159]. Local blood flow immediately increases access for cells to the area which possibly is about to be invaded by bacteria or other agents from the environment that may be harmful to the organism as a whole. Without actual puncture, the skin's physiological system sounds "all clear" and the response, subsides in a time frame of 60 min or so. If the nociceptive stimulus results in an actual puncture of the skin, a further phase is added to the triple response, first in terms of degree of the response (a more pronounced and prolonged dermal response) and second in terms of the actual likelihood of pathogen access. Physiologically the skin has increased blood flow and already recruited immunologically active cells before any bacteria gain access— inoculum size is smaller and easier to manage. Even small wounds need repairing— the inflammatory phase of wound healing runs from the response phase. The more pronounced the tissue trauma, the greater the need for defense against pathogens and the greater the innate response.

11.6.2.1   *What Happens in the Skin Puncture Scenario?*   The skin in the normal situation has by its structure, barrier functions that are an integral part of the innate immune system [13,160]. It also has sensibility functions that constitute an interface to the surrounding environment but do not induce an innate response. Microprovocation in the form of damage from water of dry air or mild tensides and solvents induces response of a homeostatic type, for example, maintenance or thickening of the 10 μm thick stratum corneum. A mild nociceptive (sharp) stimulus gives a short-term response with the erythematous part of the response mediated chiefly by an axon reflex mechanism that allows the reactivity to spread to a larger area than that actually provoked [159]. The most common illustration of this response in clinical care is seen during type I allergy prick testing in the form of the negative (diluent) control. In contact urticaria, for example, to methyl nicotinate [161], the same response is induced without mechanical puncture but through direct effects after percutaneous penetration on keratinocytes, mast cells, or endothelial cells. When the skin is actually punctured, not only the erythematous response but also an increasing component of inflammatory response is invoked reflecting participation of the innate immune system [162] with a time course that is longer, in the order of days. These types of injury are, at least initially, not associated with microbial invasion. The needle stick situation is often seen in the clinical scenario. In clinical research, cutaneous microdialysis (which allows study of local production and temporal resolution of inflammatory mediators in living skin) involves insertion of the microdialysis catheter into the dermis [163]. Microdialysis studies of the time immediately after catheter insertion in the skin demonstrate histamine release and numerous other inflammatory mediators are also certainly produced, all heightening preparedness in the organism for possible bacterial invasion [164]. While the epidermis is often the focus of skin reactivity, dermal responsiveness can be pronounced. In microdialysis it has been shown that the needle stick provocation of the dermis in the absence of epidermal stimulation results in the production of IL-1b, IL-6, and IL-8 over a 12–18 h time period (Figure 11.6) [165].

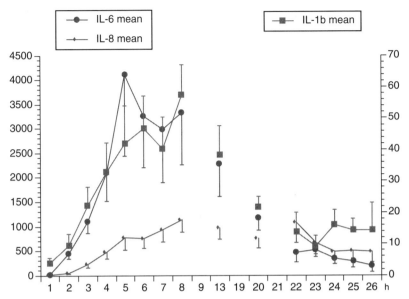

Figure 11.6   Cytokine production during 24 h after insertion of a microdialysis catheter into normal dermis. Cytokine production in the normal forearm skin of 10 subjects after insertion of a microdialysis catheter (means and 1 SD). Units are pg/mL. Measurement of seven other cytokines showed absent or very low levels (IL-10, IL-5, IL-4, and IFN-γ) or sporadic low levels (IL-2, GM-CSF, and TNF-α) (data from Ref. 165).

This sterile provocation thus produces a response in the absence of bacteria, but can be considered as a preemptive response to "danger" in anticipation of risk for microbial invasion and a preparation for wound healing. Conceptually, this form of inflammatory response has been termed "nonmicrobial inflammation" [166] and has been of interest in basic research studies of innate reactivity. With a more pronounced injury with or without an epidermal defect, the spectrum of response moves from reactivity to a more classical example of the wound healing process that follows the innate reactivity and takes days to weeks to resolve [1,167].

11.6.3   Altered Response to Minimal Trauma: The Skin Pathergy Test and Behcet's Disease

An example of altered reactivity to minimal trauma is provided by the pathergy reaction that occurs classically in Behcet's disease (BD). Behcet's disease is a multisystem disease of unknown etiology with a clinical grouping of ocular, oral, genital, and other manifestations. In addition, characteristic lesions, often pustular, can be seen after trauma, for example, after needle puncture. The provocation of skin pathergy is achieved by the skin pathergy test (SPT) in which a minimal puncturing trauma is performed on the skin and the response noted [168]. A positive SPT is one criterion in the diagnosis and classification of Behcet's disease. Defects in innate immune mechanisms have been reported in this complex disease [169–171] and it seems likely that at least part of the pathogenesis of the disease involves aberrant innate immune responsiveness. In normal individuals, naked eye observation of the course of events over 96 h after full thickness penetration of the skin by a bleeding time lancet show the reaction and repair stages of erythema, crust formation, formation of new keratin layer, and finally healing [162]. Quantification of the erythematous phase of the response was done using laser Doppler perfusion imaging. Figure 11.7 shows quantification of such a provocation using tissue viability imaging (TiVi) that is a newer alternative for the quantification of blood in the skin and thus the dynamics of erythematous reactions [172].

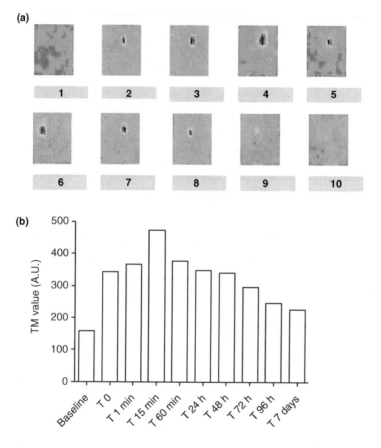

Figure 11.7 (a) Tissue viability imaging: a polarization spectroscopy technique has been used to produce serial images of the erythematous component of a minimal, full-thickness wound protocol [162] induced by a bleeding time lancet with dimensions 1 mm broad and 2 mm depth on ventral forearm skin. Timepoints are (1) baseline, (2) immediately after wound, (3) at 1 min, (4) at 15 min, (5) at 60 min, (6) at 24 h, (7) at 48 h, (8) at 72 h, (9) at 96 h, and (10) at 7 days. (b) The histogram shows the amount of blood in regions of interest around the site of the wound over 7 days illustrating the immediate axon reflex component and the more extended wound healing course. (*See the color version of this figure in Color Plate section.*)

It is proposed that this bleeding time lancet injury model may be useful in quantitative documentation of the SPT in BD that is uncommon and some other inflammatory diseases in which skin pathergy has been reported, notably inflammatory bowel disease and hematological disease [173–175]. Systematic performance of the SPT may be a clinical tool that allows the assessment of the reactive status of an individual at a specific point in time, which may be of importance not only at the time of diagnosis but also in the follow-up of disease activity and adequacy of therapy.

11.6.4   Other Types of Skin Reactivity and Diseases with Innate Immune Mechanisms

Mechanical trauma can invoke dermal reactivity [176]. Roles for innate immunity are postulated for a number of diseases and for a number of common reactivities. The reaction to ultraviolet B with erythema is a universal, though dose variable, phenomenon in many organisms, including humans [177]. Clinically contact dermatitis is classified as allergic or irritant. In adaptive, type IV, contact allergy reactivity, it is postulated that innate and adaptive mechanisms react in unison [178] with the innate reactivity setting the scene for the acquisition of the adaptive response to an agent. In fact, many allergens (e.g., dinitrochlorobenzene and Kathon) are also irritants. Diverse mechanisms underlie irritant dermatitis [168,179,180], but some irritant reactions have been shown to utilize TLRs in their induction of inflammation [181]. Thus, the irritant contact dermatitis, at least in some situations, is considered to involve innate immune responsivity. Psoriasis research has shown that innate immune mechanisms are involved in the disease's pathogenesis [111,125]. The occurrence of the Koebner phenomenon in which trauma to the skin is followed by the occurrence of psoriasis in the same area connects to the reactivity to minimal trauma that is an innate capacity of human skin but that can be subject to variability that can manifest as disease.

11.6.5   Variability

That UVB-induced erythema is individually variable and is a manifestation of phenotype is generally accepted. Fitzpatrick type I skin reacts more vigorously to erythema than a type III skin. Also, in reactivity to irritants, some individuals have sensitive skin and others more hardy skin. There are differences in reactivity between irritants. Low thresholds to irritation from sodium lauryl sulfate, for instance, are not always indicative of low thresholds of reactivity to other irritants. Thus, in the epicutaneous test, there is no feasible "negative" control in the form of a reliable irritant (nonallergic) reaction that can be universally used. A striking feature of the erythema in the previously mentioned minimal trauma wound model—based on a 1 mm wide and 2 mm deep penetrating injury that resulted in initial bleeding, axon reflex erythema followed by a longer lasting erythema, crust formation, formation of new keratin layer, and finally healing—was its variability between individuals while intraindividual variability was less marked [162]. Variability within an individual can also be seen temporally—variability from one occasion to another. Such variability has as yet no known association with disease activity but it has as yet not been systematically studied. Individual variability in skin reactivity and healing capacity after trauma is an important clinical issue. The various aspects of reactivity can be seen as an expression of phenotype. Recognizing and characterizing phenotype at a whole organism level in the clinical situation are relevant challenges in the establishment of functional evidence for the demonstration of genetic polymorphisms.

11.6.6 Pathogenetic Issues

The term "nonmicrobial inflammation" coined in basic research publications can be seen as an overbridging heading for inflammatory mechanisms not induced by microbes but possibly by using the same signaling at a membrane level as bacterial pathogens [7,166]. Detailed knowledge at a molecular level about inflammatory response to nonmicrobial inflammation/trauma is being generated in recent studies *in vitro* and in animal models [7,169,181,182] and genotypic polymorphisms are suggested that may allow better characterization/selection of individual subjects [168,183]. Another important issue in innate reactivity is the development of virulence factors in a microorganism. Changes in bacteria that are potential pathogens to an actual pathogen can modulate innate reactivity [166] with nonmicrobial (sterile) inflammation being the preparatory step taken by the tissue to prepare defense. Many challenges remain but there are possibly helpful clues from the clinical workplace— for instance, the well-known observation that atopic eczema is often secondarily infected and psoriasis usually not, despite having just as much barrier damage.

11.7 IMMUNITY AND ITCH OF SENSITIVE SKIN

Itch is not only a common symptom in many inflammatory skin disorders but also an associated phenomenon during acute or chronic stress episodes in life [142]. Indeed, even healthy persons suffer regularly from spontaneous itch or temporarily have a lower itch threshold. Refractory itch is also a major problem in neuropathic and psychogenic syndromes [184]. Itch can be a manifestation of systemic disease, for instance, in hepatic disease, renal failure, and polycythemia rubra vera [185,186]. Pruritus or itch can be defined as the strong impulse to scratch or even the urge to scratch [187]. This is the main distinguishing feature of itch in comparison to pain, which can also be triggered at distinctive nociceptors in the upper layers of the skin and transitional mucosa such as the lips and genitor–anal mucosa. How itch relates to the innate immune system in the skin is summarized below. We emphasize on the role that stress plays in the elicitation of itch.

11.7.1 Pathogenesis

11.7.1.1 The Cells

Mast Cells Pruritus is related to the release of histamine from mast cells in the skin, for example, in urticaria, or as a result of insect bites. Histamine used as a positive control in the intradermal prick tests to screen for allergy to atopic antigens typically causes an itchy, red edematous papule (wheal and flare reaction).

This reaction is predominantly mediated by C-fibers. Histamine acts on a specific subgroup of mechano-insensitive C-fibers (called the CMi(his +) units) that are also sensitive to other endogenous mediators, such as prostaglandins and acetylcholine, and capsaicin [187]. In prurigo nodularis patients, spontaneously active such CMi(his +) nerve units were found [188]. The histamine-related wheal and flare reaction is mediated by the H1 receptors in the walls of venoles and the release of calcitonin gene-related peptide (CGRP) from the axon collaterals of excited CMi(his +) units [189].

However, histamine does not explain all types of itch, since there are several clinical itch states that are not influenced by depletion of histamine (atopic itch, uremic itch, and itch in liver failure). Also, many pathological forms of pruritus are not accompanied by the wheal and flare reactions and are probably histamine independent. An experimental nonhistaminergic pruritus animal model caused by reaction on a plant ingredient mucunain, a peptidase acting at the proteinase-activated receptor 4 (PAR-4), identified the presence and involvement of polymodal nociceptors (CMH units) [187].

It is clear that the knowledge on the neuronal mechanism of pruritus is far from complete and is an actively developing research field of great importance toward the development of highly sought effective therapy.

Mast cells as one of the cell types acting as protagonists in the innate skin immunity fulfill their role through proximity with blood vessels and peripheral nerve fibers. It is a central cell in the emerging field of neuro-endocrino-immunology research in the skin. Neuroendocrine stress messengers such as hormones (corticotrophin-releasing hormone (CRH), adrenocorticotropic hormone (ACTH), pro-opiomelanocortin (POMC) and splice products such as melanocyte-stimulating hormone), growth factors (nerve growth factor, neurotrophin-4, stem cell factor through tyrosine kinase receptors (Trks)), and neuropeptides (substance P via its neurokinin-1 (NK1) receptor on mast cells, calcitonin gene-related peptide (CGRP), vasoactive intestinal peptide (VIP), neurotensin, hemokinin A, and pituitary adenylate cyclase-activating polypeptide (PACAP)) activate the mast cell toward release of its downstream mediators. These are histamine, heparin, kinins, proteases (chymase and tryptase), leukotrienes, prostaglandins, vascular endothelial growth factor, nerve growth factor, nitric oxide, substance P, vasoactive intestinal peptide, corticotropin-releasing hormone, and several cytokines (e.g., TNF-α and TGF-β). Mast cell-derived TNF enhances T cell activation, and the proteases activate proteinase-activated receptors on sensory neurons, which in turn release more substance P. Also, keratinocytes and dermal endothelial cells express PAR-2 that may create a positive feedback signal toward mast cells, enhancing the stress-induced and neurogenic inflammation equally through release of, among others, NGF and substance P [142,190].

Macrophages, NK Cells, and Dendritic Cells   Not only the mast cell is under the influence of signals from sensory peripheral nerves. The release of peripheral neuropeptides, including CRH, substance P, and CGRP, also causes activation of macrophages, B cells and T cells, and keratinocytes, all expressing CRH receptors for CRH and neurokinin-1 and neurokinin-2 receptors for substance P. The effect of CGRP on the innate immune system is still contradictory, as its direct effect on dendritic cells seems inhibiting its activation. Substance P also increases NK cell activity and migration *in vitro* and stimulates the release of CXCL8 (see also in psoriasis) and CCL2 from leukocytes.

It is interesting to note that several immune cells, including mast cells, monocytes, and dendritic cells, can also produce the neuromediators, for example, substance P, VIP, and CRH. Monocytes/macrophages are also strong producers of NGF and brain-derived neurotrophic factor (BDNF) [190]. Linking this latter fact to the clinical, it is worth mentioning that BDNF gene polymorphisms, with higher BDNF serum levels, were found in Chinese atopic dermatitis patients [191].

11.7.1.2 The Components: The Neuroendocrine Pathways It is clear that in the induction of the inflammatory (itch) response in the skin, both glucocorticoids and catecholamines, as the hormones and neurotransmitters of the hypothalamo–pituitary–adrenal (HPA) axis, in the sympathetic and parasympathetic nervous system play a modulatory role in the influence of the peripheral nervous system on immune cells. Dhabhar [192] comments on these axes in a very thorough manner, describing the immunoenhancing effects of the acute stress response and also pointing to the fact that knowledge is scarce with regard to the fact that paradoxically stress also exacerbates certain inflammatory disorders and itch.

The work of Buske-Kirschbaum [193] is in that respect very interesting as it shows that patients suffering from atopy (and often uncontrollable itch) have an altered stress response. Atopic patients show an HPA axis dysfunction, with hyporesponsive reduced cortisol responses to stress in adult atopic dermatitis patients, leading to proinflammatory responses including more itch.

In conclusion, it is now known that many immune cells possess the molecular tools to be responsive to neural factors, which are the receptors for neurotransmitters and neuromediators, and neurohormones. However, much more study is needed to know all cell types of the immune system at the same level of depth and the relevance of the neural modulation of the immune response.

11.7.2 Treatment

The novelties in treatment mainly lie in the newly discovered nonhistaminergic mechanisms in itch. To date, more than 20 neuromediators have been described in the skin [190]. The emerging knowledge sheds further light on future perspectives in research, and even more importantly, highlights novel therapeutic strategies.

Blocking substance P-mediated effects such as itch is studied in trials using NK1R antagonists (e.g., spantide II), after showing that scratching behavior reduced in a mouse dermatitis model using tachykinin NK1 antagonists [194]. Very recently, Duval and Dubertret [195] reported on the positive effect of aprepitant, an oral neurokinin-1 receptor antagonist used as antiemetic agent after chemotherapy, on pruritus in three cases with Sézary syndrome.

Capsaicin (*trans*-8-methyl-*N*-vanillyl-6-nonenamide) 0.025–0.3% cream is derived from chilli peppers and triggers the release of substance P from C nociceptors, which desensitizes nerve fibers. Moreover, the involvement in pruritus of the recently discovered histamine 4 receptor (H4R) [196] was supported by the observations that

H4R antagonists inhibit itch [197]. Also, PAR-2 antagonists or serine protease inhibitors are promising [198].

Finally, not so much at pharmacological level, it will be inevitable to counter the role that stress plays in a number of disease and overall outcomes of treatments. Dhabhar [192] exhaustively describes the effects of stress as a major factor during diagnosis, treatment, and follow-up of most diseases as stress-induced changes in immune cell numbers and function affect results. Educational programs offering techniques that enhance the individual potential to cope with stress should therefore be introduced in the classical treatment schemes of atopic dermatitis, psoriasis, and so on.

Several concepts of educational and behavioral interventions have been reported for a variety of skin diseases. The nursing program "Coping with Itch" described by Van Os-Medendorp et al. [199] led to a reduction in the frequency of itching and scratching and to a reduction of catastrophizing and helpless coping in patients with chronic pruritic skin diseases during the period immediately following the intervention. Standard medical treatment was continued along with the intervention, and the program seemed to have a favorable cost-effectiveness ratio for several months. Educational programs for children and adolescents with atopic dermatitis are also reported to be effective in the long-term management of the disease [200].

11.8 FROM THEORY TO LAB BENCH TO CLINICAL SCENARIO

Modern basic research technique allows investigation of innate immune mechanisms at a molecular level. Hypotheses generated by these data need testing in a clinical research scenario. A broader knowledge of skin reactivity in health will allow a more sure delineation of aberrant reactivity. New skin physiological (bioengineering) assessment techniques may represent an opportunity to broaden the study of innate reactive (nonmicrobial inflammation) and wound healing mechanisms in clinical materials and more rapidly take basic research findings at a molecular level to clinical research platforms. Cutaneous microdialysis especially when coupled to "endpoint biopsy" allows the study of inflammatory mediator production—the molecules that mediate "cell talk."

As conceptual development progresses, information from research into inflammation prior to the advent of modern techniques can be reviewed and placed into context. This context can be expected to have closer relevance to the clinical scenario than basic research. After all the human body has changed little over thousands of years—just our understanding of it. The old-fashioned phenomenological research on inflammation still has relevance in further extending that knowledge.

11.9 SUMMARY: TAKE HOME MESSAGE

The word innate literally means inborn and natural. Thus, in a broad sense, all reactive and defense mechanisms that do not have the features of adaptive immunity are, by default, of possible innate immune relevance. There is not only a need for continued basic research to delineate the details of specific mechanisms but there is also the need for clinical research to establish pathogenic proof of concept. Innate immunity is by its nature multifactorial involving physical, soluble, chemical, and cellular reactive barriers. Each of these has a number of components and may, if overwhelmed, induce the adaptive immune system. Aging effects are variable with a minimal change or a deterioration in response occurring with increased age. Various diseases affect the innate immunity of the skin in different ways. For instance, the physical epidermal barrier is impaired in psoriasis, but this autoimmune disease is, by nature, associated with an increased soluble, chemical, and cellular activity. In contrast, in alopecia areata, the stratum corneum function appears to be not greatly affected but the limited barrier function due to hairs is lost. This autoimmune hair follicle disease arises in part from T cell activation and action on the follicles. Obviously, direct damage results in a wound healing response, as observed after wounding of skin, sun damage, and allergen exposure. Pruritus is not a straightforward condition with histamine release, mast cells, and cytokines often involved. Much remains to be elucidated but efforts are evident in a large number of international laboratories.

ACKNOWLEDGMENTS

We would like to thank Florence Sjögren and Joakim Henricson for their assistance in illustrations provided in this chapter. We thank the NHMRC (Australia) for their support.

REFERENCES

1. Clark R, Kupper T. Old meets new: the interaction between innate and adaptive immunity. *J. Invest. Dermatol.* 2005;125(4):629–637.
2. Roth RR, James WD. Microbiology of the skin: resident flora, ecology, infection. *J. Am. Acad. Dermatol.* 1989;20(3):367–390.
3. Trowbridge JM, Gallo RL. Dermatan sulfate: new functions from an old glycosaminoglycan. *Glycobiology* 2002;12(9):117R–125R.
4. Rose MJ, Page C. Glycosaminoglycans and the regulation of allergic inflammation. *Curr. Drug Targets Inflamm. Allergy* 2004;3(3):221–225.
5. Termeer C, Benedix F, Sleeman J, Fieber C, Voith U, Ahrens T, Miyake K, Freudenberg M, Galanos C, Simon JC. Oligosaccharides of Hyaluronan activate dendritic cells via Toll-like receptor 4. *J. Exp. Med.* 2002;195(1):99–111.
6. Fraser JR, Laurent TC, Laurent UB. Hyaluronan: its nature, distribution, functions and turnover. *J. Intern. Med.* 1997;242(1):27–33.
7. Yamasaki K, Muto J, Taylor KR, Cogen AL, Audish D, Bertin J, Grant EP, Coyle AJ, Misaghi A, Hoffman HM et al. NLRP3/cryopyrin is necessary for interleukin-1beta (IL-1beta) release in response to Hyaluronan, an endogenous trigger of inflammation in response to injury. *J. Biol. Chem.* 2009;284(19):12762–12771.
8. Barreda DR, Hanington PC, Belosevic M. Regulation of myeloid development and function by colony stimulating factors. *Dev. Comp. Immunol.* 2004;28(5):509–554.
9. Travers P, Walport M, Shlomchik M. *Immunobiology*, 5th ed. New York: Garland Science, 2001.
10. Moore KW, de Waal Malefyt R, Coffman RL, O'Garra A. Interleukin-10 and the interleukin-10 receptor. *Annu. Rev. Immunol.* 2001;19: 683–765.
11. Fulop T, Seres I. Signal transduction changes in granulocytes and lymphocytes with aging. *Immunol. Lett.* 1994;40:259–268.
12. Medzhitov R. Toll-like receptors and innate immunity. *Nat. Rev. Immunol.* 2001;1(2):135–145.

13. Braff MH, Bardan A, Nizet V, Gallo RL. Cutaneous defense mechanisms by antimicrobial peptides. *J. Invest. Dermatol.* 2005;125(1):9–13.

14. Palaniyar N, Nadesalingam J, Reid KB. Pulmonary innate immune proteins and receptors that interact with Gram-positive bacterial ligands. *Immunobiology* 2002;205(4–5):575–594.

15. Goodarzi H, Trowbridge J, Gallo RL. Innate immunity: a cutaneous perspective. *Clin. Rev. Allergy Immunol.* 2007;33(1–2):15–26.

16. Rottem M, Mekori YA. Mast cells and autoimmunity. *Autoimmun. Rev.* 2005;4(1):21–27.

17. Galli SJ, Tsai M, Piliponsky AM. The development of allergic inflammation. *Nature* 2008; 454(7203):445–454.

18. Raulet DH. Interplay of natural killer cells and their receptors with the adaptive immune response. *Nat. Immunol.* 2004;5(10):996–1002.

19. Liu CC, Walsh CM, Young JD. Perforin: structure and function. *Immunol. Today* 1995;16(4):194–201.

20. Liu CC, Persechini PM, Young JD. Perforin and lymphocyte-mediated cytolysis. *Immunol. Rev.* 1995;146:145–175.

21. Sato K, Hida S, Takayanagi H, Yokochi T, Kayagaki N, Takeda K, Yagita H, Okumura K, Tanaka N, Taniguchi T et al. Antiviral response by natural killer cells through TRAIL gene induction by IFN-alpha/beta. *Eur. J. Immunol.* 2001;31(11):3138–3146.

22. Bendelac A, Savage PB, Teyton L. The biology of NKT cells. *Annu. Rev. Immunol.* 2007;25:297–336.

23. Joyce S. CD1d and natural T cells: how their properties jump-start the immune system. *Cell. Mol. Life Sci.* 2001;58(3):442–469.

24. Barker JN, Mitra RS, Griffiths CE, Dixit VM, Nickoloff BJ. Keratinocytes as initiators of inflammation. *Lancet* 1991;337(8735):211–214.

25. Pivarcsi A, Nagy I, Koreck A, Kis K, Kenderessy-Szabo A, Szell M, Dobozy A, Kemeny L. Microbial compounds induce the expression of pro-inflammatory cytokines, chemokines and human beta-defensin-2 in vaginal epithelial cells. *Microbes Infect.* 2005;7(9–10):1117–1127.

26. Akira S, Hemmi H. Recognition of pathogen-associated molecular patterns by TLR family. *Immunol. Lett.* 2003;85(2):85–95.

27. Szolnoky G, Bata-Csorgo Z, Kenderessy AS, Kiss M, Pivarcsi A, Novak Z, Nagy Newman K, Michel G, Ruzicka T, Marodi L et al. A mannose-binding receptor is expressed on human keratinocytes and mediates killing of *Candida albicans. J. Invest. Dermatol.* 2001;117(2):205–213.

28. Hawlisch H, Kohl J. Complement and Toll-like receptors: key regulators of adaptive immune responses. *Mol. Immunol.* 2006;43(1–2):13–21.

29. Song PI, Park YM, Abraham T, Harten B, Zivony A, Neparidze N, Armstrong CA, Ansel JC. Human keratinocytes express functional CD14 and Toll-like receptor 4. *J. Invest. Dermatol.* 2002;119(2): 424–432.

30. Pivarcsi A, Bodai L, Rethi B, Kenderessy-Szabo A, Koreck A, Szell M, Beer Z, Bata-Csorgoo Z, Magocsi M, Rajnavolgyi E et al. Expression and function of Toll-like receptors 2 and 4 in human keratinocytes. *Int. Immunol.* 2003;15(6):721–730.

31. Kawai K, Shimura H, Minagawa M, Ito A, Tomiyama K, Ito M. Expression of functional Toll-like receptor 2 on human epidermal keratinocytes. *J. Dermatol. Sci.* 2002;30(3):185–194.

32. Baker BS, Ovigne JM, Powles AV, Corcoran S, Fry L. Normal keratinocytes express Toll-like receptors (TLRs) 1,2 and 5: modulation of TLR expression in chronic plaque psoriasis. *Br. J. Dermatol.* 2003;148(4):670–679.

33. Ali H, Panettieri RA, Jr. Anaphylatoxin C3a receptors in asthma. *Respir. Res.* 2005;6:19.

34. Oppenheim JJ, Biragyn A, Kwak LW, Yang D. Roles of antimicrobial peptides such as defensins in innate and adaptive immunity. *Ann. Rheum. Dis.* 2003;62 (Suppl. 2): ii17–ii21.

35. Ganz T. Defensins: antimicrobial peptides of innate immunity. *Nat. Rev. Immunol.* 2003;3(9): 710–720.

36. Biragyn A, Ruffini PA, Leifer CA, Klyushnenkova E, Shakhov A, Chertov O, Shirakawa AK, Farber JM, Segal DM, Oppenheim JJ et al. Toll-like receptor 4-dependent activation of dendritic cells by beta-defensin 2. *Science* 2002;298(5595):1025–1029.

37. Niyonsaba F, Iwabuchi K, Matsuda H, Ogawa H, Nagaoka I. Epithelial cell-derived human beta-defensin-2 acts as a chemotaxin for mast cells through a pertussis toxin-sensitive and phospholipase C-dependent pathway. *Int. Immunol.* 2002;14(4):421–426.

38. Niyonsaba F, Ogawa H, Nagaoka I. Human beta-defensin-2 functions as a chemotactic agent for tumour necrosis factor-alpha-treated human neutrophils. *Immunology* 2004;111(3):273–281.

39. De Y, Chen Q, Schmidt AP, Anderson GM, Wang JM, Wooters J, Oppenheim JJ, Chertov O. LL-37, the neutrophil granule- and epithelial cell-derived cathelicidin, utilizes formyl peptide receptor-like 1 (FPRL1) as a receptor to chemoattract human peripheral blood neutrophils, monocytes, and T cells. *J. Exp. Med.* 2000;192(7):1069–1074.

40. Gyurko R, Boustany G, Huang PL, Kantarci A, Van Dyke TE, Genco CA, Gibson FC, 3rd. Mice lacking inducible nitric oxide synthase demonstrate impaired killing of *Porphyromonas gingivalis. Infect. Immun.* 2003;71(9):4917–4924.

41. Matsubara M, Harada D, Manabe H, Hasegawa K. *Staphylococcus aureus* peptidoglycan stimulates granulocyte macrophage colony-stimulating factor production from human epidermal keratinocytes via mitogen-activated protein kinases. *FEBS Lett.* 2004;566(1–3):195–200.

42. Midorikawa K, Ouhara K, Komatsuzawa H, Kawai T, Yamada S, Fujiwara T, Yamazaki K, Sayama K, Taubman MA, Kurihara H et al. *Staphylococcus aureus* susceptibility to innate antimicrobial peptides, beta-defensins and CAP18, expressed by human keratinocytes. *Infect. Immun.* 2003;71(7):3730–3739.

43. Wollina U, Kunkel W, Bulling L, Funfstuck C, Knoll B, Vennewald I, Hipler UC. *Candida albicans*-induced inflammatory response in human keratinocytes. *Mycoses* 2004;47(5–6):193–199.

44. Homey B, Alenius H, Muller A, Soto H, Bowman EP, Yuan W, McEvoy L, Lauerma AI, Assmann T, Bunemann E et al. CCL27–CCR10 interactions regulate T cell-mediated skin inflammation. *Nat. Med.* 2002;8(2):157–165.

45. Barker JN, Jones ML, Mitra RS, Crockett-Torabe E, Fantone JC, Kunkel SL, Warren JS, Dixit VM, Nickoloff BJ. Modulation of keratinocyte-derived interleukin-8 which is chemotactic for neutrophils and T lymphocytes. *Am. J. Pathol.* 1991;139(4):869–876.

46. Parham P. *The Immune System.* New York: Garland Science, 2000.

47. Roitt I, Brostoff J, Male D, Roth D. *Immunology,* 7th ed. Saint Louis: Mosby, 2006.

48. Wolff K, Goldsmith LA, Katz SI, Gilchrest BA, Paller A, Leffell DJ. *Fitzpatrick's Dermatology in General Medicine,* 7th ed. McGraw-Hill Professional, 2007.

49. Girardi M. Cutaneous perspectives on adaptive immunity. *Clin. Rev. Allergy Immunol.* 2007; 33(1–2):4–14.

50. Gomez CR, Boehmer ED, Kovacs EJ. The aging innate immune system. *Curr. Opin. Immunol.* 2005; 17(5):457–462.

51. Mishto M, Santoro A, Bellavista E, Bonafe M, Monti D, Franceschi C. Immunoproteasomes and immunosenescence. *Ageing Res. Rev.* 2003;2(4):419–432.

52. Plackett TP, Boehmer ED, Faunce DE, Kovacs EJ. Aging and innate immune cells. *J. Leukoc. Biol.* 2004;76(2):291–299.

53. Fulop T, Larbi A, Douziech N, Fortin C, Guerard KP, Lesur O, Khalil A, Dupuis G. Signal transduction and functional changes in neutrophils with aging. *Aging Cell* 2004;3(4):217–226.

54. Weiskopf D, Weinberger B, Grubeck-Loebenstein B. The aging of the immune system. *Transpl. Int.* 2009;22(11):1041–1050.

55. Nomellini V, Gomez CR, Kovacs EJ. Aging and impairment of innate immunity. *Contrib. Microbiol.* 2008;15:188–205.

56. O'Mahony L, Holland J, Jackson J, Feighery C, Hennessy TP, Mealy K. Quantitative intracellular cytokine measurement: age-related changes in proinflammatory cytokine production. *Clin. Exp. Immunol.* 1998;113(2):213–219.

57. Franceschi C, Bonafe M, Valensin S, Olivieri F, De Luca M, Ottaviani E, De Benedictis G. Inflamm-aging: an evolutionary perspective on immunosenescence. *Ann. N. Y. Acad. Sci.* 2000;908:244–254.

58. Tercedor J, Lopez-Hernandez B, Rodenas JM, Delgado-Rodriguez M, Cerezo S, Serrano-Ortega S. Multivariate analysis of cutaneous markers of aging in chronic hemodialyzed patients. *Int. J. Dermatol.* 1995;34(8):546–550.

59. Chatta GS, Andrews RG, Rodger E, Schrag M, Hammond WP, Dale DC. Hematopoietic progenitors and aging: alterations in granulocytic precursors and responsiveness to recombinant human G-CSF, GM-CSF, and IL-3. *J. Gerontol.* 1993;48(5):M207–M212.

60. Butcher SK, Chahal H, Nayak L, Sinclair A, Henriquez NV, Sapey E, O'Mahony D, Lord JM. Senescence in innate immune responses: reduced neutrophil phagocytic capacity and CD16 expression in elderly humans. *J. Leukoc. Biol.* 2001;70(6):881–886.

61. Biasi D, Carletto A, Dell'Agnola C, Caramaschi P, Montesanti F, Zavateri G, Zeminian S, Bellavite P, Bambara LM. Neutrophil migration, oxidative metabolism, and adhesion in elderly and young subjects. *Inflammation* 1996;20(6):673–681.

62. Hajishengallis G. Too old to fight? Aging and its Toll on innate immunity. *Mol. Oral Microbiol.* 2010; 25(1):25–37.

63. Wenisch C, Patruta S, Daxbock F, Krause R, Horl W. Effect of age on human neutrophil function. *J. Leukoc. Biol.* 2000;67(1):40–45.

64. Alvarez E, Ruiz-Gutierrez V, Sobrino F, Santa-Maria C. Age-related changes in membrane lipid composition, fluidity and respiratory burst in rat peritoneal neutrophils. *Clin. Exp. Immunol.* 2001; 124(1):95–102.

65. Yuli I, Tamonga A, Snyderman R. Chemoattractant receptor functions in human polymorphonuclear leukocytes are divergently altered by membrane fluidizers. *Proc. Natl. Acad. Sci. USA* 1982;79:5906–5910.

66. Emanuelli G, Lanzio M, Anfossi T, Romano S, Anfossi G, Calcamuggi G. Influence of age on polymorphonuclear leukocytes *in vitro*: phagocytic activity in healthy human subjects. *Gerontology* 1986;32(6):308–316.

67. Lloberas J, Celada A. Effect of aging on macrophage function. *Exp. Gerontol.* 2002; 37(12):1325–1331.

68. Plowden J, Renshaw-Hoelscher M, Engleman C, Katz J, Sambhara S. Innate immunity in aging: impact on macrophage function. *Aging Cell* 2004;3(4):161–167.

69. Zissel G, Schlaak M, Muller-Quernheim J. Age-related decrease in accessory cell function of human alveolar macrophages. *J. Investig. Med.* 1999;47(1):51–56.

70. Herrero C, Sebastian C, Marques L, Comalada M, Xaus J, Valledor AF, Lloberas J, Celada A. Immunosenescence of macrophages: reduced MHC class II gene expression. *Exp. Gerontol.* 2002; 37(2–3):389–394.

71. Kirschmann DA, Murasko DM. Splenic and inguinal lymph node T cells of aged mice respond differently to polyclonal and antigen-specific stimuli. *Cell Immunol.* 1992;139(2):426–437.

72. Albright JW, Albright JF. Ageing alters the competence of the immune system to control parasitic infection. *Immunol. Lett.* 1994;40(3):279–285.

73. Mancuso P, McNish RW, Peters-Golden M, Brock TG. Evaluation of phagocytosis and arachidonate metabolism by alveolar macrophages and recruited neutrophils from F344xBN rats of different ages. *Mech. Ageing Dev.* 2001;122(15):1899–1913.

74. Renshaw M, Rockwell J, Engleman C, Gewirtz A, Katz J, Sambhara S. Cutting edge: impaired Toll-like receptor expression and function in aging. *J. Immunol.* 2002;169(9):4697–4701.

75. Beharka AA, Wu D, Han SN, Meydani SN. Macrophage prostaglandin production contributes to the age-associated decrease in T cell function which is reversed by the dietary antioxidant vitamin E. *Mech. Ageing Dev.* 1997;93(1–3):59–77.

76. Goodwin JS, Messner RP. Sensitivity of lymphocytes to prostaglandin E2 increases in subjects over age 70. *J. Clin. Invest.* 1979;64(2):434–439.

77. Gosain A, DiPietro LA. Aging and wound healing. *World J. Surg.* 2004;28(3):321–326.

78. Barbul A, Regan MC. Immune involvement in wound healing. *Otolaryngol. Clin. North Am.* 1995; 28(5):955–968.

79. Danon D, Kowatch MA, Roth GS. Promotion of wound repair in old mice by local injection of macrophages. *Proc. Natl. Acad. Sci. USA* 1989;86(6):2018–2020.

80. Swift ME, Burns AL, Gray KL, DiPietro LA. Age-related alterations in the inflammatory response to dermal injury. *J. Invest. Dermatol.* 2001;117(5):1027–1035.

81. Steger MM, Maczek C, Grubeck-Loebenstein B. Morphologically and functionally intact dendritic cells can be derived from the peripheral blood of aged individuals. *Clin. Exp. Immunol.* 1996; 105(3):544–550.

82. Lung TL, Saurwein-Teissl M, Parson W, Schonitzer D, Grubeck-Loebenstein B. Unimpaired dendritic cells can be derived from monocytes in old age and can mobilize residual function in senescent T cells. *Vaccine* 2000;18(16):1606–1612.

83. Agrawal A, Agrawal S, Gupta S. Dendritic cells in human aging. *Exp. Gerontol.* 2007;42(5): 421–426.

84. Fadok VA, Bratton DL, Konowal A, Freed PW, Westcott JY, Henson PM. Macrophages that have ingested apoptotic cells *in vitro* inhibit proinflammatory cytokine production through autocrine/paracrine mechanisms involving TGF-beta, PGE2, and PAF. *J. Clin. Invest.* 1998;101(4):890–898.

85. Grolleau-Julius A, Harning EK, Abernathy LM, Yung RL. Impaired dendritic cell function in aging leads to defective antitumor immunity. *Cancer Res.* 2008;68(15):6341–6349.

86. Del Prete A, Vermi W, Dander E, Otero K, Barberis L, Luini W, Bernasconi S, Sironi M, Santoro A, Garlanda C et al. Defective dendritic cell migration and activation of adaptive immunity in PI3Kgamma-deficient mice. *EMBO J.* 2004;23(17):3505–3515.

87. Sansoni P, Cossarizza A, Brianti V, Fagnoni F, Snelli G, Monti D, Marcato A, Passeri G, Ortolani C, Forti E et al. Lymphocyte subsets and natural killer cell activity in healthy old people and centenarians. *Blood* 1993;82(9):2767–2773.

88. Facchini A, Mariani E, Mariani AR, Papa S, Vitale M, Manzoli FA. Increased number of circulating Leu 11 + (CD 16) large granular lymphocytes and decreased NK activity during human ageing. *Clin. Exp. Immunol.* 1987;68(2):340–347.

89. Mariani E, Mariani AR, Meneghetti A, Tarozzi A, Cocco L, Facchini A. Age-dependent decreases of NK cell phosphoinositide turnover during spontaneous but not Fc-mediated cytolytic activity. *Int. Immunol.* 1998;10(7):981–989.

90. Solana R, Mariani E. NK and NK/T cells in human senescence. *Vaccine* 2000;18(16):1613–1620.

91. Dubey DP, Husain Z, Levitan E, Zurakowski D, Mirza N, Younes S, Coronell C, Yunis D, Yunis EJ. The MHC influences NK and NKT cell functions associated with immune abnormalities and lifespan. *Mech. Ageing Dev.* 2000;113(2):117–134.

92. Faunce DE, Palmer JL, Paskowicz KK, Witte PL, Kovacs EJ. CD1d-restricted NKT cells contribute to the age-associated decline of T cell immunity. *J. Immunol.* 2005;175(5):3102–3109.

93. Ishimoto Y, Tomiyama-Miyaji C, Watanabe H, Yokoyama H, Ebe K, Tsubata S, Aoyagi Y, Abo T. Age-dependent variation in the proportion and number of intestinal lymphocyte subsets, especially natural killer T cells, double-positive CD4+ CD8+ cells and B220 + T cells, in mice. *Immunology* 2004;113(3):371–377.

94. Berzins SP, McNab FW, Jones CM, Smyth MJ, Godfrey DI. Long-term retention of mature NK1.1 + NKT cells in the thymus. *J. Immunol.* 2006;176(7):4059–4065.

95. DelaRosa O, Tarazona R, Casado JG, Alonso C, Ostos B, Pena J, Solana R. Valpha24 + NKT cells are decreased in elderly humans. *Exp. Gerontol.* 2002;37(2–3):213–217.

96. Peralbo E, DelaRosa O, Gayoso I, Pita ML, Tarazona R, Solana R. Decreased frequency and proliferative response of invariant Valpha24Vbeta11 natural killer T (iNKT) cells in healthy elderly. *Biogerontology* 2006;7(5–6):483–492.

97. Peralbo E, Alonso C, Solana R. Invariant NKT and NKT-like lymphocytes: two different T cell subsets that are differentially affected by ageing. *Exp. Gerontol.* 2007;42(8):703–708.

98. Faunce DE, Palmer JL. The Effects of Age on CD1d-Restricted NKT Cells and Their Contribution to the Age-Associated Decline of T Cell Immunity. New York: Springer Press, 2008.

99. Poynter ME, Mu HH, Chen XP, Daynes RA. Activation of NK1.1 + T cells *in vitro* and their possible role in age-associated changes in inducible IL-4 production. *Cell Immunol.* 1997;179(1):22–29.

100. Mocchegiani E, Malavolta M. NK and NKT cell functions in immunosenescence. *Aging Cell* 2004; 3(4):177–184.

101. Mocchegiani E, Giacconi R, Cipriano C, Gasparini N, Bernardini G, Malavolta M, Menegazzi M, Cavalieri E, Muzzioli M, Ciampa AR et al. The variations during the circadian cycle of liver CD1d-unrestricted NK1. 1 + TCR gamma/delta + cells lead to successful ageing. Role of metallothionein/IL-6/gp130/PARP-1 interplay in very old mice. *Exp. Gerontol.* 2004;39(5):775–788.

102. Tsukahara A, Seki S, Iiai T, Moroda T, Watanabe H, Suzuki S, Tada T, Hiraide H, Hatakeyama K, Abo T. Mouse liver T cells: their change with aging and in comparison with peripheral T cells. *Hepatology* 1997;26(2):301–309.

103. Buchau AS, Gallo RL. Innate immunity and antimicrobial defense systems in psoriasis. *Clin. Dermatol.* 2007;25(6):616–624.

104. Langewouters AM, van Erp PE, de Jong EM, van de Kerkhof PC. Lymphocyte subsets in peripheral blood of patients with moderate-to-severe versus mild plaque psoriasis. *Arch. Dermatol. Res.* 2008;300(3):107–113.

105. Nestle FO. *Psoriasis*. Basel: Karger, 2008.

106. Nestle FO, Kaplan DH, Barker J. Psoriasis. *N. Engl. J. Med.* 2009;361(5):496–509.

107. Gelfand JM, Neimann AL, Shin DB, Wang X, Margolis DJ, Troxel AB. Risk of myocardial infarction in patients with psoriasis. *JAMA* 2006;296(14):1735–1741.

108. Gelfand JM, Troxel AB, Lewis JD, Kurd SK, Shin DB, Wang X, Margolis DJ, Strom BL. The risk of mortality in patients with psoriasis: results from a population-based study. *Arch. Dermatol.* 2007;143(12):1493–1499.

109. Gisondi P, Tessari G, Conti A, Piaserico S, Schianchi S, Peserico A, Giannetti A, Girolomoni G. Prevalence of metabolic syndrome in patients with psoriasis: a hospital-based case-control study. *Br. J. Dermatol.* 2007;157(1):68–73.

110. Peternel S, Kastelan M. Immunopathogenesis of psoriasis: focus on natural killer T cells. *J. Eur. Acad. Dermatol. Venereol.* 2009;23(10):1123–1127.

111. Prpic-Massari L, Kastelan M. Innate and acquired immunity in psoriasis. *Arch. Dermatol. Res.* 2009;301(2):195–196.

112. Bos JD, de Rie MA, Teunissen MB, Piskin G. Psoriasis: dysregulation of innate immunity. *Br. J. Dermatol.* 2005;152(6):1098–1107.

113. Wrone-Smith T, Mitra RS, Thompson CB, Jasty R, Castle VP, Nickoloff BJ. Keratinocytes derived from psoriatic plaques are resistant to apoptosis compared with normal skin. *Am. J. Pathol.* 1997; 151(5):1321–1329.

114. Di Cesare A, Di Meglio P, Nestle FO. The IL-23/Th17 axis in the immunopathogenesis of psoriasis. *J. Invest. Dermatol.* 2009;129(6):1339–1350.

115. Cameron AL, Kirby B, Fei W, Griffiths CE. Natural killer and natural killer-T cells in psoriasis. *Arch. Dermatol. Res.* 2002;294(8):363–369.

116. van der Vliet HJ, von Blomberg BM, Nishi N, Reijm M, Voskuyl AE, van Bodegraven AA, Polman CH, Rustemeyer T, Lips P, van den Eertwegh A.J. et al. Circulating V(alpha24$^+$) Vbeta11$^+$ NKT cell numbers are decreased in a wide variety of diseases that are characterized by autoreactive tissue damage. *Clin. Immunol.* 2001;100(2):144–148.

117. Boehncke WH, Sterry W. Psoriasis—a systemic inflammatory disorder: clinic, pathogenesis and therapeutic perspectives. *J. Dtsch. Dermatol. Ges.* 2009;7(11):946–952.

118. Prinz JC. The role of T cells in psoriasis. *J. Eur. Acad. Dermatol. Venereol.* 2003;17(3):257–270.

119. Clark RA, Fuhlbrigge RC. Immunology and skin disease 2009: frontiers in cutaneous immunology. *J. Invest. Dermatol.* 2009;129(8):1849–1851.

120. Harder J, Bartels J, Christophers E, Schroder JM. Isolation and characterization of human beta-defensin-3, a novel human inducible peptide antibiotic. *J. Biol. Chem.* 2001;276(8):5707–5713.

121. Ong PY, Ohtake T, Brandt C, Strickland I, Boguniewicz M, Ganz T, Gallo RL, Leung DY. Endogenous antimicrobial peptides and skin infections in atopic dermatitis. *N. Engl. J. Med.* 2002;347(15): 1151–1160.

122. Curry JL, Qin JZ, Bonish B, Carrick R, Bacon P, Panella J, Robinson J, Nickoloff BJ. Innate immune-related receptors in normal and psoriatic skin. *Arch. Pathol. Lab. Med.* 2003;127(2):178–186.

123. Matzinger P. The danger model: a renewed sense of self. *Science* 2002;296(5566):301–305.

124. Pasch M, Bos JD, Asghar SS. Activation of complement in psoriasis. *Clin. Exp. Dermatol.* 1998; 23(4):189–190.

125. Nickoloff BJ. Cracking the cytokine code in psoriasis. *Nat. Med.* 2007;13(3):242–244.

126. Austin LM, Ozawa M, Kikuchi T, Walters IB, Krueger JG. The majority of epidermal T cells in psoriasis vulgaris lesions can produce type 1 cytokines, interferon-gamma, interleukin-2, and tumor necrosis factor-alpha, defining TC1 (cytotoxic T lymphocyte) and TH1 effector populations: a type 1 differentiation bias is also measured in circulating blood T cells in psoriatic patients. *J. Invest. Dermatol.* 1999;113(5):752–759.

127. Lew W, Bowcock AM, Krueger JG. Psoriasis vulgaris: cutaneous lymphoid tissue supports T-cell activation and "Type 1" inflammatory gene expression. *Trends Immunol.* 2004;25(6):295–305.

128. Wilson NJ, Boniface K, Chan JR, McKenzie BS, Blumenschein WM, Mattson JD, Basham B, Smith K, Chen T, Morel F et al. Development, cytokine profile and function of human interleukin 17-producing helper T cells. *Nat. Immunol.* 2007;8(9):950–957.

129. Zaba LC, Fuentes-Duculan J, Eungdamrong NJ, Abello MV, Novitskaya I, Pierson KC, Gonzalez J, Krueger JG, Lowes MA. Psoriasis is characterized by accumulation of immunostimulatory and Th1/Th17 cell-polarizing myeloid dendritic cells. *J. Invest. Dermatol.* 2009;129(1):79–88.

130. Arican O, Aral M, Sasmaz S, Ciragil P. Serum levels of TNF-alpha, IFN-gamma, IL-6, IL-8, IL-12, IL-17, and IL-18 in patients with active psoriasis and correlation with disease severity. *Mediators Inflamm.* 2005;2005(5):273–279.

131. Sugiyama H, Gyulai R, Toichi E, Garaczi E, Shimada S, Stevens SR, McCormick TS, Cooper KD. Dysfunctional blood and target tissue CD4$^+$CD25high regulatory T cells in psoriasis: mechanism underlying unrestrained pathogenic effector T cell proliferation. *J. Immunol.* 2005;174(1):164–173.

132. Jullien D, Prinz JC, Langley RG, Caro I, Dummer W, Joshi A, Dedrick R, Natta P. T-cell modulation for the treatment of chronic plaque psoriasis with efalizumab (Raptiva): mechanisms of action. *Dermatology* 2004;208(4):297–306.

133. Ortonne JP, Prinz JC. Alefacept: a novel and selective biologic agent for the treatment of chronic plaque psoriasis. *Eur. J. Dermatol.* 2004;14(1):41–45.

134. Gisondi P, Girolomoni G. Biologic therapies in psoriasis: a new therapeutic approach. *Autoimmun. Rev.* 2007;6(8):515–519.

135. Boehncke WH, Prinz J, Gottlieb AB. Biologic therapies for psoriasis: a systematic review. *J. Rheumatol.* 2006;33(7):1447–1451.

136. Leonardi CL, Kimball AB, Papp KA, Yeilding N, Guzzo C, Wang Y, Li S, Dooley LT, Gordon KB. Efficacy and safety of ustekinumab, a human interleukin-12/23 monoclonal antibody, in patients with psoriasis: 76-week results from a randomised, double-blind, placebo-controlled trial (PHOENIX 1). *Lancet* 2008;371(9625):1665–1674.

137. Saurat JH, Stingl G, Dubertret L, Papp K, Langley RG, Ortonne JP, Unnebrink K, Kaul M, Camez A. Efficacy and safety results from the randomized controlled comparative study of adalimumab vs. methotrexate vs. placebo in patients with psoriasis (CHAMPION). *Br. J. Dermatol.* 2008;158(3): 558–566.

138. McDonagh AJ, Tazi-Ahnini R. Epidemiology and genetics of alopecia areata. *Clin. Exp. Dermatol.* 2002;27(5):405–409.

139. Wolff K, Richard J, Suurmond D. *Fitzpatrick's Color Atlas and Synopsis of Clinical Dermatology.* London: McGraw-Hill, 2005.

140. Gip L, Lodin A, Molin L. Alopecia areata: a follow-up investigation of outpatient material. *Acta Derm. Venereol.* 1969;49(2):180–188.

141. Kos L, Conlon J. An update on alopecia areata. *Curr. Opin. Pediatr.* 2009;21(4):475–480.

142. Arck P, Paus R. From the brain–skin connection: the neuroendocrine-immune misalliance of stress and itch. *Neuroimmunomodulation* 2006;13(5–6):347–356.

143. Harrist TJ, Ruiter DJ, Mihm MC, Jr., Bhan AK. Distribution of major histocompatibility antigens in normal skin. *Br. J. Dermatol.* 1983;109(6):623–633.

144. Brocker EB, Echternacht-Happle K, Hamm H, Happle R. Abnormal expression of class I and class II major histocompatibility antigens in alopecia areata: modulation by topical immunotherapy. *J. Invest. Dermatol.* 1987;88(5):564–568.

145. Abbas AK, Lichtman AH. *Basic Immunology.* Philadelphia: Saunders, 2006.

146. Gilhar A, Ullmann Y, Berkutzki T, Assy B, Kalish RS. Autoimmune hair loss (alopecia areata) transferred by T lymphocytes to human scalp explants on SCID mice. *J. Clin. Invest.* 1998;101(1): 62–67.

147. Kalish RS, Johnson KL, Hordinsky MK. Alopecia areata: autoreactive T cells are variably enriched in scalp lesions relative to peripheral blood. *Arch. Dermatol.* 1992;128(8):1072–1077.

148. van den Boorn JG, Konijnenberg D, Dellemijn TA, van der Veen JP, Bos JD, Melief CJ, Vyth-Dreese FA, Luiten RM. Autoimmune destruction of skin melanocytes by perilesional T cells from vitiligo patients. *J. Invest. Dermatol.* 2009;129(9):2220–2232.

149. Delamere FM, Sladden MM, Dobbins HM, Leonardi-Bee J. Interventions for alopecia areata. *Cochrane Database Syst. Rev.* 2008; (2): CD004413.

150. Luggen P, Hunziker T. High-dose intravenous corticosteroid pulse therapy in alopecia areata: own experience compared with the literature. *J. Dtsch. Dermatol. Ges.* 2008;6(5):375–378.

151. Rokhsar CK, Shupack JL, Vafai JJ, Washenik K. Efficacy of topical sensitizers in the treatment of alopecia areata. *J. Am. Acad. Dermatol.* 1998;39 (5 Part 1): 751–761.

152. Tosti A, Guidetti MS, Bardazzi F, Misciali C. Long-term results of topical immunotherapy in children with alopecia totalis or alopecia universalis. *J. Am. Acad. Dermatol.* 1996;35 (2 Part 1): 199–201.

153. Fernandez-Guarino M, Harto A, Garcia-Morales I, Perez-Garcia B, Arrazola JM, Jaen P. Failure to treat alopecia areata with photodynamic therapy. *Clin. Exp. Dermatol.* 2008;33(5):585–587.

154. Kaelin U, Hassan AS, Braathen LR, Yawalkar N. Treatment of alopecia areata partim universalis with efalizumab. *J. Am. Acad. Dermatol.* 2006;55(3):529–532.

155. Price VH, Hordinsky MK, Olsen EA, Roberts JL, Siegfried EC, Rafal ES, Korman NJ, Altrabulsi B, Leung HM, Garovoy MR et al. Subcutaneous efalizumab is not effective in the treatment of alopecia areata. *J. Am. Acad. Dermatol.* 2008;58(3):395–402.

156. Strober BE, Siu K, Alexis AF, Kim G, Washenik K, Sinha A, Shupack JL. Etanercept does not effectively treat moderate to severe alopecia areata: an open-label study. *J. Am. Acad. Dermatol.* 2005;52(6):1082–1084.

157. Posten W, Swan J. Recurrence of alopecia areata in a patient receiving etanercept injections. *Arch. Dermatol.* 2005;141(6):759–760.

158. Chaves Y, Duarte G, Ben-Said B, Tebib J, Berard F, Nicolas JF. Alopecia areata universalis during treatment of rheumatoid arthritis with anti-TNF-alpha antibody (adalimumab). *Dermatology* 2008;217(4):380.

159. Wardell K, Naver HK, Nilsson GE, Wallin BG. The cutaneous vascular axon reflex in humans characterized by laser Doppler perfusion imaging. *J. Physiol.* 1993;460:185–199.

160. Elias PM, Choi EH. Interactions among stratum corneum defensive functions. *Exp. Dermatol.* 2005;14(10):719–726.

161. Boelsma E, Anderson C, Karlsson AM, Ponec M. Microdialysis technique as a method to study the percutaneous penetration of methyl nicotinate through excised human skin, reconstructed epidermis, and human skin *in vivo*. *Pharm. Res.* 2000;17(2):141–147.

162. Varol AL, Anderson CD. A minimally invasive human *in vivo* cutaneous wound model for the evaluation of innate skin reactivity and healing status. *Arch. Dermatol. Res.* 2010;302(5):383–393.

163. Anderson C, Andersson T, Wardell K. Changes in skin circulation after insertion of a microdialysis probe visualized by laser Doppler perfusion imaging. *J. Invest. Dermatol.* 1994;102(5):807–811.

164. Anderson C, Andersson T, Andersson RG. *In vivo* microdialysis estimation of histamine in human skin. *Skin Pharmacol.* 1992;5(3):177–183.

165. Sjogren F, Anderson C. Sterile trauma to normal human dermis invariably induces IL1beta, IL6 and IL8 in an innate response to "danger". *Acta Derm. Venereol.* 2009;89(5):459–465.

166. Barton GM. A calculated response: control of inflammation by the innate immune system. *J. Clin. Invest.* 2008;118(2):413–420.

167. Singer AJ, Clark RA. Cutaneous wound healing. *N. Engl. J. Med.* 1999;341(10):738–746.

168. Varol A, Seifert O, Anderson CD. The skin pathergy test: innately useful? *Arch. Dermatol. Res.* 2010;302(3):155–168.

169. Meylan E, Tschopp J, Karin M. Intracellular pattern recognition receptors in the host response. *Nature* 2006;442(7098):39–44.

170. Do JE, Kwon SY, Park S, Lee ES. Effects of vitamin D on expression of Toll-like receptors of monocytes from patients with Behcet's disease. *Rheumatology (Oxford)* 2008;47(6):840–848.

171. Nara K, Kurokawa MS, Chiba S, Yoshikawa H, Tsukikawa S, Matsuda T, Suzuki N. Involvement of innate immunity in the pathogenesis of intestinal Behcet's disease. *Clin. Exp. Immunol.* 2008;152(2):245–251.

172. O'Doherty J, Henricson J, Anderson C, Leahy MJ, Nilsson GE, Sjoberg F. Sub-epidermal imaging using polarized light spectroscopy for assessment of skin microcirculation. *Skin Res. Technol.* 2007;13(4):472–484.

173. Dwarakanath AD, Yu LG, Brookes C, Pryce D, Rhodes JM. 'Sticky' neutrophils, pathergic arthritis, and response to heparin in pyoderma gangrenosum complicating ulcerative colitis. *Gut* 1995;37(4):585–588.

174. Fox LP, Geyer AS, Husain S, Grossman ME. Bullous pyoderma gangrenosum as the presenting sign of fatal acute myelogenous leukemia. *Leuk. Lymphoma* 2006;47(1):147–150.

175. Callen JP, Jackson JM. Pyoderma gangrenosum: an update. *Rheum. Dis. Clin. North Am.* 2007;33(4):787–802, vi.

176. Ryan TJ. Biochemical consequences of mechanical forces generated by distention and distortion. *J. Am. Acad. Dermatol.* 1989;21(1):115–130.

177. Feldmeyer L, Keller M, Niklaus G, Hohl D, Werner S, Beer HD. The inflammasome mediates UVB-induced activation and secretion of interleukin-1beta by keratinocytes. *Curr. Biol.* 2007;17(13):1140–1145.

178. Watanabe H, Gaide O, Petrilli V, Martinon F, Contassot E, Roques S, Kummer JA, Tschopp J, French LE. Activation of the IL-1beta-processing inflammasome is involved in contact hypersensitivity. *J. Invest. Dermatol.* 2007;127(8):1956–1963.

179. de Jongh CM, Lutter R, Verberk MM, Kezic S. Differential cytokine expression in skin after single and repeated irritation by sodium lauryl sulphate. *Exp. Dermatol.* 2007;16(12):1032–1040.

180. Willis CM, Stephens CJ, Wilkinson JD. Selective expression of immune-associated surface antigens by keratinocytes in irritant contact dermatitis. *J. Invest. Dermatol.* 1991;96(4):505–511.

181. Taylor KR, Yamasaki K, Radek KA, Di Nardo A, Goodarzi H, Golenbock D, Beutler B, Gallo RL. Recognition of hyaluronan released in sterile injury involves a unique receptor complex dependent on Toll-like receptor 4, CD44, and MD-2. *J. Biol. Chem.* 2007;282(25):18265–18275.

182. Mariathasan S, Monack DM. Inflammasome adaptors and sensors: intracellular regulators of infection and inflammation. *Nat. Rev. Immunol.* 2007;7(1):31–40.

183. Alayli G, Aydin F, Coban AY, Sullu Y, Canturk F, Bek Y, Durupinar B, Canturk T. T helper 1 type cytokines polymorphisms: association with susceptibility to Behcet's disease. *Clin. Rheumatol.* 2007;26(8):1299–1305.

184. Yosipovitch G, Samuel LS. Neuropathic and psychogenic itch. *Dermatol. Ther.* 2008;21(1):32–41.

185. Davis M. Cholestasis and endogenous opioids: liver disease and exogenous opioid pharmacokinetics. *Clin. Pharmacokinet.* 2007;46(10):825–850.

186. Dyachenko P, Shustak A, Rozenman D. Hemodialysis-related pruritus and associated cutaneous manifestations. *Int. J. Dermatol.* 2006;45(6):664–667.

187. Handwerker HO. Microneurography of pruritus. *Neurosci. Lett.* 2010;470(3):193–196.

188. Schmelz M, Hilliges M, Schmidt R, Orstavik K, Vahlquist C, Weidner C, Handwerker HO, Torebjork HE. Active "itch fibers" in chronic pruritus. *Neurology* 2003;61(4):564–566.

189. Steinhoff M, Bienenstock J, Schmelz M, Maurer M, Wei E, Biro T. Neurophysiological, neuro-immunological, and neuroendocrine basis of pruritus. *J. Invest. Dermatol.* 2006;126(8): 1705–1718.

190. Cevikbas F, Steinhoff A, Homey B, Steinhoff M. Neuroimmune interactions in allergic skin diseases. *Curr. Opin. Allergy Clin. Immunol.* 2007;7(5):365–373.

191. Ma L, Gao XH, Zhao LP, Di ZH, McHepange UO, Zhang L, Chen HD, Wei HC. Brain-derived neurotrophic factor gene polymorphisms and serum levels in Chinese atopic dermatitis patients. *J. Eur. Acad. Dermatol. Venereol.* 2009;23(11):1277–1281.

192. Dhabhar FS. Enhancing versus suppressive effects of stress on immune function: implications for immunoprotection and immunopathology. *Neuroimmunomodulation* 2009;16(5):300–317.

193. Buske-Kirschbaum A. Cortisol responses to stress in allergic children: interaction with the immune response. *Neuroimmunomodulation* 2009;16(5):325–332.

194. Ohmura T, Hayashi T, Satoh Y, Konomi A, Jung B, Satoh H. Involvement of substance P in scratching behaviour in an atopic dermatitis model. *Eur. J. Pharmacol.* 2004;491(2–3):191–194.

195. Duval A, Dubertret L. Aprepitant as an antipruritic agent? *N. Engl. J. Med.* 2009;361(14):1415–1416.

196. Bell JK, McQueen DS, Rees JL. Involvement of histamine H4 and H1 receptors in scratching induced by histamine receptor agonists in Balb C mice. *Br. J. Pharmacol.* 2004;142(2):374–380.

197. Dunford PJ, Williams KN, Desai PJ, Karlsson L, McQueen D, Thurmond RL. Histamine H4 receptor antagonists are superior to traditional antihistamines in the attenuation of experimental pruritus. *J. Allergy Clin. Immunol.* 2007;119(1):176–183.

198. Akiyama T, Carstens MI, Carstens E. Excitation of mouse superficial dorsal horn neurons by histamine and/or PAR-2 agonist: potential role in itch. *J. Neurophysiol.* 2009;102(4):2176–2183.

199. van Os-Medendorp H, Ros WJ, Eland-de Kok PC, Kennedy C, Thio BH, van der Schuur-van der Zande A, Grypdonck MH, Bruijnzeel-Koomen CA. Effectiveness of the nursing programme 'Coping with itch': a randomized controlled study in adults with chronic pruritic skin disease. *Br. J. Dermatol.* 2007;156(6):1235–1244.

200. Staab D, Diepgen TL, Fartasch M, Kupfer J, Lob-Corzilius T, Ring J, Scheewe S, Scheidt R, Schmid-Ott G, Schnopp C et al. Age related, structured educational programmes for the management of atopic dermatitis in children and adolescents: multicentre, randomised controlled trial. *BMJ* 2006;332(7547):933–938.

CHAPTER *12*

EPIDERMIS AS A SHIELD FROM RADIATION AND OXIDATIVE STRESS

Giuseppe Valacchi

Department of Biomedical Sciences, University of Siena, Siena, Italy

12.1 STRATUM CORNEUM AS FIRST DEFENSE AGAINST THE OUTDOOR ENVIRONMENT

The skin consists of two main layers: the epidermis and the dermis. The dermis is superficial to the subcutaneous fat tissue and is reachable by blood capillaries. Dermal fibroblasts synthesize a complex extracellular matrix containing collagenous and elastic fibers. The epidermis contains mostly keratinocytes that rise to the skin surface as they differentiate progressively to form the nonnucleated corneocytes that consist of the superficial part of the epidermis, the stratum corneum (SC). The SC comprises a unique two-compartment system of structural, nonnucleated cells (corneocytes) embedded in a lipid-enriched intercellular matrix, forming stacks of bilayers that are rich in ceramides, cholesterol, and free fatty acids. SC functions as a physio-chemical barrier to protect and prevent water loss from the epidermis, maintaining its integrity, and to provide protection from the environment by producing antioxidant molecules that interact with reactive oxygen species (ROS) or their by-products to eliminate or minimize their deleterious effects. The SC supports the absorption of liposoluble compounds and promotes the penetration of lipophilic molecules. There are several ways how molecules can penetrate in the SC such as intercellular (penetration between the corneocytes), transcellular (penetration through the keratinized corneocytes), intrafollicular (penetration through hair follicles), and polar (penetration between polar pores) [1]. Physiochemical factors that regulate penetration include molecular mass, concentration, solubility, partition coefficient, pH variations, cosolvents, temperature, and enhancers.

Because of its critical location, the SC is a major interface between the body and the environment and provides a biological barrier against an array of chemical and physical environmental pollutants. Due to the constant exposure to oxidants including

Innate Immune System of Skin and Oral Mucosa: Properties and Impact in Pharmaceutics, Cosmetics, and Personal Care Products, First Edition. Nava Dayan and Philip W. Wertz.
© 2011 John Wiley & Sons, Inc. Published 2011 by John Wiley & Sons, Inc.

ultraviolet (UV) radiation and other environmental pollutants such as diesel fuel exhaust, cigarette smoke (CS), halogenated hydrocarbons, heavy metals, and O_3 (one of the most toxic of these compounds) [2], the SC can be defined as our first defense against the outdoor environment.

12.2 ENVIRONMENTAL STRESSORS AND CUTANEOUS TISSUES

Living organisms are continuously exposed to environmental pollutants. Depending on their state, pollutants can be taken up by ingestion, inhalation, or contact with the skin. Because the skin is an interface between the body and the environment, it is chronically exposed to several forms of stress such as UV and other environmental oxidants such as CS and O_3. UVB and to a lesser degree UVA induce various skin pathological conditions, including erythema, edema, hyperplasia, "sunburn cell" formation, photoaging, and photocarcinogenesis. There is abundant information that ROS such as hydroxyl radicals are involved in UV-induced skin damage, both by direct effects of UV and by subsequent phagocyte infiltration and activation. Oxidative environmental pollutants such as CS, O_3, and oxides of nitrogen, which have been studied in the respiratory tract [3], also represent a potential oxidant stress to the skin.

In order of importance, the skin is the second most frequent route by which chemicals can enter into the body. The skin is the major target of liquid and gaseous pollutants, and although the pollutants that react with the cutaneous tissues are several, in this chapter we will focus on those that have been reported in the literature with more emphasis, such as UV radiation and O_3.

12.3 ULTRAVIOLET RADIATION

UV radiation is a well-characterized oxidative stressor and it is well known that oxidative stress contributes to skin carcinogenesis [4]. Solar UV radiation represents electromagnetic energy between 100 and 400 nm and includes vacuum UV, UVC, UVB, and UVA [5,6]. Vacuum UV (100–200 nm) and UVC (200–290 nm) are absorbed by the atmosphere; therefore, their biological effects are not measured [5]. UVB (290–320 nm) and to a lesser degree UVA (320–400 nm) induce a multitude of pathological conditions. Therefore, acute and chronic exposure to UV has been linked to several skin pathologies, such as photodermatoses and photocarcinogenesis, skin inflammation including erythema, edema, hyperplasia, "sunburn cell" formation, and photoaging via the production of ROS [7].

UV-induced inflammation is the result of increased blood flow and infiltration of leukocytes, such as macrophages and neutrophils into the skin. The inflammatory cells in turn produce ROS that further drive damage to lipids, proteins, and DNA that further promotes reactive oxygen stress in the skin. As a result, this high production of ROS has been shown to cause gene mutations and drive tumor progression [4].

One accepted hypothesis for the genesis of skin pathologies due to exposure to UV is that such exposure causes the formation of free radicals, reactive oxygen, and nitrogen species and mobilization of transition metal ions [8]. Furthermore, UV radiation also increases the activity of enzymes such as xanthine oxidase, increasing the production of superoxide and hydrogen peroxide [9].

If the flux of ROS is high and antioxidant regeneration becomes a limiting factor, antioxidants will be depleted, resulting in an imbalance between oxidants and antioxidants. The consequences of such imbalance may be involved in the pathogenesis of photodamage. UV-induced oxidative stress causes three biological events in skin, including inflammation, gene mutation, and photoimmunosuppression. However, the underlying mechanisms of UV-induced changes in SC barrier function are not completely clear. A prime mechanism of UVA- and UVB-induced damage to cutaneous tissues is thought to be the peroxidation of lipids and depletion of antioxidant levels.

12.4   INTERACTION BETWEEN SKIN AND UV

In the normal epidermis, absorption is the dominant process over most of the optical spectrum. In the UV wavelengths below 300 nm, strong absorption by proteins, melanin, urocanic acid, and DNA occurs. For wavelengths of 320–1200 nm, absorption by melanin dominates epidermal optical properties. In the dermis, strong wavelength-dependent scattering by collagen fibers occurs. Optical penetration through the dermis is largely dominated by scattering, which varies inversely with wavelength.

Different wavelengths of UV have different biological effects. The reaction pattern and the time course of UV-mediated acute inflammatory reaction (sun burn) are wavelength dependent [10]. Furthermore, the effects of UV on immune system, photoaging, and photocarcinogenesis show wavelength dependencies most likely for the different capacity of UV to penetrate into the skin layers and also for the specific reaction cascades initiated by a specific wavelength band.

UVC is almost completely absorbed in the SC. UVB radiations are absorbed in the epidermis by target structures such as nucleic acids, proteins, and polyunsaturated lipids causing epidermal cell damage, while UVA primarily causes dermal injury by inducing oxidative stress in human skin cells [11]. The effects of UVA seem to be mediated not only by endogenous photosensitizers such as flavins, tryptophan and tyrosine, ubiquinones, porphyrins, NADH and NADPH, nucleosides, and iron–sulfur clusters [12] but also by exogenous photosensitizers derived from environmental pollution, compounds derived from plant, and some cosmetic products. Phototoxicity of UVA is oxygen dependent and involves generation of ROS. In contrast, UVB-induced erythema and pigment response showed no oxygen dependency [13], although endogenous glutathione protects against UVA- and UVB-induced cytotoxic effects in human skin fibroblasts indicating that antioxidants can anyway scavenge oxidizing and electrophilic photointermediates and confirming their importance in defending the skin from exogenous stressors.

12.5 FREE RADICAL FORMATION BY UV RADIATION

EPR spectroscopy has evidenced the formation of free radicals in skin after UV exposure. Some of these free radical species are derived from melanin [14]. Indirect evidence for the formation of free radical species (hydroxyl, superoxide anion, and peroxyl radical) by UV is provided by spin trapping experiments in animal and human skin. The formation of radical is characterized by the reaction of activated photosensitizer directly with a substrate molecule via electron or hydrogen atom transfer with the formation of free radicals. This reaction may involve the formation of superoxide anion radical by electron transfer from an excited photosensitizer to oxygen. Superoxide anion may also be generated by the reaction of oxygen with the sensitizer anion radical that is produced through the first reaction.

Tissue/cell damage can then be a consequence of the formation of hydroxyl radicals derived from metal ion-catalyzed reaction of superoxide anion radical and its dismutation product hydrogen peroxide.

Another possible reaction is when the energy is transferred from the excited state of a photosensitizer to the ground state of oxygen to produce singlet oxygen. If the concentration and reaction rate of a reductant with the triplet-state compound is sufficiently high, the direct reduction pathway will predominate over that producing singlet oxygen.

Different antioxidants have different rate constants with reactive oxidants, they are present in distinct cellular microdomains, and their regeneration involves different mechanisms.

It has been shown that after just single exposure to UV, regardless of A or B, the permeability barrier function of the skin diminished [15], most likely as a consequence of lipid peroxidation. Recent reports have shown that at low doses of UV irradiation, antioxidants of the SC are dramatically depleted, specifically 50% of human α-tocopherol [16]. This evident susceptibility of the vitamin E in the SC was speculated to be due to the absence of coantioxidants in the SC. The barrier α-tocopherol depletion and the subsequent oxidation of lipid and proteins were believed to be very sensitive biomarkers for oxidative stress induced by O_3 and UV [17]. Protein oxidation has been shown to be inversely correlated with vitamin E [16] and free thiol gradient in the human skin [15].

In general, the outermost part of the skin, the epidermis, contains higher antioxidant concentration than the dermis [18]. In the lipophilic phase, α-tocopherol is the most prominent antioxidant, while vitamin C and GSH have the highest abundance in the cytosol.

12.6 OZONE: ANOTHER STRESSOR FOR SKIN TISSUES

Not only the UV radiation but also the gaseous oxidants such as O_3 are able to induce oxidative stress in the skin. Oxidative damage produced by O_3 could not only affect the structural integrity of the SC by compromising antioxidant defenses and inducing oxidative damage to lipids but also the proteins [19–21].

Ozone is naturally present in the atmosphere surrounding the earth. The molecule is composed of three oxygen atoms and has a molecular weight of 48 kDa. Ozone arises from chemical reactions in the atmosphere through the action of sunlight on oxygen molecules. It is generally understood that although O_3 is not a radical species *per se*, the toxic effects of O_3 are mediated through free radical reactions and they are achieved directly by the oxidation of biomolecules to give classical radical species (hydroxyl radical) or by driving the radical-dependent production of cyto-toxic, nonradical species (aldehydes) [22].

Furthermore, the formation of the oxidation products characteristic of damage from free radicals have been shown to be prevented by the addition of the antioxidants vitamin E and C, although the mechanism is not fully understood. The target specificity of O_3 toward specific compounds together with its physicochemical properties of fairly low aqueous solubility and diffusibility must be taken into account when a target tissue like the skin is exposed to O_3.

When the skin was separated into upper epidermis, lower epidermis, papillary dermis, and dermis, O_3 induced a significant depletion of tocopherols and ascorbate followed by an increase in the lipid peroxidation measured as malondialdehyde (MDA) content. O_3 is known to react readily with biomolecules and does not penetrate through the cells; therefore, it was hypothesized that O_3 mainly reacts within the SC [23]. This hypothesis was further supported whereby hairless mice were exposed to several O_3 doses for 2 h. This increased in oxidative stress-depleted SC lipophilic (tocopherols) and hydrophilic (ascorbate, urate, and GSH) antioxidants upon O_3 exposure. This was accompanied by a rise in lipid peroxidation, an indicator of oxidative stress [24].

Carbonyl formation has been used as a marker of oxidative stress and has been found in the upper layer of the SC and in whole skin homogenates exposed to environmental insults. Keratin 10 was shown to be the main protein oxidized and increased oxidation was seen from the lower SC to the upper level. This protein oxidation gradient was inversely correlated with the gradient of the antioxidant vitamin E. Studies have also shown that protein oxidation can be quenched by antioxidants such as tocopherol and thiols. Interestingly, the keratin in SC contained dramatically more carbonyl groups than the keratin present in keratinocytes, indi-cating that the baseline levels of keratin oxidation are considerably higher in the SC compared to that in the epidermal layers.

Proinflammatory marker cyclooxygenase-2 (COX-2) expression along with heat shock protein (HSP)-32 was detected in hairless mice when exposed to O_3 [25], as also shown with the UV exposure.

As it was hypothesized, O_3 does not penetrate the cells but oxidizes available antioxidants and reacts instantaneously with polyunsaturated fatty acids (PUFAs) to form ROS, such as hydrogen peroxide and a mixture of heterogeneous LOPs including lipoperoxyl radicals, hydroperoxides, malonyldialdeyde, isoprostanes, the ozonide radical, $O_3^{\bullet-}$ [26], and alkenals, particularly 4-hydroxy-2,3-*trans*-nonenal, HNE [27,28]. As cholesterol is a component of the upper layer of the skin and because its double bond is readily attacked by O_3, it can give rise to biologically active oxysterols [29].

Using a spin trapping technique, the formation of radicals in the SC upon exposure to O_3 was detected. The spin adduct could arise from an alkoxyl radical formed during lipid peroxidation. Furthermore, lipid radicals ($L^{\bullet}$) are generated in epidermal homogenates that have been exposed to environmental stressors. The organic free radical $L^{\bullet}$ reacts with O_2, forming peroxyl radical $LOO^{\bullet}$ and hydro-lipoperoxides (LOOH). Transition metals and in particular iron play a key role in the reactions of LOOH and in the subsequent generation of alkoxyl radicals ($RO^{\bullet}$ can amplify the lipid peroxidation process).

Moreover, the toxicity is certainly augmented by the presence of NO_2, CO, SO_2, and particles (PM10). On this basis, it clearly appears how the O_3-generated ROS and LOPs at the tissue level, after being only partly quenched by the antioxidants, will act as cell signals able to activate transcription factors such as nuclear factor-kappa B (NF-κB), NO synthase, and some protein kinases, thus enhancing the synthesis and release of proinflammatory cytokines (TNF-α, IL-1, IL-8, IFN-γ, and TGF-β) and the possible formation of nitrating species. With a possible increasing inflow into the cutaneous tissues of neutrophils and activated macrophages, a vicious circle will start, perpetuating the production of an excess of ROS including hypochlorous acid, LOPs, isoprostanes, tachykinins, cytokines, and proteases, which will self-maintain the inflammation after O_3 exposure.

12.7 UV AND OZONE

The skin is continuously exposed to several oxidative stressors simultaneously in life, which most likely will result in an additive if not synergistic effect. The SC is most exposed to environmental sunlight and is the main cutaneous oxidation target of atmospheric O_3, a major part of photochemical smog. This damage affects many molecules and structures and could lead to DNA alteration and generation of a local oxidative stress and can ultimately lead to skin cancer [30].

While UV radiation penetrates into the epidermis (UVB) or into the dermis (UVA) and is known to induce the release of tissue-degrading enzymes even at suberythemal levels, O_3 oxidizes biological systems only at the surface. Therefore, since O_3 and UV cooperatively damage SC components, they exert an additive effect on the cutaneous tissues. Data have suggested that UV irradiation compromises the skin barrier. O_3 may enhance this phenomenon by perturbing SC lipid constituents, which are known to be critical determinants of the barrier function.

Products of O_3-induced lipid oxidation penetrate the outer skin barrier and affect the constituents of the deeper epidermis. This can lead to the activation of redox-sensitive transcription factor such as NF-κB that regulates a variety of proinflammatory cytokines. On the other hand, NF-κB activation has also been implicated in the expression of collagenases by solar simulated UV radiation and in cutaneous responses to wounding. UV radiation has been shown to compromise the skin barrier. Since O_3 enhances UV-induced oxidation in the SC, it cannot be excluded that O_3 also potentially enhances other UV effects such as photoaging [31].

In fact, one of the few studies that evaluated a possible additive/synergistic effect of pollutants/stressors on skin has shown that UV and O_3 had an additive effect on antioxidant depletion (vitamin E), and this can lead to an additive effect on the biological skin responses to stressors [32].

This effect demonstrates that O_3 and UV radiation, two common sources of environmental oxidant stressors, exhibit additive effects in terms of oxidative damage to the skin barrier.

12.8   SKIN DEFENSE

12.8.1   Antioxidant Molecules

To protect itself against oxidative stress, the skin is equipped with an elaborate system of antioxidant substances and enzymes that includes a network of redox-active antioxidants. Antioxidant enzymes include but are not limited to glutathione reductases and peroxidases, superoxide dismutases (SODs), and catalase. These enzymes interact with the low molecular weight antioxidant substances such as vitamin E isoforms, vitamin C, GSH, and ubiquinol [33]. α-Tocopherol, the major biologically active vitamin E homologue, is generally regarded as the most important lipid-soluble antioxidant in human tissues. Besides its protection against lipid peroxidation, vitamin E is necessary to stabilize lipid bilayers, which may also be of relevance for SC lipid bilayers. Using tape-stripping-based sampling and HPLC-assisted detection, a sharp gradient was found with high levels of α-tocopherol in the lower SC and sharply decreasing concentrations toward the surface in human arm skin [33].

Thiele et al. [16] demonstrated that inherent vitamin E in human SC is relatively depleted on the surface and increases with SC depth. In fact, a single dose of solar simulated UV light (0.75 MED) depleted human SC α-tocopherol by almost 50% and murine SC α-tocopherol by 85% [16].

The high susceptibility of SC vitamin E to UV may be, at least in part, due to a lack of coantioxidants in the SC. *In vitro* ubiquinol-10 protects α-tocopherol from photooxidation by recycling mechanisms [34]. As has been previously reported, there is a lack of lipophilic antioxidant ubiquinol-9 in the SC of hairless mice [24], compared to the levels found in the whole epidermis and dermis of hairless mice [35]. Similarly, no detectable amounts of ubiquinol-10, the human equivalent of this antioxidant, were found in human SC (detection limit: 0.1 pmol), whereas its concentration in full-thickness human epidermis is similar to α-tocopherol [18]. Although in UV-irradiated murine skin homogenates, ascorbate, the major hydrophilic coantioxidant, can recycle photooxidized α-tocopherol [36,37], in murine and human SC the levels of ascorbate are very low compared to that in the epidermal and dermal tissues, which is not surprising because the SC is a very hydrophobic tissue. Thus, SC appears to lack any antioxidants that are known to recycle vitamin E, potentially explaining the susceptibility of SC vitamin E to oxidative stress.

Of interest is the fact that α-tocopherol in murine SC is depleted by UV exposure, although the formation of lipid peroxidation is not as evident as the antioxidant depletion. *In vitro* studies examining low-density lipoprotein oxidation show that lipid peroxidation occurs when vitamin E is almost completely depleted and that linoleic acid is depleted during this process [38,39]. Although linoleic acid accounts for only 1.4% of human SC free fatty acids [40], its presence is critical because essential fatty acid deficiency in rats causes severe barrier abnormalities [41]. Thus, minor amounts of lipid peroxidation of polyunsaturated fatty acids may still have severe pathophysiological consequences.

Of note, a vitamin E gradient in human SC has been shown with lowest tocopherol concentrations at the surface and the highest concentrations in the deepest SC layers. In human epidermis, the ratio of α-tocopherol to γ-tocopherol is about 10–1 [18]. The tocopherol gradient in human SC appears to reflect a depletion of tocopherols in surface layers and this could be a consequence of the following: (i) The irradiance of UV at the absorption maximum of α-tocopherol (around 295 nm) is highest at the outer surface and decreases within the SC [42]. (ii) The oxygen partial pressure (pO_2) decreases gradually from the outer to the inner SC layers as a result of the high diffusion resistance [43] and thus is inversely correlated with the α-tocopherol concentrations within the SC. Because the presence of oxygen is needed for the induction of UV-induced generation of ROS, this might contribute to the increasing α-tocopherol depletion toward the outer SC layers. (iii) The percutaneous penetration of most molecules, among them noxious, oxidizing xenobiotics, follows a gradient within the SC with highest concentrations in the outer layers [44]. Oxidation of α-tocopherol by such exogenous oxidants would therefore also be higher in the outer SC. Besides its protection against lipid peroxidation, vitamin E stabilizes lipid bilayer structures [45,46], which may also be of relevance for SC lipid physiology; remarkably, the degree of disorder and the amount of lipids decrease over the outer cell layers of human SC [47]. Thus, low levels of SC vitamin E are associated with a high degree of SC lipid disorder.

α-Tocopherol protection against UVB-induced lipid peroxidation is a consequence of both its ability to scavenge peroxyl radicals and its UVB absorbance resulting in a sunscreen effect [48]. Both mechanisms would provide photoprotection in adjacent epidermal layers. Hence, the presence of α-tocopherol in the human SC and its distribution gradient appear to be of major relevance, especially because its absorption maximum is very similar to the action spectrum for UV-induced erythema and carcinogenesis of hairless mice with a flat peak at 293 nm. In addition to its antioxidant properties, α-tocopherol was reported to act as a human skin penetration enhancer, resulting from its interactions with the gel-phase interstitial lipid region of the SC [49]. *In vitro* evidence exists that α-tocopherol modulates the fluidity and permeability of lipid bilayer membranes [50]. Consequently, depletion of inherent SC α-tocopherol could affect the barrier function of human SC.

Furthermore, the concentrations of ascorbate (water-soluble antioxidant) detected in human SC are lowest in the outer SC and increases almost 10-fold in the lower SC, however still between one and two orders of magnitude lower than epidermal ascorbate concentrations. Urate concentrations within human SC have been shown to be distributed more evenly than ascorbate and tocopherols, its concentration in the upper SC was more than 100-fold higher than ascorbate. Similar gradients with highest levels in basal SC layers were found for ascorbate, glutathione, and uric acid in the SC of the untreated hairless mouse [51].

As mentioned earlier, SC layers move up in time as a part of the physiological turnover and are replaced by newly differentiated keratinocytes. Therefore, the superficial layer has been exposed longer to chronic oxidative stress than a deeper layer and the distribution of antioxidants in the SC follows a gradient with higher concentrations in deeper layers [51]. In the lipophilic phase, tocopherol is the most prominent antioxidant, while vitamin C and GSH have the highest abundance in the cytosol. These antioxidant defenses remove and/or absorb ROS from the skin [52].

12.8.2 Enzymes

Although many antioxidant enzymes have been shown to be present in cutaneous tissues, superoxide dismutase and catalase are considered as major antioxidant enzymes in the SC. The dismutation of superoxide by SOD results in the production of hydrogen peroxide, which is subsequently converted to water and oxygen through a reaction that is catalyzed by catalase. An imbalance in the ratio of antioxidant enzymes may thus contribute to an excessive accumulation of ROS, increasing oxidative stress and damage. Different types of SOD can be discerned, depending on the redox-active metal at the catalytic site. Cu/Zn SOD is localized mainly in the cytosol and nucleus, whereas Mn SOD is located in the mitochondria, which may suggest a different functionality. Catalase is a tetrameric, heme-containing redox enzyme. It neutralizes hydrogen peroxide to water and oxygen and thereby prevents excessive hydrogen peroxide buildup. Catalase is located intracellularly within the mitochondria and the peroxisomes. The enzymatic activity of SOD and catalase is about 2.3- and 8-fold higher in epidermis compared to that in the dermis [18]. Low catalase activity levels have been measured in several skin disorders such as vitiligo [53], physical urticaria [54], and in human epitheliomas [55]. In all these skin disorders, the decreased catalase activity might be considered as a very sensitive marker for the increased susceptibility of the skin to external stimuli [54]. It is well documented that the catalase activity is lower after an acute dose of UVA. This has been demonstrated in mouse skin [18,56] as well as in human skin fibroblasts [57,58] and keratinocytes [59]. Chronic UVA exposure suppressed the catalase activity in hairless mouse skin [60], whereas acute or chronic UVB irradiation had no effect on the catalase activity in mice [61]. After an acute dose of UVA, the catalase activity in mouse skin recovered slowly [18].

Guarrera et al. [62] measured the catalase activity in SC with tape stripping technique and demonstrated a linear increase of the catalase activity in human SC from the surface down to layer 4. Using a larger cross section of the SC down to layer 20, Thiele et al. showed a decrease in both SOD and catalase activity toward the skin surface. A constant value is measured approximately from layer 10 onward [16]. Further results on pooled tape strippings of the human SC also showed increasing activities with depth over the first 10 layers for the enzymes β-glucocerebrosidase, acid phosphatase, and phospholipase A2 [63]. Analogous observations were published with respect to several nonenzymatic antioxidants, showing the existence of a redox gradient across the SC with decreasing vitamin E [16], vitamin C, uric acid, and glutathione concentrations [51] toward the skin surface. Several reasons for the existence of such a gradient have been suggested: (i) The outer layers of the skin are exposed to high loads of different kinds of environmental sources of ROS, such as UV light, air pollution, and ozone in the presence of relatively high concentrations of oxygen. It can therefore be expected that the oxidative damage to proteins and other biomolecules is higher toward the outer layers of the SC. This has been demonstrated for tape strippings where an increase in keratin oxidation was observed toward the outer layers of the SC [64]. (ii) In the case of catalase, its activity can also most probably be lost by a mechanism of direct photodestruction ([18], and our observation), which will also contribute to the gradient. (iii) Interestingly, a reversed activity gradient is observed for the trypsin- or chymotrypsin-like activities over the first 10 layers of the SC with higher activity toward the surface [63]. These proteases are supposed to be involved in the desquamation process and are presumably quite resistant to the oxidative stress that leads to the activation of the other enzymes. It can therefore be suggested that a gradual enzymatic proteolysis of the antioxidant enzymes by these proteases may also partly contribute to their deactivation toward the SC surface.

An interesting study on the use of sunbed for tanning has confirmed the loss of catalase activity in the SC upon exposure to UV light. The same study has observed a seasonal variation in the enzymatic activity of catalase, with low activities in summer, especially at sun-exposed sites, and high activities in winter. On the other hand, the activity of SOD is not affected, confirming that the ratio of catalase to SOD is also dramatically lower in summer compared to that in winter in the upper layers of the human SC. It can therefore be expected that a reduction in the ratio of catalase to SOD may lead to a local overproduction of hydrogen peroxide and thus an increase in oxidative stress. This is in accordance with studies showing a depletion of the antioxidant enzyme expression, especially in the SC and epidermis concomitant with increased protein oxidation, mainly in the dermis [65], suggesting that the UV-induced oxidative damage in human skin might partly occur via the formation of hydrogen peroxide.

This oxidative damage to the SC not only affects antioxidant levels in the SC but might also induce deeper cellular responses in the cutaneous tissue via an indirect mechanism in which second messengers activate the stress responses [66].

The loss in catalase activity upon sun exposure is at least partly compensated by the activity of glutathione peroxidase (GSH-Px), which is also capable of neutralizing hydrogen peroxide. There seem to be some functional differences, however, between catalase and GSH-Px in human dermal fibroblasts [67]: GSH-Px mainly shields the cell from damage at high hydrogen peroxide concentrations, whereas catalase protects from oxidative stress at relatively low hydrogen peroxide concentrations and acts as a primary defense mechanism. Furthermore literature data suggest that in the epidermis, the enzymatic activity of GSH-Px is much lower than that of catalase [18,68].

It has also been shown that the deactivation of catalase could be mimicked by exposure to a source of broadband UVA, whereas UVB did not affect the catalase activity while SOD activity is not affected by the irradiation. The decrease in catalase activity after UVA irradiation has been well documented both *in vitro* and in animals [18,56–58]. *In vitro* experiments have revealed that the dose-dependent decline in catalase activity is mainly due to direct photodestruction [18] in which the heme group, which absorbs at 410 nm, might be involved.

12.8.3 Melatonin

Because of its broad antioxidant and radical scavenger properties [69], melatonin may act as a protective agent against UV radiation-induced damage in the skin. Clinical studies indicated that melatonin can prevent sun damage. In fact, melatonin increases cell viability in UV-irradiated fibroblasts by counteracting the formation of polyamine levels and the accumulation of MDA while decreasing apoptosis cells [70]. Melatonin has also been shown to protect against UV light-induced damage in human leuko-cytes. In this cell model, melatonin significantly suppresses the formation of ROS leading consecutively to an increased rate of cell survival when applied to the cells prior to UV irradiation. In fact, melatonin exhibited stronger radical-scavenging properties than vitamin C and Trolox [71,72]. Given the antioxidant effects of melatonin, it could have a role in skin biology, where its short plasma half-life and low molecular weight suggest that it could be useful as a constituent of sun-protective creams. It has been reported that intraperitoneal administration of melatonin at physiological levels to pinealectomized rats undergoing skin surgery can reduce MDA and NO levels in the skin, while GSH, GSH-Px, and SOD are increased, compared to nontreated pinealectomized animals [73]. Furthermore, treatment of animals with melatonin led the postinjury GSH levels to be increased significantly and lipid peroxidation to be significantly decreased in skin homogenates. Melatonin is a strong radical scavenger directed especially against hydroxyl radicals, which are thought to be the most damaging effectors produced during UV. Therefore, melatonin is an important player for the skin defense against environmental stressors in not only the suppression but also the promotion of skin carcinogenesis stages [74].

12.9 CONCLUDING REMARKS

Individuals are constantly exposed to environmental pollutants such as UV and O_3 and it is not possible to protect ourselves from these stressors; therefore, it is important to understand the full extent and molecular mechanisms involved in the apparent additive or even synergistic effect of these stressors in causing skin cellular damage. The use of antioxidants to inhibit photooxidative toxicity has been suggested to be an important strategy in preventing and treating photodamage. However, the clinical data on antioxidant treatments do not yet convincingly show that dietary monotherapy is of significant therapeutic value in protection from acute or chronic photodamage.

REFERENCES

1. Pouillot A, Dayan N, Polla AS, Polla LL, Polla BS. The stratum corneum: a double paradox. *J. Cosmet. Dermatol.* 2008;7(2):143–148.
2. Athar M. Oxidative stress and experimental carcinogenesis. *Indian J. Exp. Biol.* 2002;40(6):656–667.

3. Reddy SP. The antioxidant response element and oxidative stress modifiers in airway diseases. *Curr. Mol. Med.* 2008;8(5):376–383.

4. de Gruijl FR, Rebel H. Early events in UV carcinogenesis: DNA damage, target cells and mutant p53 foci. *Photochem. Photobiol.* 2008;84(2):382–387.

5. Morison WL, Kerker BJ, Tunnessen WW, Farmer ER. Disseminated hypopigmented keratoses. *Arch. Dermatol.* 1991;127(6):848–850.

6. Goldsmith LA, DeYoung LM, Falciano V, Ballaron SJ, Akers W. Inhibition of human epidermal transglutaminases *in vitro* and *in vivo* by tyrosinamidomethyl dihydrohaloisoxazoles. *J. Invest. Dermatol.* 1991;97(1):156–158.

7. Halliday GM. Inflammation, gene mutation and photoimmunosuppression in response to UVR-induced oxidative damage contributes to photocarcinogenesis. *Mutat. Res.* 2005;571(1–2): 107–120.

8. Hruza LL, Pentland AP. Mechanisms of UV-induced inflammation. *J. Invest. Dermatol.* 1993; 100(1):35S–41S.

9. Deliconstantinos G, Villiotou V, Stavrides JC. Alterations of nitric oxide synthase and xanthine oxidase activities of human keratinocytes by ultraviolet B radiation: potential role for peroxynitrite in skin inflammation. *Biochem. Pharmacol.* 1996;51(12):1727–1738.

10. Diffey BL, Farr PM, Oakley AM. Quantitative studies on UVA-induced erythema in human skin. *Br. J. Dermatol.* 1987;117(1):57–66.

11. Dubertret L. UVA and oxidative stress. *Eur. J. Dermatol.* 1996;6:236–237.

12. Kütting B, Drexler H. Evaluation of skin-protective means against acute and chronic effects of ultraviolet radiation from sunlight. *Curr. Probl. Dermatol.* 2007;34:87–97.

13. Auletta M, Gange RW, Tan OT, Matzinger E. Effect of cutaneous hypoxia upon erythema and pigment responses to UVA, UVB, and PUVA (8-MOP + UVA) in human skin. *J. Invest. Dermatol.* 1986;86(6):649–652.

14. Seagle BL, Rezai KA, Gasyna EM, Kobori Y, Rezaei KA, Norris JR, Jr., Time-resolved detection of melanin free radicals quenching reactive oxygen species. *J. Am. Chem. Soc.* 2005;127(32):11220–11221.

15. Haratake A, Uchida Y, Schmuth M, Tanno O, Yasuda R, Epstein JH, Elias PM, Holleran WM. UVB-induced alterations in permeability barrier function: roles for epidermal hyperproliferation and thymocyte-mediated response. *J. Invest. Dermatol.* 1997;108(5):769–775.

16. Thiele JJ, Traber MG, Packer L. Depletion of human stratum corneum vitamin E: an early and sensitive *in vivo* marker of UV induced photo-oxidation. *J. Invest. Dermatol.* 1998;110(5):756–761.

17. Thiele JJ. Oxidative targets in the stratum corneum: a new basis for antioxidant strategies. *Skin Pharmacol. Appl. Skin Physiol.* 2001;14(Suppl. 1): 87–91.

18. Shindo Y, Witt E, Han D, Epstein W, Packer L. Enzymic and non-enzymic antioxidants in epidermis and dermis of human skin. *J. Invest. Dermatol.* 1994;102(1):122–124.

19. Thiele JJ, Friesleben HJ, Fuchs J, Ochsendorf FR. Ascorbic acid and urate in human seminal plasma: determination and interrelationships with chemiluminescence in washed semen. *Hum. Reprod.* 1995;10(1):110–115.

20. Thiele JJ, Traber MG, Re R, Espuno N, Yan LJ, Cross CE, Packer L. Macromolecular carbonyls in human stratum corneum: a biomarker for environmental oxidant exposure? *FEBS Lett.* 1998;422(3): 403–406.

21. Uppu RM, Cueto R, Squadrito GL, Pryor WA. What does ozone react with at the air/lung interface? Model studies using human red blood cell membranes. *Arch. Biochem. Biophys.* 1995;319 (1):257–266.

22. Pryor WA. Mechanisms of radical formation from reactions of ozone with target molecules in the lung. *Free Radic. Biol. Med.* 1994;17(5):451–465.

23. Thiele JJ, Schroeter C, Hsieh SN, Podda M, Packer L. The antioxidant network of the stratum corneum. *Curr. Probl. Dermatol.* 2001;29:26–42.

24. Thiele JJ, Traber MG, Polefka TG, Cross CE, Packer L. Ozone-exposure depletes vitamin E and induces lipid peroxidation in murine stratum corneum. *J. Invest. Dermatol.* 1997;108(5):753–757.

25. Valacchi G, Fortino V, Bocci V. The dual action of ozone on the skin. *Br. J. Dermatol.* 2005;153(6): 1096–1100.

26. Chen LC, Qu Q. Formation of intracellular free radicals in guinea pig airway epithelium during *in vitro* exposure to ozone. *Toxicol. Appl. Pharmacol.* 1997;143(1):96–101.

27. Hamilton RF, Jr., Li L, Eschenbacher WL, Szweda L, Holian A. Potential involvement of 4-hydroxynonenal in the response of human lung cells to ozone. *Am. J. Physiol.* 1998;274 (1 Part 1): L8–L16.

28. Kirichenko A, Li L, Morandi MT, Holian A. 4-Hydroxy-2-nonenal-protein adducts and apoptosis in murine lung cells after acute ozone exposure. *Toxicol. Appl. Pharmacol.* 1996; 141(2):416–424.

29. Smith LL. Oxygen, oxysterols, ouabain, and ozone: a cautionary tale. *Free Radic. Biol. Med.* 2004;37(3):318–324.

30. Cadet J, Sage E, Douki T. Ultraviolet radiation-mediated damage to cellular DNA. *Mutat. Res.* 2005;571(1–2):3–17.

31. Burke KE, Wei H. Synergistic damage by UVA radiation and pollutants. *Toxicol. Ind. Health* 2009;25(4–5):219–224.

32. Valacchi G, Weber SU, Luu C, Cross CE, Packer L. Ozone potentiates vitamin E depletion by ultraviolet radiation in the murine stratum corneum. *FEBS Lett.* 2000;466(1):165–168.

33. Packer L, Valacchi G. Antioxidants and the response of skin to oxidative stress: vitamin E as a key indicator. *Skin Pharmacol. Appl. Skin Physiol.* 2002;15(5):282–290.

34. Stoyanovsky DA, Osipov AN, Quinn PJ, Kagan VE. Ubiquinone-dependent recycling of vitamin E radicals by superoxide. *Arch. Biochem. Biophys.* 1995;323(2):343–351.

35. Shindo Y, Witt E, Packer L. Antioxidant defense mechanisms in murine epidermis and dermis and their responses to ultraviolet light. *J. Invest. Dermatol.* 1993;100(3):260–265.

36. Kagan V, Witt E, Goldman R, Scita G, Packer L. Ultraviolet light-induced generation of vitamin E radicals and their recycling: a possible photosensitizing effect of vitamin E in skin. *Free Radic. Res. Commun.* 1992;16(1):51–64.

37. Kitazawa M, Podda M, Thiele J, Traber MG, Iwasaki K, Sakamoto K, Packer L. Interactions between vitamin E homologues and ascorbate free radicals in murine skin homogenates irradiated with ultraviolet light. *Photochem. Photobiol.* 1997;65(2):355–365.

38. Esterbauer H, Wäg G, Puhl H. Lipid peroxidation and its role in atherosclerosis. *Br. Med. Bull.* 1993;49(3):566–576.

39. Lodge JK, Sadler PJ, Kus ML, Winyard PG. Copper-induced LDL peroxidation investigated by 1H-NMR spectroscopy. *Biochim. Biophys. Acta* 1995;1256(2):130–140.

40. Wertz PW, Downing DT. Metabolism of linoleic acid in porcine epidermis. *J. Lipid Res.* 1990;31(10):1839–1844.

41. Hansen HS, Jensen B. Essential function of linoleic acid esterified in acylglucosylceramide and acylceramide in maintaining the epidermal water permeability barrier: evidence from feeding studies with oleate, linoleate, arachidonate, columbinate and alpha-linolenate. *Biochim. Biophys. Acta* 1985;834(3):357–363.

42. Anderson RR, Parrish JA. The optics of human skin. *J. Invest. Dermatol.* 1981;77(1):13–19.

43. Hatcher ME, Plachy WZ. Dioxygen diffusion in the stratum corneum: an EPR spin label study. *Biochim. Biophys. Acta* 1993;1149(1):73–78.

44. Rougier A, Rallis M, Krien P, Lotte C. *In vivo* percutaneous absorption: a key role for stratum corneum/vehicle partitioning. *Arch. Dermatol. Res.* 1990;282(8):498–505.

45. Lucy JA. Functional and structural aspects of biological membranes: a suggested structural role for vitamin E in the control of membrane permeability and stability. *Ann. N. Y. Acad. Sci.* 1972;203:4–11.

46. Stillwell W, Ehringer W, Wassall Sr., Interaction of alpha-tocopherol with fatty acids in membranes and ethanol. *Biochim. Biophys. Acta* 1992;1105(2):237–244.

47. Bommannan D, Potts RO, Guy RH. Examination of stratum corneum barrier function *in vivo* by infrared spectroscopy. *J. Invest. Dermatol.* 1990;95(4):403–408.

48. Kramer KA, Liebler DC. UVB induced photooxidation of vitamin E. *Chem. Res. Toxicol.* 1997;10(2):219–224.

49. Trivedi A. Percutaneous absorption of tritium-gas-contaminated pump oil. *Health Phys.* 1995; 69(2):202–209.

50. Srivista S, Phadke RS, Govil G, Rao CNR. Fluidity, permeability, and antioxidant behaviour of model membranes incorporated with α-tocopherol and vitamin E acetate. *Biochim. Biophys. Acta* 1983;734:353–362.

51. Weber SU, Thiele JJ, Cross CE, Packer L. Vitamin C, uric acid, and glutathione gradients in murine stratum corneum and their susceptibility to ozone exposure. *J. Invest. Dermatol.* 1999;113(6): 1128–1132.

52. Moysan A, Morlière P, Marquis I, Richard A, Dubertret L. Effects of selenium on UVA-induced lipid peroxidation in cultured human skin fibroblasts. *Skin Pharmacol.* 1995;8(3):139–148.

53. Schallreuter KU. Successful treatment of oxidative stress in vitiligo. *Skin Pharmacol. Appl. Skin Physiol.* 1999;12(3):132–138.

54. Briganti S, Cristaudo A, D'Argento V, Cassano N, Turbino L, Guarrera M, Vena G, Picardo M. Oxidative stress in physical urticarias. *Clin. Exp. Dermatol.* 2001;26(3):284–288.

55. Rabilloud T, Asselineau D, Miquel C, Calvayrac R, Darmon M, Vuillaume M. Deficiency in catalase activity correlates with the appearance of tumor phenotype in human keratinocytes. *Int. J. Cancer* 1990;45(5):952–956.

56. Fuchs J, Huflejt ME, Rothfuss LM, Wilson DS, Carcamo G, Packer L. Acute effects of near ultraviolet and visible light on the cutaneous antioxidant defense system. *Photochem. Photobiol.* 1989;50(6): 739–744.

57. Moysan A, Marquis I, Gaboriau F, Santus R, Dubertret L, Morlière P. Ultraviolet A-induced lipid peroxidation and antioxidant defense systems in cultured human skin fibroblasts. *J. Invest. Dermatol.* 1993;100(5):692–698.

58. Shindo Y, Hashimoto T. Time course of changes in antioxidant enzymes in human skin fibroblasts after UVA irradiation. *J. Dermatol. Sci.* 1997;14(3):225–232.

59. Punnonen K, Puntala A, Ahotupa M. Effects of ultraviolet A and B irradiation on lipid peroxidation and activity of the antioxidant enzymes in keratinocytes in culture. *Photodermatol. Photoimmunol. Photomed.* 1991;8(1):3–6.

60. Okada K, Takahashi Y, Ohnishi K, Ishikawa O, Miyachi Y. Time-dependent effect of chronic UV irradiation on superoxide dismutase and catalase activity in hairless mice skin. *J. Dermatol. Sci.* 1994;8(3):183–186.

61. Iizawa O, Kato T, Tagami H, Akamatsu H, Niwa Y. Long-term follow-up study of changes in lipid peroxide levels and the activity of superoxide dismutase, catalase and glutathione peroxidase in mouse skin after acute and chronic UV irradiation. *Arch. Dermatol. Res.* 1994;286(1):47–52.

62. Guarrera M, Ferrari P, Rebora A. Catalase in the stratum corneum of patients with polymorphic light eruption. *Acta Derm. Venereol.* 1998;78(5):335–336.

63. Redoules D, Tarroux R, Assalit MF, Peri JJ. Characterisation and assay of five enzymatic activities in the stratum corneum using tape-strippings. *Skin Pharmacol. Appl. Skin Physiol.* 1999;12(4):182–192.

64. Thiele JJ, Hsieh SN, Briviba K, Sies H. Protein oxidation in human stratum corneum: susceptibility of keratins to oxidation *in vitro* and presence of a keratin oxidation gradient *in vivo*. *J. Invest. Dermatol.* 1999;113(3):335–339.

65. Sander CS, Chang H, Salzmann S, Müller CS, Ekanayake-Mudiyanselage S, Elsner P, Thiele JJ. Photoaging is associated with protein oxidation in human skin *in vivo*. *J. Invest. Dermatol.* 2002;118(4):618–625.

66. Valacchi G, van der Vliet A, Schock BC, Okamoto T, Obermuller-Jevic U, Cross CE, Packer L. Ozone exposure activates oxidative stress responses in murine skin. *Toxicology* 2002;179(1–2):163–170.

67. Masaki H, Okano Y, Sakurai H. Differential role of catalase and glutathione peroxidase in cultured human fibroblasts under exposure of H_2O_2 or ultraviolet B light. *Arch. Dermatol. Res.* 1998;290(3): 113–118.

68. Rhie G, Shin MH, Seo JY, Choi WW, Cho KH, Kim KH, Park KC, Eun HC, Chung JH. Aging- and photoaging-dependent changes of enzymic and nonenzymic antioxidants in the epidermis and dermis of human skin *in vivo*. *J. Invest. Dermatol.* 2001;117(5):1212–1217. Erratum in *J. Invest. Dermatol.* 2002;118(4):741.

69. Tan DX, Reiter RJ, Manchester LC, Yan MT, El-Sawi M, Sainz RM, Mayo JC, Kohen R, Allegra M, Hardeland R. Chemical and physical properties and potential mechanisms: melatonin as a broad spectrum antioxidant and free radical scavenger. *Curr. Top. Med. Chem.* 2002;2(2):181–197.

70. Lee KS, Lee WS, Suh SI, Kim SP, Lee SR, Ryoo YW, Kim BC. Melatonin reduces ultraviolet-B induced cell damages and polyamine levels in human skin fibroblasts in culture. *Exp. Mol. Med.* 2003;35(4):263–268.

71. Fischer TW, Scholz G, Knöll B, Hipler UC, Elsner P. Melatonin suppresses reactive oxygen species in UV-irradiated leukocytes more than vitamin C and trolox. *Skin Pharmacol. Appl. Skin Physiol.* 2002;15(5):367–373.

72. Fischer TW, Scholz G, Knöll B, Hipler UC, Elsner P. Melatonin suppresses reactive oxygen species induced by UV irradiation in leukocytes. *J. Pineal Res.* 2004;37(2):107–112.

73. Gurlek A, Aydogan H, Parlakpinar H, Bay-Karabulut A, Celik M, Sezgin N, Acet A. Protective effect of melatonin on random pattern skin flap necrosis in pinealectomized rat. *J. Pineal Res.* 2004;36(1):58–63.

74. Kumar CA, Das UN. Effect of melatonin on two stage skin carcinogenesis in Swiss mice. *Med. Sci. Monit.* 2000;6(3):471–475.

CHAPTER 13

THE IMPACT ON THE SKIN'S INNATE IMMUNITY BY COSMETIC PRODUCTS APPLIED TO THE SKIN AND SCALP

Rudranath Persaud and Thomas Re

Safety Evaluation, L'Oreal USA, Inc., Clark, NJ

13.1   INTRODUCTION

Innate immunity refers to the nonspecific pathogen resistance mechanisms that offer protection to the host in conjunction with adaptive or acquired immunity. It is composed of four types of defensive barriers: anatomical, physiological, phagocytic, and inflammatory. Anatomical barriers include the skin and mucous membranes; physiological barriers are temperature and low pH; phagocytic barriers involve the various cell types that ingest and digest microorganisms; and inflammatory barriers pertain to a migration of serum proteins and phagocytic cells to an area of tissue damage and infection.

Intact skin functions as a mechanical barrier that prevents the entry of microorganisms into the host. It consists of two distinct layers: the outer layer or epidermis and a thicker inner layer or the dermis. The epidermis is made up of many layers of tightly packed simple squamous epithelial cells and is infiltrated with the hydrophobic protein keratin. The upper layers of the epidermis are composed of dead squamous cells that lose their shape and eventually slough off constantly being replenished by the lower living tissue. The dermis is composed of connective tissue and includes the blood vessels, hair follicles, and sebaceous and sweat glands. The sebaceous glands produce and secrete sebum, an oily substance consisting of lactic acid and fatty acids. These acids maintain the pH of the skin surface between 3.0 and 5.0 that is acidic enough to impede the growth of microbes. The skin therefore provides both an anatomic barrier and an acid mantle that are involved in innate immunity by preventing both the entry and growth of pathogens. Damage to the skin can result in an inflammatory process, including the release of mediator substances such as interleukins and the recruitment of phagocytic cells.

Innate Immune System of Skin and Oral Mucosa: Properties and Impact in Pharmaceutics, Cosmetics, and Personal Care Products, First Edition. Nava Dayan and Philip W. Wertz.
© 2011 John Wiley & Sons, Inc. Published 2011 by John Wiley & Sons, Inc.

13.2 ALTERATIONS IN BARRIER INTEGRITY AND FUNCTION

Generally cosmetic and personal care products such as color makeup and moisturizing lotions are formulated to be mild with no significant cause of skin adverse reactions. However, some cosmetic products such as skin peels, hair bleaches, and hair relaxers can be more aggressive and may alter the properties of the skin or scalp that could potentially interfere with innate immune function.

Professional peels are products used by dermatologists in their offices to reduce hyperpigmentation and fine lines or wrinkles. The active ingredients in peels generally include glycolic acid, salicylic acid [1], and other related materials. The mechanism of action of these agents is exfoliation that promotes rejuvenation of the skin. Depending on the type and concentration of active ingredients, the process of exfoliation can remove from one to several layers of skin cells. Mild exfoliating agents are known as surface peels and may include products available to consumers for home use. Higher concentrations and more aggressive agents cause a deeper exfoliation. The peels of this nature could compromise the integrity of the skin and alter its barrier function, resulting in an increase susceptibility to invasion by microbes. Deeper peels are generally applied by dermatologists or aestheticians working in the controlled environment of an office or professional spa.

Hair bleaches are cosmetic products that are available both on retail and for professional use by hairdressers. The purpose of using hair bleaches is twofold: to give hair a lighter color and to prepare it for the application of a dye. Persulfates, ammonia, and hydrogen peroxide are some of the major ingredients used as bleaching actives. One of the major safety concerns following the use of hair bleaches is irritation of the scalp and adjacent skin areas that the product may come in contact with. Extensive scalp contact with persulfates can cause an immediate irritant reaction manifested as burning and redness [2]. Severe irritation can potentially lead to breaks in the skin providing a portal for microorganisms. Professional bleaching products intended for salon use are classified as on-scalp (milder formulations) products for application close to the hair root and off-scalp products that are more aggressive in their bleaching potential. Products for home use are generally milder but may not provide the same amount of "lift" or bleaching.

Hair relaxers are products also available on retail to the consumer and for professional use. Hair relaxers are used to straighten tightly curled or "kinky" hair and are extensively used in the African–American community. There are two approaches that can be implemented: first, a reducer/oxidant technology; second, an alkaline technology. The latter is more common and the active material is usually a base and can include the hydroxides of sodium, potassium, lithium, or guanidine/calcium carbonate. The hydroxides, particularly lithium, are more aggressive and are generally used in a professional hair salon environment. The combination of guanidine and calcium carbonate to generate an alkaline environment is more often used for home products. Due to the physicochemical properties of these compounds, there is possibility of irritation and if misused, corrosion of the scalp and surrounding skin. This would then potentially lead to breakages in the skin, thereby disrupting its integrity with potential invasion by pathogenic microbes that can cause inflammatory reactions and even wounds.

The stratum corneum is made up of a keratin protein network embedded within a lipid matrix. The isoelectric point of keratin is about 5 pH and the effective pK_a of the fatty acids within the lipid matrix is about 7 pH. This indicates that changes in topical pH can influence the properties of the stratum corneum. Skin cleansing with surfactants alters the pH of proteins and lipids within the stratum corneum leading to protein swelling and lipid rigidity, effects that are more marked at a pH of 10 than at a pH of 6.5 [3]. These changes in the structure of the skin, therefore, lead to a compromised barrier and interfere with its function. Again, the result here may be invasion by pathogenic microorganisms and inflammation.

The hydration of the skin is essential for the maintenance of its intact barrier function and for making it soft, flexible, smooth, and healthy. In addition, the human face is covered by a lipid film sebum, secreted by the sebaceous glands, that keeps the face supple and moist. A high hydration and low sebum secretion are considered optimal for skin. An excess of sebum secretion could make the skin surface very oily and can promote acne. Cosmetic products moisturize the skin surface and at the same time reduce sebum secretion, for example, products that include nicotinamide as an ingredient. The mechanism postulated involves a disruption in the transport of sebum by an alteration of the duct that connects the sebaceous gland to the skin surface. Such personal care regimens for human facial skin can provide the balance necessary to maintain an intact and effective barrier [4].

13.3   CHANGES IN SKIN pH

More aggressive topical products applied to skin and hair can temporary change the normal pH of skin and scalp influencing the growth of resident pathogenic microbes. An increase in such growth rate can elevate the risk of infection to the user of these types of products.

Professional peels are acidic and can have a pH value as low as 1.0. As the pH of skin is in the range of 3.0–5.0 that reduces the growth of most microbes, a pH change to more acidic can potentially increase the growth of pathogens that thrive better under acidic conditions. This can therefore increase the risk for infection.

Hair bleaches are formulated to have an acidic pH generally above 3.0 and below 4.0. Since the natural pH of skin is between 3.0 and 5.0, hair bleaches would not be anticipated to alter the growth of microorganisms on the scalp and skin.

The more common hair relaxers utilize an alkaline technology formulated with various bases. These products therefore have a basic pH in the range of 11.0–13.6. The temporary change of the skin's pH from acidic to basic could lead to increased growth of microbes on the skin and coupled with the irritation and possible breakage of skin may lead to invasion of these pathogenic opportunistic microbes.

The acidic pH of the skin's surface is essential for the growth conditions of both the resident and transient microflora. The resident microflora includes the Gram-positive bacteria. Examples of Gram-negative resident bacteria that are of limited distribution on the skin are *Propionibacterium, Corynebacterium, Brevibacterium, Staphylococcus, Micrococcus, Kytococcus, Dermatococcus,* and *Kocuria* spp. and *Acinetobacter* spp. The other type of prevalent resident on the skin is the yeast *Malassezia furfur* [5]. *S. epidermidis* represents more than 80% of the total microflora of areas such as the arms, legs, and lower torso. The skin provides the appropriate environment for the resident microflora that in turn prevents the colonization of harmful bacteria, thereby strengthening the barrier function [6]. It seems the skin microflora may have a role in the development and maintenance of appropriate immunity. The hypothesis is that the natural acquisition and nurturing of the normal microflora of young children may modulate the immune system in a way that it responds to certain allergens ensuring their elimination rather than producing delayed hypersensitivity [5]. In an 8-week study, the cleansing of the skin of the forehead and the forearm repeatedly with an alkali synthetic detergent preparation influences both the skin surface pH and the bacterial resident flora. The bacterial counts at both sites correlated with the pH. These findings implied that changes in pH resulting from using personal care products can influence both the skin surface pH and the microflora [7].

13.4   MODULATION OF INFLAMMATORY RESPONSES

A product with a pH ≤ 2.0 and ≥ 11.5 can be considered a corrosive without *in vivo* confirmatory testing [8]. The alkaline hair relaxers therefore fall within this category. The potential damage to skin can therefore trigger an inflammatory response where there is recruitment of serum proteins with antibacterial activity and migration of phagocytic cells into the affected area. In one case study, the loss of skin integrity manifested as irritant contact dermatitis with clinical signs of an inflammatory response after the use of a hair relaxer was also complicated by an infection from *S. aureus* [9].

13.5   SAFE APPLICATION OF COSMETICS

The products described in this chapter can all be designed and used in a way that they reduce or minimize the potential damage to skin and scalp. Professional skin peels are only used at intervals of two or more weeks, depending upon the depth of peel and the anticipated clinical outcome and are generally done under the care or direction of a dermatologist. For acid peels, neutralizers can be used to stop the activity as needed. For home products, the concentration and nature of the peeling agents are designed to produce a minimal surface peel. Hair bleaches are designed and labeled for on- or off-scalp use with clearly defined application times. Bleaching products are advised to be usually used every 4–6 weeks to avoid irritation and minimize hair breakage. Scalp protectants such as petrolatum are generally used with hair relaxers to minimize skin exposure. Timing of the relaxation process is critical and is clearly defined on the labeling. Care should be taken to prevent overexposure of consumers to these products. Professionals such as hairdressers and aestheticians are required to wear approved protective equipment such as gloves during application of these products.

In conclusion, most cosmetic and personal care products are formulated and tested to be mild and free of irritation to the dermatological normal consumer. More aggressive products can be used safely both at home and in professional environment provided the adequate label instructions are provided and followed.

REFERENCES

1. Oresajo C, Yatskayer M, Hansenne I. Clinical tolerance and efficacy of capryloyl salicylic acid peel compared to a glycolic acid peel in subjects with fine lines/wrinkles and hyperpigmented skin. *J. Cosmet. Dermatol.* 2008;7:259–262.
2. Fisher AA, Dooms-Goossens A. Persulfate hair bleach reactions: cutaneous and respiratory manifestations. *Arch. Dermatol.* 1976;112:1407–1409.
3. Amanthapadmanabhan KP, Lips A, Vincent C, Meyer F, Caso S, Johnson A, Subramanyan K, Vethamuthu M, Rattinger G, Moore DJ. pH-induced alterations in stratum corneum properties. *Int. J. Cosmet. Sci.* 2003;25:103–112.
4. Cheng Y, Dong Y, Wang J, Dong M, Zou Y, Ren D, Yang X, Li M, Schrader A, Rohr M, Liu W. Moisturizing and anti-sebum secretion effects of cosmetic application on human facial skin. *J. Cosmet. Sci.* 2009;60:7–14.
5. Holland KT, Bojar AB. Cosmetics: what is their influence on the skin microflora? *Am. J. Clin. Dermatol.* 2002;3:445–449.
6. Lambers H, Piessens S, Bloem A, Finkel P. Natural skin surface pH is on the average below 5, which is beneficial for its resident flora. *Int. J. Cosmet. Sci.* 2006;28:359–370.
7. Korting HC, Greiner K, Hubner K, Hamm G. Changes in skin pH and resident flora by washing with synthetic detergent preparations at pH 5.5 and 8.5. *J. Soc. Cosmet. Chem.* 1991;42:147–158.
8. Scientific Committee on Consumer Products. *The SCCP's Notes of Guidance for the Testing of Cosmetic Ingredients and Their Safety Evaluation*, 6th revision, 2006.
9. Kaur BJ, Singh H, Lin-Greenburg L. Irritant contact dermatitis complicated by deep-seated *Staphylococcal* infection caused by a hair relaxer. *J. Natl. Med. Assoc.* 2002;94:121–123.

CHAPTER 14

UV-INDUCED IMMUNOSUPPRESSION OF SKIN

Roger L. McMullen

International Specialty Products, Wayne, NJ

The skin is a unique organ equipped with an arsenal of cells that are able to launch an immune response in the event of attack by a foreign pathogen. The field of photoimmunology, concerned with the effects of solar radiation on the immune system, is still a blossoming discipline of research with abundant possibilities for new discoveries. In the past 40 years, a solid foundation was laid by many dedicated researchers who embarked on a journey to the unknown world of photoimmunology. There are, however, questions that still remain unanswered, especially in regard to the molecular mechanisms responsible for UV-induced immunosuppression. It has been well established that UV-induced immunosuppression begins with the action of photoreceptors, namely, keratinocyte DNA and *trans*-urocanic acid, and also with lipid peroxidation, which lead to a series of successive molecular signaling events that mediate the immune response. As a result of or in conjunction with these processes, Langerhans cells may either undergo apoptosis (programmed cell death) or their antigen presenting function could be compromised. A hallmark of UV-induced immunosuppression is the activation of T regulatory cells, which are specialized T cells that suppress the immune response. In this chapter, we will review the basic knowledge we have in the field of photoimmunology and establish some points of reference for the mechanisms responsible for UV-induced immunosuppression.

14.1 HISTORICAL PERSPECTIVE

Prior to the 1970s, the skin was not considered the intricate organ that we are so familiar with today. In fact, it was not until the early 1970s that we began to identify skin as a lymphoid organ [1]. Later on, skin was accepted as an integral component of the immune system and at first was denominated as skin associated lymphoid tissue (SALT) until later when it was given its present day designation of skin immune system (SIS) [2–4]. The origin of photoimmunology is most often credited to Michael Fisher and Margaret Kripke for their revolutionary work on mice models

Innate Immune System of Skin and Oral Mucosa: Properties and Impact in Pharmaceutics, Cosmetics, and Personal Care Products, First Edition. Nava Dayan and Philip W. Wertz.
© 2011 John Wiley & Sons, Inc. Published 2011 by John Wiley & Sons, Inc.

in the 1970s [5–8]. Researchers in Professor Kripke's laboratory demonstrated that UVB irradiation suppressed immune system function, which is now known to play an integral role in the development of skin cancer (see Figure 14.1). In their experiments, mice were subjected to UVB radiation causing them to develop tumors. The tumors from these mice were transplanted into non-immune suppressed mice (i.e., not exposed to UVB radiation or any other agent that could cause immunosuppression) and mice that were immune suppressed (given immunosuppressive drugs or subjected to subcarcinogenic doses of UV—both capable of suppressing the immune system). Their findings were revolutionary in as much as that tumors could not survive in the normal mice (non-immune suppressed), but were able to flourish in immune-suppressed mice. In addition, their studies demonstrated that UV-induced tumors in skin are highly antigenic (stimulate the production of antibodies), as opposed to other tumors, and are rejected by transplant recipients if their immune system is not compromised. These studies provided a definitive link between photocarcinogenesis and immunity, resulting in the birth of a new field of photobiology, photoimmunology. The amount of research focused on UV irradiation and its effects on the immune system is colossal. One need not look any further than the number of periodicals that publish a significant amount of this research, such as *Photodermatology, Photoimmunology & Photomedicine, Photochemistry and Photobiology, Photochemical and Photobiological Sciences*, and *Journal of Photochemistry and Photobiology B: Biology* in addition to the many dermatological and immunological research journals (e.g., *Journal of Investigative Dermatology, Journal of Immunology*, etc.) that also publish many studies related to solar radiation and the skin immune system.

14.2 INTERACTION OF SOLAR IRRADIATION WITH SKIN

The interaction of light with skin consists of reflection, scattering, and absorption. In terms of reflection, depending on the local geometry of the skin surface only a small fraction of the incident light undergoes reflection. However, anywhere from 93% to 96% of the incident light may be scattered or absorbed by endogenous chromophores [9]. As the outermost organ of the body, the skin is in constant contact with solar radiation. UV, visible, and infrared radiation reaching the surface of the Earth is able to interact with the cutaneous system. In terms of biological insult, UV light is of particular concern, which is often further categorized as UVA 320–400 nm, UVB 290–320 nm, and UVC 200–290 nm. Wavelengths of light greater than 290 nm reach the surface of the Earth and interact with the skin in various manners. Thus, wavelengths less than 290 nm (UVC) are filtered by ozone (O_3), which is present in the stratosphere, hence rendering protection to land inhabitants of the Earth. Historically, UVB radiation was thought to be very detrimental to the integrity of the skin since it is directly absorbed by nucleic acid bases resulting in DNA mutations. Moreover, due to its higher energy rays, UVB was typically the recipient of more attention in the literature as there was great concern about its potential deleterious effects. On the other hand, the amount of UVA that reaches the Earth's surface is much greater than that of UVB. Thus, it has

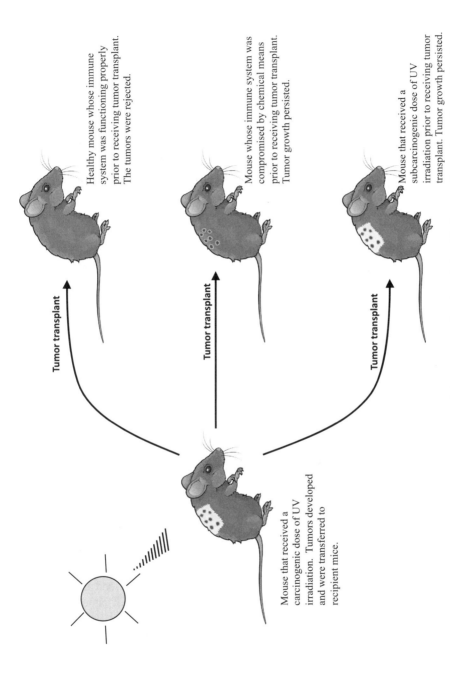

Figure 14.1   Initial experiments conducted by Margaret L. Kripke demonstrating the relationship between immunity and cancer development.

been recognized that the role played by UVA in causing damage to the skin is also of substantial concern. In fact, in more recent years, the deleterious effects of UVA have been realized and it is now well recognized that exposure to UVA results in photosensitization reactions in the skin, which leads to free radical damage that plays a pivotal role in photoimmunosuppression.

An important matter when discussing the interactions of light with the skin is an understanding of the penetration capabilities of the different segments of the electromagnetic spectrum into the skin. For example, longer wavelength light, such as that found in the visible region of the spectrum, is able to penetrate deep into the dermis. On the other hand, UVA radiation is typically limited to the upper levels of the dermis while UVB reaches only the epidermal layers. When taken into this perspective and with the knowledge of a particular cell type or chromophore location, we can better understand the outcomes ensuing from exposure to the different bands of electromagnetic radiation.

14.2.1 Chromophores in Skin

There are a plethora of chromophores present in human skin ranging from cellular DNA to the forms of hemoglobin present in the vascular network [9–11]. These molecules absorb electromagnetic radiation in the UVB, UVA, and visible region of the spectrum. Table 14.1 contains a list of the most common chromophores found in the skin along with pertinent information, such as the absorption maxima and the anatomical or cellular location. In most reviews written on the subject of UV-induced immunosuppression, epidermal DNA and *trans*-urocanic acid are awarded the most attention. While these two chromophores are, presumably, the most important mediators of UV-induced immunosuppression, we should also consider deleterious actions that may be mediated by other chromophores present in skin. We will discuss the contributions of DNA and *trans*-urocanic acid in another section of this chapter.

14.2.2 UV-Induced Alterations in Skin

In order for solar irradiation to induce a response in biological tissues, it is necessary for some type of photochemical reaction to take place. The skin contains many chromophores that absorb light in the UVB, UVA, and visible regions of the electromagnetic spectrum. Typically, UVB light is thought to be most damaging to nucleic acids (nucleotide bases) followed by proteins (tryptophan, phenylalanine, and tyrosine) and other chromophores (e.g., antioxidants). In more recent years, significant attention has been given to UVA irradiation as findings shed light on the vulnerability of skin to these wavelengths of light. The mechanism of damage induced by UVA irradiation has been associated with free radical reactions, resulting from photosensitization of a chromophore, ultimately leading to the production of reactive oxygen species (ROS) or reactive nitrogen species (RNS), which damage the structural components of skin (e.g., lipid peroxidation). It should also be noted that UVA irradiation is responsible for damage to nucleic acids.

TABLE 14.1   Selected Chromophores Present in Skin

Chromophore	λ_{max}	Location
Nucleotides		
AMP	259	The nucleotides form the structural backbone of nucleic acids and can be found in the nuclei and mitochondria of epidermal and dermal cells
GMP	252	
CMP	271	
UMP	262	
GMP	267	
Amino acids		
Tryptophan	280	The amino acids are found in cellular and extracellular proteins in the dermis and epidermis
Tyrosine	275	
Phenylalanine	257	
Cystine		
Pigment molecules		
Eumelanin/pheomelanin	UV/visible	The melanins are mostly found in the lower strata of the epidermis
Lipofuscins	UV/visible	Lipofuscins can be found in the secretory tubule of sweat glands
β-Carotene	Visible	Epidermis
Porphyrin-related compounds		
Hemoglobin	Visible	All compounds in this class are found in vascular vessels in the dermis
Oxyhemoglobin	Visible	
Bilirubin	Visible	
Cofactors		
NAD(P)H	340	Ubiquitous in the cell
Flavins (FMN^+, FAD^+)	300–500	Ubiquitous in the cell
Cross-linking amino acids		
Pyridine derivatives	UVA	Extracellular matrix proteins
Miscellaneous		
Quinones	UVA/UVB	Dermis/epidermis
Pterins	UVA	
7-Dehydrocholesterol	UVB	Stratum basale/stratum spinosum
trans-Urocanic acid	UVA/UVB	Stratum corneum

As only 5% of incident UV radiation that strikes the Earth surface is UVB, there has been tremendous interest in elucidating the effects of UVA on skin, which constitutes 95% of the incident UV radiation. Unlike UVB, less photons of UVA are absorbed by DNA and, thus, DNA photoproducts are not formed to as great an extent as a result of exposure to UVA radiation. It has been found that UVA induces a response from endogenous photosensitizers in skin, such as porphyrins and flavins, in which several different pathways lead to oxidative damage to skin. Once exposed to UVA, a photosensitizer becomes excited to a triplet electronic energy state, thereby allowing it to react with other molecules ultimately resulting in the formation of free radical species. In the field of photoimmunology, most studies are concerned with the harmful effects of UVB radiation. Recently, several studies have illuminated the significance of UVA in photoimmunosuppression. We elaborate further on this subject in Section 14.2.3.

14.2.3 Immediate Manifestations of Ultraviolet Irradiation Damage to Skin

There are several well-documented effects that occur immediately after exposure to UV radiation, which refers to a timescale on the order of minutes to days. These include an increase in epidermal thickness, deleterious effects on immune system function, increase in vitamin D synthesis, suntan (increased pigmentation), immediate pigment darkening, and sunburn (erythema) [12]. An increase in epidermal thickness and melanin production is thought to be a defense mechanism against subsequent sun exposure. The action spectrum for sun tanning shows that UVB is primarily responsible for the induced effect; however, UVA and visible light also contribute to tanning [12]. Erythema, on the other hand, is primarily caused by UVB radiation and is characterized by reddening, swelling, and pain in the skin. The reddening results from vasodilation, while swelling is caused by vasopermeability [12]. In addition, sunburned skin is often elevated in temperature due to increased blood flow to the region.

14.2.4 UV-Induced Signaling Cascades

It is well documented that UV light plays a key role in the induction of signaling pathways in skin. This results in ligand-independent activation of cell surface receptors, such as membrane-bound growth factor and cytokine receptors. The activation of these receptors results in signal transduction cascades, which ultimately lead to the activation of transcription factors. Thus, the upregulation or downregulation of a particular gene is affected by external stress factors, such as UV irradiation. In the event of an immune response, numerous cytokines are secreted by keratinocytes and other resident immune cells, which act as an outpost of the immune system. Often, the secreted cytokines function as proinflammatory agents; however, they may also be associated with cell growth or proliferation, which aid in the repair and homeostasis of the skin [13]. As already discussed, cytokines are also able to carry out an immune suppressive role. The interleukin (IL) family constitutes the bulk of cytokines encountered; however, cytokines from the interferon family, tumor necrosis factor (TNF), chemokines, and various growth factors equally perform critical functions in the skin.

As noted, keratinocytes immediately release numerous cytokines as part of the inflammatory response leading to the interaction with and recruitment of other immune cells. An illustration of some of the cytokine pathways that are likely to be followed in the event of UV insult is provided in Figure 14.2. Langerhans cells

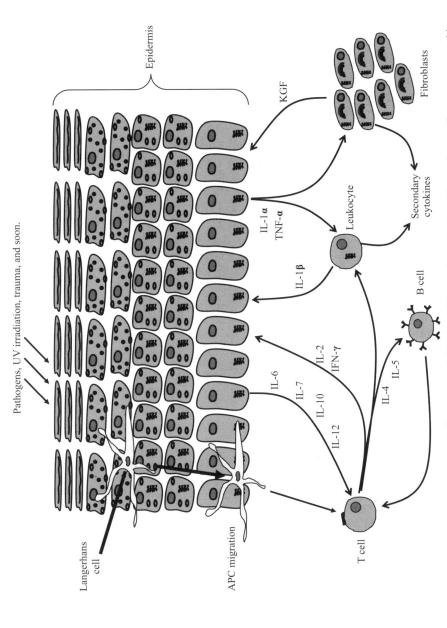

Figure 14.2 Signaling pathways associated with inflammation of skin. In addition to the activation of Langerhans cells, numerous cytokines are secreted by keratinocytes, which interact with receptors on leukocytes and fibroblasts. In turn, the activated cells generate cytokines resulting in multidirectional cellular signaling cascades. Adapted from B.E. Rich and T.S. Kupper [14].

begin their APC migration to T cells (if not first sent into an apoptotic state), while keratinocytes secrete primary cytokines (IL-1α or TNF-α), which perturb the other cells (leukocytes, fibroblasts, keratinocytes, etc.), resulting in the production of more primary cytokines. As a consequence, T cells secrete cytokines that interact with B cells or keratinocytes [14]. Figure 14.2 provides just a sample of a selected number of signaling mechanisms that are activated during the immune response. The signaling cascade goes back and forth between the various cell types and is extremely complex in nature. Still, many efforts are underway to elucidate and better understand signaling pathways and their activation or impairment by UV irradiation. These signaling mechanisms are believed to allow UV-induced systemic immunosuppression to occur in which exposure at one site will allow suppression to occur at a distant site that has not been irradiated [15].

Since we are mostly concerned about immunosuppression, it is worth noting that several cytokines are notorious for immunosuppressive activities. For example, IL-10, transforming growth factor-β (TGF-β), and α-melanocyte stimulating hormone (α-MSH) function in different capacities as immune suppressive cytokines. IL-10 may be secreted by leukocytes (T or B cells), mast cells, or keratinocytes. It functions as an immunosuppressive agent by impeding the expression of other cytokines such as IL-1, IL-12, and TNF-α as well as major histocompatibility (MHC) class II molecules (on the surface of phagocytes) [13]. TGF-β serves as an immunosuppressive instrument by preventing the growth of certain cell types while at the same time triggering the growth of others. TGF-β is known to inhibit the mobilization of phagocytes and the proliferation of T cells [13]. Keratinocyte, fibroblast, and melanocyte proliferation and differentiation can be regulated by α-MSH. It can behave in an immunosuppressive manner through downregulation of CD86, an important costimulatory molecule on the surface of monocytes and macrophages. For more details about cytokines in the skin, the reader may see Burbach et al. [13].

14.2.5 Photocarcinogenesis

Cancer refers to a disease that results from the overproliferation of mutant cells (neoplasm), which can be benign (remaining at the original site) or malignant in which case they can spread to distant sites of the body. Carcinogenesis, at the molecular level, begins with genes in which there are defects in the DNA. Defects in DNA are typically caused by exposure to chemical carcinogens, physical mutagens (irradiation), or in some cases, viruses. The DNA mutations are normally repaired by cellular repair mechanisms, such as nucleotide excision repair. However, throughout the lifetime of an organism, mutations augment eventually leading to cellular and tissue deformity. In many cases, the protein p53 is implicated in carcinogenesis. The wild-type p53 is a tumor suppressive protein that regulates the cell cycle and is known as the guardian of the genome. Mutations in the gene (TP53) that encodes p53 protein ultimately result in the protein's inability to regulate apoptosis, leading to carcinogenesis.

There are three different types of skin cancer and consist of basal cell carcinoma, squamous cell carcinoma, and malignant melanoma. The last of this group is the most dangerous and less frequent type of skin cancer—only 5% of the diagnosed skin cancers [16]. Melanoma can be found anywhere there is pigmentation—it is essentially cancer of the melanocytes, and it is able to metastasize to nearby blood vessels and lymph [16]. As may be inferred from the names, basal cell carcinoma and squamous cell carcinoma arise from keratinocytes of the basal layer and the stratum spinosum. These two types of skin cancer are much more common than malignant melanoma, however, much less threatening as they are less likely to metastasize before detection.

In our understanding of cutaneous cancer development, there are two pathways for the induction of cancer [17]. The first pathway is associated with direct DNA mutations (discussed above) or a free radical-induced DNA damage mechanism. Upon exposure to UV, cellular events include DNA damage, induction of p53- and p53-regulated proteins, cell cycle arrest, DNA repair, and apoptosis [17]. In the event of p53 genetic mutations, cellular proliferation will take place resulting in the formation of a neoplasm. An alternative pathway occurs during immunosuppression. DNA damage still occurs; however, rather than follow the p53 mutation route, immunosuppression alone is enough to allow neoplasm growth. While a definitive link between UV-induced immunosuppression and photocarcinogenesis may seem obscure, it has been shown that treatment with agents that inhibit UV-induced immunosuppression also impede photocarcinogenesis. Such treatments consist of antibodies to *cis*-urocanic acid, cyclooxygenase inhibitors, sunscreens, and the green tea polyphenol $(-)$-epigallocatechin-3-gallate [15].

14.2.6   Chromophores Involved in Photoimmunosuppression

In Section 14.2.1, we identified numerous chromophores present in skin to summarize other possible light-induced interactions, which could play some role in immuno-modulation. Regardless, out of the chromophores shown in Table 14.1, only epidermal DNA and *trans*-urocanic acid have been shown definitively to partake in UV-induced immunosuppression. While *trans*-urocanic acid is found in high concentrations in the stratum corneum, DNA resides in the lower layers of the epidermis. Considering the morphology of skin, both chromophores are ideal targets for UVB irradiation, which can reach as deep as the upper layers of the dermis. These points are in keeping with the action spectrum for photoimmunosuppression, which shows the largest peak in the UVB region [18]. Further work is pending to determine the UVA contribution to the action spectrum for immunosuppression.

14.2.6.1   DNA   It has been well established that DNA damage occurs when skin is exposed to UV radiation. This occurs through the process of light absorption by the base portion of the nucleotides, which is attached to the ribose unit that forms the backbone of DNA. Since maximum absorption of DNA occurs in the UVB region (ca. 260 nm), the shorter wavelength light (290–320 nm) that reaches the terrestrial surface is the most deleterious to the structural integrity of DNA. As a result of UVB absorption, DNA cross-links are formed between adjacent nucleotide residues in DNA. The two most common photoproducts are cyclobutane pyrimidine dimers (CPDs) and pyrimidine (6-4) pyrimidone photoadducts (see Figure 14.3).

DNA damage occurs in keratinocytes and resident immune cells (especially Langerhans cells) of the skin. Keratinocytes suffering from DNA damage are known to secrete cytokines that mediate immune function, both locally and systemically [20]. Immune cells, such as Langerhans cells, that undergo DNA damage experience decreased antigen presentation capabilities. Therefore, they are unable to carry out their duty of migrating to draining lymph nodes and presenting antigens to T cells. However, it has been reported that migrating APCs have been tested and found not to contain CPDs [21]. Thus, we would be led to believe that these cells were able to repair DNA *en route* and another force is responsible for poor antigen presentation. The reader is advised that this is a matter of disagreement in the literature. There are accounts in which it is reported that APCs with damaged DNA can be found in the draining lymph nodes after their migration from skin [19].

Overall, the mechanism of damaged DNA-mediated immunosuppression is still an active area of investigation with hopes of discerning a more direct connection between the formation of CPDs and the immunosuppressive action. The most convincing evidence of a link between CPDs and immunomodulation is provided in a review by de Gruijl [21]. In cases where the existing levels of CPDs are decreased (repaired), immune function is not compromised, whereas CPDs left unrepaired result in immunosuppressive behavior. (Note that these studies were conducted by employing the contact hypersensitivity (CHS) model—see Section 14.6.) Interestingly, it is noted that repair of pyrimidine (6-4) pyrimidone photoadducts is not immunomodulatory. Thus, CPDs are presumed to be the predominantly damaged DNA form that mediates immune function. Other evidence lies in studies where treatment with a DNA excision-repair enzyme (T4 endonuclease V) resulted in normal immune function [4].

14.2.6.2 *trans-Urocanic Acid*

Filaggrin (filament aggregating protein) is a protein rich in histidine and arginine that plays an integral role in the arrangement of keratin fibrils of epidermal cells as they undergo differentiation. Once its job of condensing keratin filaments is accomplished—in the upper layers of the epidermis—it is digested by protease enzymes resulting in the formation of smaller molecules, which constitute the natural moisturizing factor (NMF). One of these constituents is *trans*-urocanic acid, which accumulates in the stratum corneum. Numerous studies have shown that *trans*-urocanic acid is intimately involved in UV-induced immunosuppression. Upon exposure to UV radiation, *trans*-urocanic acid undergoes a photoisomerization reaction, converting it to the immunomodulating form, *cis*-urocanic acid. While a great deal of work has deepened our understanding of the importance of the role carried out by *cis*-urocanic acid in photoimmunosuppression, the precise mechanism of its action has yet to be elucidated.

The importance of *trans*-urocanic acid in UV-induced immunosuppression was first realized from tape-stripping studies in mice, which demonstrated that inhibition of UVB-induced immunosuppression could be impeded by removal of the stratum corneum. Thus, removal of the *trans*-urocanic acid along with the stratum corneum prevented CHS responses from occurring [22]. Similar studies were carried out in which *cis*-urocanic acid treatment was administered resulting in immunosuppression (using delayed type hypersensitivity (DTH) as a model—see Section 14.6) [22]. Likewise, treatment of mice with anti-*cis*-urocanic acid antibodies in combination with UVB irradiation inhibited immunosuppression [22]. Overall, the general conclusion in the literature is that *cis*-urocanic acid is capable of suppressing CHS and DTH.

Structurally, *cis*-urocanic acid is similar to serotonin. For this reason, it is not surprising that *cis*-urocanic acid can bind to serotonin receptors (5HT1 and 5HT2a), which are present in T cells, B cells, and dendritic cells [22]. There has been a considerable interest in the photoimmunology community to discern a possible role played by the serotonin receptors in UV-induced immunosuppression [15].

14.3 KEY MECHANISMS INVOLVED IN UV-INDUCED IMMUNOSUPPRESSION

Numerous molecular and cellular events occur in the skin as a result of exposure to UV irradiation. As mentioned previously, the onset of immunosuppression occurs as a result of the absorption of light by a chromophore present in the skin. The most studied and well-characterized photochemical events involved in UV-induced immunosuppression are based on absorption of light by *trans*-urocanic acid in the stratum corneum and DNA found in the epidermis (most likely in the basal layer). Many of the ensuing molecular events, that is, after chromophore absorption, have yet to be elucidated. Some of the other pivotal molecular mechanisms involved in UV-induced immunosuppression include cytokines, prostaglandins, and transcription factors. Cytokines, which are largely secreted by keratinocytes in response to UV irradiation, play a major role in the activation/recruitment of immune cells.

At this point in time, the onset of immunosuppression by UV light is best characterized by four independent, but possibly interrelated, processes involving photoreceptors in skin (DNA and *trans*-urocanic acid), lipid peroxidation, and dysfunctional or apoptotic Langerhans cells [19]. As shown in Figure 14.3, keratinocyte DNA can undergo cross-linking as a result of UV exposure to form, for example, cyclobutane pyrimidine dimers. Significant evidence has accumulated, which demonstrates that cytokines are released as a result of DNA damage. The cytokine, IL-10, is the most notorious, probably due to its immunosuppressive behavior. The conversion of *trans*-urocanic acid to *cis*-urocanic acid, and its subsequent migration from the stratum corneum to deeper tissues, is also accepted as one of the critical events necessary for UV-induced immunosuppression to take place. Although the mode of action of *trans*-urocanic acid is still not completely understood, it does play a role by impeding the migration and antigen presentation of Langerhans cells to T lymphocytes. In addition to impaired antigen presenting cell function, Langerhans cells may undergo apoptosis upon UV exposure. Lipid peroxidation also plays an important role in the induction of UV-induced immunosuppression. Free radical species (ROS or RNS) are formed as a result of UV irradiation exposure and can have profound effects on skin health and the skin immune system. An event provoked by lipid peroxidation is the expression of platelet

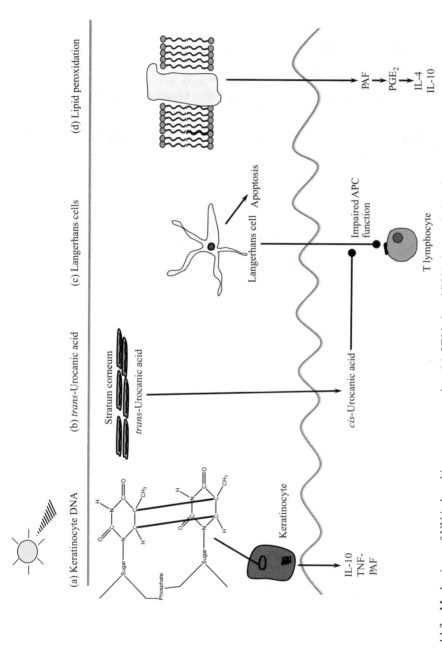

Figure 14.3 Mechanisms of UV-induced immunosuppression. (a) UV-induced DNA damage in keratinocytes resulting in the formation of cyclobutane pyrimidine dimers, or possibly another damaged form of DNA, results in keratinocyte secretion of cytokines (IL-10 and TNF-α) and PAF. (b) *trans*-Urocanic acid in the stratum corneum can undergo conversion to the *cis* isomeric form followed by migration to lower tissues where it interferes, by a yet unknown mechanism, with the antigen presentation by Langerhans cells to T lymphocytes. (c) Langerhans cells may undergo apoptosis or suffer impaired antigen presentation capabilities. (d) UV irradiation results in free radical species, which can cause lipid peroxidation. Such events eventually lead to generation of PAF and PGE$_2$, which result in further downstream events that produce IL-4 and IL-10. Adapted from J. Leitenberger et al. [19].

activating factor (PAF), which is secreted by keratinocytes as a result of oxidative stress and binds to membrane receptors in mast cells, monocytes, and other keratinocytes. Such an undertaking activates prostaglandin synthesis leading further to the secretion of IL-4 and IL-10 [23]. More than 10 years ago, it was shown that a series of cytokines (prostaglandin E_2, IL-4, and IL-10—in the respective order) are released due to lipid peroxidation and are in part responsible for the ensuing immunosuppression [24].

14.4 EFFECT OF UV IRRADIATION ON VARIOUS CELLULAR COMPONENTS OF THE IMMUNE SYSTEM

The immune system is composed of a complex system of cells, organs, and tissues that protect the organism against invasion by foreign pathogens. Various cell types with unique immunological functions are either present or may be deployed to the skin in the event when an immunological defense strike is necessary. The inflammatory cells— neutrophils, eosinophils, basophils, mast cells, and macrophages—may undergo UV-induced reactions, which affect their ability to carry out normal immune system functions. Likewise, lymphocytes can also suffer impairment due to UV irradiation. These include B cells, T cells (T helper cells, memory T cells, cytotoxic T cells, regulatory T cells, and natural killer T cells), and natural killer (NK) cells. In the sections that follow, we will review some studies that have shed light on the susceptibility of various cell types to UV irradiation.

14.4.1 Mast Cells

Most well known for their role in allergy responses, mast cells contain granules, which contain copious amounts of histamine and heparin. It is the secretion of such compounds that provides the symptoms of the allergic response [25]. Cutaneous mast cells are found in the dermis, where they are preferentially located adjacent to capillaries, lymphatics, nerves, and appendages [26]. While the role of cis-urocanic acid was well established in the 1990s, it was not until several years later that it was accepted that a contributing role is played by mast cells in UV-B-induced immunosuppression [27]. This phenomenon was demonstrated with mast cell-deficient mice that did not undergo immunosuppression when exposed to UVB or treated with cis-urocanic acid [28]. At this point in time, it is believed that histamine, released by mast cells, plays an integral role in the molecular events leading to immunosuppression [28]. In fact, mast cell migration from the skin to the draining lymph nodes is believed to be cardinal in the induction of immunosuppression [29].

14.4.2 Phagocytes

Phagocytes are a category of white blood cells (leukocytes), which act on foreign invaders (bacteria, viruses, etc.) by subjecting them to a process, known as phagocytosis, in which they engulf/ingest the pathogen rendering it nonfunctional. Our immune system is bestowed with several cell types that include macrophages, neutrophils, and Langerhans/dendritic cells.

14.4.2.1 Macrophages This cell type (macrophage) is a large form of phagocyte that develops from monocytes once it migrates to tissues. It is rather long-lived and contains an arsenal of cellular machinery to conduct phagocytosis including an expansive network of the Golgi apparatus and mitochondria as well as lysosomes [30]. It also produces ROS and RNS as a defense mechanism. In addition to its role in the innate response (nonspecific), it plays a part in the cell-mediated (specific) response. After exposure to acute UV radiation, macrophages migrate via the blood to the dermis and may even reach the epidermis. Specific populations of macrophages have been identified as the migrating species; however, there appears to be limited reports in the literature that specifically identify the cell line. They also secrete anti-inflammatory cytokines, most notably IL-10, when subjected to UV radiation [23]. Surprisingly, little is known in regard to the effects of UV on macrophage activity. Several studies have shown that UVB is able to influence the activity of macrophages, both positively and negatively; however, further research should shed more light on what is really happening to UV-exposed macrophages.

14.4.2.2 Neutrophils The most abundant leukocytes in the blood stream are neutrophils—inflammatory cells that do not divide and are short-lived. Like macrophages, neutrophils infiltrate the skin as a result of UV exposure. In recent years, there has been increasing attention given to neutrophils with respect to their role during skin exposure to UV irradiation—especially in terms of photoaging [31–34]. It is universally accepted that matrix metalloproteinases (MMPs) are responsible for the breakdown of fibrous proteins of the dermis, such as collagen and elastin [35–38]. Present belief is based on the school of thought that fibroblasts are primarily responsible for the secretion of these connective tissue degradative enzymes. An alternative to this thinking was put forth by Rijken et al. who found that neutrophils secrete greater amounts of MMP-1, MMP-9, and elastase than fibroblasts (2005, 2006). Before any conclusions can be drawn, further studies must be conducted on the effects of UV irradiation on neutrophil behavior.

14.4.2.3 Langerhans/Dendritic Cells Langerhans cells serve as sentinels of the immune system, which patrol the epidermis, process foreign antigens, and return to lymph node tissue to present the antigen to T helper cells so that the appropriate antibody can be generated [39]. In addition to their dendritic nature, Langerhans cells are also characterized by large Birbeck granules located within the cell structure. Langerhans cell activity is affected by UV irradiation—most notably its migration to the draining lymph nodes upon UVB exposure. In addition, the number of active Langerhans cells, and their morphological structure, is also affected by UVB irradiation [40]. Keratinocytes, mast cells, and macrophages secrete TNF as a result of UVB exposure [22]. TNF is believed to be the principal signal received by Langerhans cells directing them to migrate to the draining lymph nodes [22]. Other targets of UVB are the surface cell receptors of Langerhans cells,

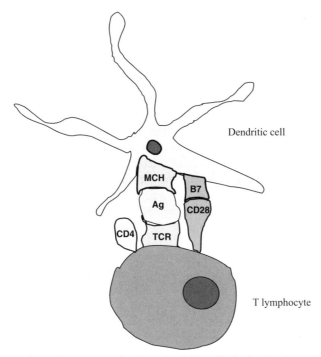

Figure 14.4   Antigen (Ag) presentation by a dendritic cell (Langerhans) to a T lymphocyte (CD4$^+$) by its receptor (TCR). UV irradiation impairs or downregulates the expression of MHC II molecules resulting in the failed antigen presentation by the dendritic cell. The costimulatory surface molecules, B7 located on the surface of dendritic cells and CD28 on T lymphocytes, are also necessary for proper antigen presentation to take place. Adapted from Thomas Schwarz [41].

such as MHC class II, adenosine triphosphatase (ATPase), intercellular adhesion molecule-1 (ICAM-1), and B7 (see Figure 14.4) [40,41]. Langerhans cells are also known to undergo DNA damage when exposed to UVB—Langerhans cells with damaged DNA have even been found in the draining lymph nodes [19]. Ultimately, damaged Langerhans cells can undergo apoptosis. DNA damage could also lead to a cellular signaling cascade, which could alter the activity of other cells or activate transcription factors. UVB also increases B cell activity (in the draining lymph nodes), which impedes antigen presentation to T cells [22].

14.4.3   Basophils and Eosinophils

Basophils and eosinophils are leukocytes that circulate in the blood and can be recruited to tissues, especially during inflammation. Both cell types are granulo-cytes—a type of white blood cell that contains granules in its cytoplasm—and represent a small fraction of the overall leukocyte population. Basophils are actually derived from eosinophils and share some features with mast cells, such as the secretion of histamine responsible for allergy symptoms [42]. Very little attention has been given to basophils and eosinophils in relation to UV irradiation—most likely because both cell types usually circulate in the blood rather than reside in one particular tissue area. There has been some interest in determining the effects of UVB on the ability of basophils to release histamine [43–45].

14.4.4 Lymphocytes

T cells (thymus) and B cells (bone) are lymphocytes responsible for, respectively, cell-mediated and humoral immunity. In cell-mediated immunity, immune cells patrol blood and tissues and are able to exert their influence by attacking foreign bacteria, fungi, parasites, cells that are infected by viruses, and cancer cells. In contrast, humoral immunity is associated with the ability of B cells to generate antibodies providing us with acquired immunity. There are a number of different types of T cells, which include T helper cells, memory T cells, cytotoxic T cells, regulatory T cells, and natural killer T (NKT) cells.

14.4.4.1 B Cells These are lymphocytes that reside in the lymphoid tissues, such as draining lymph nodes, spleen, and thymus, which generate antibodies against antigens (humoral response). B cells are an important component of the secondary immune response and, ultimately, are responsible for the generation of memory B cells and plasma cells. In general, B cells have not received a great deal of attention in most studies investigating photoimmunosuppression—probably due to the belief that such an event is due to the cell-mediated arm of immunity and the activity of T cells. Recent findings, however, have shed light on the involvement of B cells in the regulation of the immune response [46]. Specifically, UV irradiation was found to activate B cells in the draining lymph nodes, which in turn inhibit dendritic cell activation of T cells—a process that is believed to be mediated, to some extent, by IL-10.

14.4.4.2 T Cells As already stated, the task of T cells is paramount for the cell-mediated response. Structurally, they can be differentiated from their leukocyte counterparts (B cells and natural killer cells) by the receptor found on their surface known as T cell receptor and often abbreviated as TCR. Since there are a variety of T cell types, each is subcategorized into its own category in the following sections.

T Helper Cells (T_H Cells) As the name indicates, T_H cells aid other immunological cells in carrying out their respective functions. For example, they are responsible for the activation of macrophages and cytotoxic T cells. They also assist B cells and other T cells to proliferate after antigen binding. Thus, T_H cells play an integral role in both the humoral and the cell-mediated branches of the immune system. There are two principal types of T_H cells, $T_H 1$ and $T_H 2$, which can be distinguished by their mode of action. $T_H 1$ cells release TNF-β, INF-γ, and IL-2, which activate macrophages and play an integral role in the cell-mediated response. $T_H 2$ cells, on the other hand, secrete IL-4, IL-5, IL-10, and IL-13, which activate the humoral arm of the immune system by stimulating antibody production by B cells. UV exposure causes keratinocytes, and other cells, to release IL-10, which activates T_H2 cells thereby triggering a humoral (rather than cell-mediated) response. In addition, antigen presentation by Langerhans cells to T_H1 cells is diminished by UV. A humoral immune response, rather than cell-mediated, is favored as a result of UV irradiation in which T_H cells play a pivotal role [19].

Memory T Cells These cells are T cells that remain after a humoral response is launched, which contain a surface receptor (antibody) specific to a particular antigen. In this manner, immune memory is preserved after an antibody has been generated. While these cell types have not been the primary focus of photoimmunosuppression studies, it has been shown that UVB irradiation diminishes the immune system's ability to properly develop memory T cells (47).

Cytotoxic T Cells These cells, also known as killer T cells, attack host cells infected by viruses and tumor cells. They tightly bind to target cells at the site of MHC class I via a surface $CD8^+$ receptor. Cytotoxic T cells are able to recognize an altered MHC class I molecule, which has been altered by the binding of a foreign antigen. Although the direct effects of UV on cytotoxic T cells do not readily appear in the literature, the actions of other cells (APCs and regulatory cells) as a result of UV irradiation include the impediment of pathways leading to a cytotoxic T cell response [48].

Regulatory T Cells Historically known as suppressor T cells, regulatory T cells have been a topic of considerable debate for the past several decades [47]. In response to UV irradiation, regulatory T cells suppress the immune response, which has been mostly characterized using CHS models. There are various types of regulatory T cells, which are characterized by the cell surface receptors that it expresses, such as $CD4^+$ and $CD25^+$, which interact with other immunological cells. Regulatory T cells are also known to release IL-10 (an immunosuppressive cytokine) upon UV irradiation [49].

Natural Killer T Cells Not to be confused with natural killer cells, natural killer T cells contain an $\alpha\beta$ surface receptor in addition to some receptors that are in common with natural killer cells, thus providing it with properties from both cell lines. They represent an extremely small fraction of the overall T cell population. Overall, studies examining the behavior of natural killer T cells in the presence of UV have not been very forthcoming. On the other hand, conceivable proposals have been made about the possible significant roles played by natural killer cells in photoimmunosuppression—even to take on the role as regulatory T cells [50].

14.4.4.3 Natural Killer Cells This type of immune cell represents a relatively small portion of the circulating lymphocytes in the blood stream and can be distinguished from T cells and B cells by its lower degree of specificity in its surface receptors. Natural killer cells partake in the innate response by attacking virus-infected and tumor cells by attaching themselves to the surface of the target cell and inserting apoptosis-inducing proteins known as perforins. Natural killer cells are distinct from natural killer T cells, which represent a subcategory of T cells (see above). Relatively little data exists on the effects of UV irradiation on natural killer cells. A summary of the literature was provided by Norval and coworkers, who concluded that repeated UV exposure can lead to reduced natural killer cell activity and the number of active cells [51].

14.5 COMPARISON OF THE INVOLVEMENT OF UVA AND UVB IN PHOTOIMMUNOSUPPRESSION

Historically, most studies sought to investigate the immunosuppressive effects of UVB radiation—presumably due to the erythema action spectrum, which has a large distribution peak centered on the UVB region of the electromagnetic spectrum. Therefore, throughout most of the text when we refer to UV, we are in fact referring to UVB. In recent years, there has been an accumulation of studies investigating the effects of UVA-induced immunosuppression, which have been reviewed by Halliday and Rana [22]. As noted previously, the UVB portion of the electromagnetic spectrum falls between 290 and 320 nm and accounts for 5% of terrestrial UV radiation while UVA is light falling in the range of 320–400 nm and comprising 95% of UV radiation reaching Earth's surface. These relative contributions, of course, depend on the time of the day, latitude, season, and atmospheric conditions [22].

From a review of the literature, some general conclusions could be drawn with respect to UVA-induced immunosuppression. Both UVA and UVB impact various aspects of the immune system: primary, memory, local, and systemic. Furthermore, CHS and DTH are suppressed by UVA and UVB. Moreover, Halliday and Rana provide a systematic analysis of immunosuppression as a function of dose dependency of UVA and UVB radiation [22]. UVB radiation, in a time frame of 40 min to 5 h, was found to provide a linear dose-dependent immunosuppression (0.5–4 MED). Similar MED values of UVA radiation were also found to be immunosuppressive; however, higher doses of UVA radiation were not found to suppress immune function unless it was combined with UVB light. Using solar simulated light (UVA + UVB), it was concluded that under normal exposure conditions, UVA and UVB function synergistically and are immunosuppressive. The synergy is provided by the findings that the combined UVA and UVB are more immunosuppressive than either waveband alone. It is still unknown which chromophore is responsible for UVA-induced immunosuppression; however, it is postulated that a free radical mechanism may be the culprit. The signaling mechanisms, more than likely, are extremely complex and will require a significant amount of further research. It is important to note that both UVA and UVB affect Langerhans cell function, activate T regulatory cells, and inhibit effector and memory T cells. The reader is advised that the information in this section was garnered from a recent review by Halliday and Rana [22].

14.6 DELAYED TYPE HYPERSENSITIVITY AND CONTACT HYPERSENSITIVITY MODELS TO MONITOR PHOTOIMMUNOSUPPRESSION

During its course of action, the immune system can often become sensitized to a particular antigen, allergen, or pathogen. As a result of sensitization, any future encounter with the foreign substance will cause an exaggerated immune response even if it is a small quantity of the foreign body. Such responses are known as hypersensitivity reactions and may result in erythema, edema, and induration (hardening) of the skin. There are four classes of hypersensitivity reactions denoted as type I, II, III, and IV. Types I–III are mediated by antibodies (immunoglobins) and the reaction occurs immediately after exposure to antigen. In contrast, type IV reactions, commonly referred to as DTH reactions, are mediated by T cells (cell-mediated immunity) rather than by antibodies, and as the name indicates, the response usually does not appear right away—normally 48–72 h after exposure to antigen. Our interest in DTH stems from its utilization as a technique to monitor photoimmuno-suppression. The first phase of the technique is an induction phase in which the antigen (viral or bacterial) is injected intradermally into skin. Later (at least several days), skin is exposed to UV irradiation followed by another treatment with the antigen (elicitation phase). The subsequent antigen treatment should elicit an immune response unless, of course, UV-induced immunosuppression has occurred. A normal functioning immune system will cause DTH to occur when the skin is exposed to certain antigens. Clinically, DTH is often used as a test to determine if a patient has been previously exposed to an antigen. The antigen is injected into the skin and if DTH occurs, this indicates there is an immune recall response, which is antigen specific. The entire process is initiated and mediated by T cells (CD4$^+$ or CD8$^+$) [52]. DTH is typically assessed by subjective determination of whether or not an immune response is elicited. If the skin is first exposed to erythemal, or even suberythemal, doses of UV radiation, the immune system may not be capable of launching an attack, and DTH will not occur. This is a very unique way to monitor photoimmunosuppression. Almost all photoimmunological studies conducted on mice/humans utilize some type of DTH reaction. In summary, whether or not this reaction occurs tells us if the applied UV radiation suppresses the immune response.

The most common hypersensitivity model utilized to monitor photoimmunosuppression is CHS, which is a type IV reaction that falls under the umbrella of DTH. It is used extensively to monitor whether or not photoimmunosuppression takes place. Like other DTH reactions, it is mediated by T cells (CD4$^+$ or CD8$^+$) and requires the following sequence to take place in order for a reaction to occur: sensitization, trafficking, and elicitation [52]. The first phase, sensitization, occurs when a hapten is applied to naïve skin. (Haptens are chemical compounds, such as dinitrochlorobenzene or nickel, which produce CHS in skin.) The hapten penetrates and covalently binds with either membrane-bound or extracellular proteins. The protein–hapten complex may be taken up by APC, which then presents the complex to T cells. During later exposure to the hapten (after sensitization), the elicitation phase takes place in which the protein–hapten complex is presented by APC to memory T cells. As is the case with DTH, CHS is suppressed by UV irradiation. Most likely, this process is thought to occur due to depletion of Langerhans cells (APC) by apoptosis [52]. However, there is also evidence that demonstrates the disruption of cytokine pathways secreted by both Langerhans cells and keratino-cytes and disruption in the expression of APC costimulatory molecules ([53,54]; Ullrich, 1998).

In conclusion, both DTH and CHS are models utilized to monitor the cell-mediated immune response. Upon treatment with pathogen, antigen or hapten is taken up by Langerhans cells that is then presented to T cells resulting in the initiation of a cell-mediated response. It should be noted, however, that recent studies indicate possible involvement of natural killer cells in CHS [55]. Much of the contents of this section were garnered from a review on DTH by C. Allen Black [52].

14.7 LOCAL VERSUS SYSTEMIC IMMUNOSUPPRESSION

Normally, when conducting immunosuppression-based experiments, and using animal models, a distinction is made between local and systemic immunosuppres-sion. At the beginning of the experiment, the subject is usually sensitized to an antigen/hapten prior to any exposure to UV irradiation, which is accomplished by treating the subject epicutaneously (sometimes transdermally) with the desired agent. At a later date, after sensitization to hapten, the subject is exposed to UV irradiation followed by a second hapten treatment. Since the subject was previously exposed (sensitized) to the agent, one would expect a pronounced CHS or DTH response upon subsequent exposure. The successive treatment and radiation pro-tocol can be classified as "local" or "systemic." Local refers to the case when the UV irradiation site on the skin is the same as the first and subsequent hapten treatment. Systemic, on the other hand, would represent the situation when UV irradiation and subsequent hapten treatment are administered at a distant site to the first hapten treatment. Therefore, if in either case a CHS or DTH response occurs, it would be classified as local or systemic immunosuppression. It is believed that in the case of local immunosuppression, UV irradiation impairs the function of Langerhans cells directly (antigen presenting capability), whereas in systemic immunosuppression, cytokines that can circulate in the blood stream act as mediators that can travel to distant sites and impair the immune response [4].

14.8 ANIMAL MODELS USED TO STUDY PHOTOIMMUNOSUPPRESSION

Murine models are used almost exclusively to monitor photoimmunosuppression. Studies have shown that similar mechanisms (e.g., DTH and CHS are suppressed by UVR) take place in humans and that the chromophore contributions to UV-induced immunosuppression and the damaging effects on dendritic cells are the same in mouse and man [23]. In a typical laboratory experiment, mice are sensitized to a hapten, exposed to photoirradiation (to induced photoimmunosuppression), followed by treatment with a sensitizing agent to see whether or not an immune response occurs. If an immune response occurs—reddening or swelling of the skin—the immune system is considered to be functioning normally. This type of evaluation is normally a clinical appraisal, rather than objective measurement, of the skin's state—making this portion of the experiment a more objective assessment could certainly enhance the test. Aside from what most studies report in their methods section, there are few guidelines (to this author's knowledge) in the literature on experimental procedures for conducting photoimmunosuppression. Some guidance is provided by Ullrich and Schmitt in a chapter dedicated to the experimental details for those who are new to or are already working in the field [56]. There is also a report that found differences when comparing hairless versus haired mice in their sunscreen efficacy against photoimmunosuppression [57]. Overall, more discussion on the choice of assay and debate on the overall experimental conditions would be a welcome addition to the literature.

14.9 CONCLUDING REMARKS

Almost four decades have passed since the genesis of the field of photoimmunology. Early on, it was recognized that photocarcinogenesis and photoimmunology are intimately interrelated. Since these early days, a considerable amount of research has elucidated many of the mechanisms that occur during UV-induced immunosuppression. Initial events include the absorption of light by chromophores—termed photoreceptors—such as DNA and *trans*-urocanic acid. Likewise, damage to membrane components, resulting in lipid peroxidation, may be a concurrent or disparate pathway. Regardless, both routes are believed to lead to the release of cytokines, first and foremost by keratinocytes and also by other resident skin cells (e.g., Langerhans cells), as well as migrating immune cells. The signaling molecules, which play the most prominent role in UV-induced immunosuppression, are IL-10, TNF-α, PAF, and PGE$_2$. Cytokines interact with T cells and determine whether an immune response will be cell mediated or humoral. Another critical event, which is impaired as result of UV exposure, is the ability of Langerhans cells to migrate from the skin to the draining lymph nodes where they normally carry out antigen presentation. Numerous studies have shown that the antigen-presenting function of Langerhans cells is diminished by UV irradiation in part both due to apoptosis and due to impairment of cell function. Since the 1970s, it has been known that T regulatory cells (formerly known as T suppressor cells) are chief participants in the cellular mechanisms responsible for UV-induced immunosuppression. As a rule, UV-induced immunosuppression can be divided into two classifications depending on whether it is local or systemic. The study of UV-induced immunosuppression is almost universally carried out utilizing murine models in combination with CHS. Strong evidence indicates that the murine models are accurate and predictive of events that occur in humans as a result of UV exposure.

ACKNOWLEDGMENTS

I wish to thank my good friend and colleague, Raymond B. Clark, for his encouragement to write this manuscript and for offering useful suggestions in regard to the text. Also, many thanks to Gopi Menon, who critically reviewed the text and throughout the last several years has helped me better understand skin biology. Recognition also goes to Timothy Gillece, a good friend and coworker who always offers indispensable advice. A great debt of gratitude is also in order for Silvia Mendiola Buj, my spouse and confidant, who sacrificed much of our time together so that I could embark on a journey into the realm of photoimmunosuppression. Finally, I would like to express my appreciation to the editors, Nava Dayan and Phil Wertz, for their confidence and invitation to write this chapter.

REFERENCES

1. Fichtelius KE, Lidén S, et al. The skin—a first level lymphoid organ? *Int. Arch. Allergy* 1971;41: 13–15.
2. Wayne Streilein J. Skin-associated lymphoid tissues (SALT): origins and functions. *J. Invest. Derm.* 1983;80 (6 Suppl.): 12s–16s.
3. Bos JD, Kapsenberg ML. The skin immune system (SIS): its cellular constituents and their interactions. *Immunol. Today* 1986;7:235–240.
4. Amerio P, Carbone A, et al. UV induced skin immunosuppression. *Antiinflamm. Antiallergy Agents Med. Chem.* 2009;8:3–13.
5. Kripke ML. Antigenicity of murine skin tumors induced by ultraviolet light. *J. Natl. Cancer Inst.* 1974;53:1333–1336.
6. Kripke ML, Fisher MS. Immunologic parameters of ultraviolet carcinogenesis. *J. Natl. Cancer Inst.* 1976;57:211–215.
7. Fisher MS, Kripke ML. Systemic alteration induced in mice by ultraviolet light irradiation and its relationship to ultraviolet carcinogenesis. *Proc. Natl. Acad. Sci. USA* 1977;74:1688–1692.
8. Fisher MS, Kripke ML. Further studies on the tumor-specific suppressor cells induced by ultraviolet radiation. *J. Immunol.* 1978;121:1139–1144.
9. Anderson RR, Parrish JA. The optics of human skin. *J. Invest. Derm.* 1981;77:13–19.
10. Young AR. Chromophores in human skin. *Phys. Med. Biol.* 1997;42:789–802.
11. Wondrak GT, Jacobson MK, et al. Endogenous UVA-photosensitizers: mediators of skin photodamage and novel targets for skin photoprotection. *Photochem. Photobiol. Sci.* 2006;5:215–237.
12. Soter NA. Sunburn and suntan: immediate manifestations of photodamage. In: Gilchrest BA,editor. *Photodamage.* Cambridge, MA: Blackwell Science, 1995; pp. 12–25.
13. Burbach GJ, Ansel JC, et al. Cytokines in the skin. In: Freinkel RK, Woodley DT,editors. *The Biology of the Skin.* New York: Parthenon, 2001.
14. Rich BE, Kupper TS. Cytokines: IL-20—a new effector in skin inflammation. *Curr. Biol.* 2001;11: R531–R534.
15. Ullrich SE. Sunlight and skin cancer: lessons from the immune system. *Mol. Carcinog.* 2007; 46: 629–633.
16. Hoehn NE, Marieb EN. *Human Anatomy and Physiology.* Menlo Park, CA: Benjamin Cummings, 2010.
17. Ouhtit A, Ananthaswamy HN. A model for UV-induction of skin cancer. *J. Biomed. Biotech.* 2001;1:5–6.
18. Noonan FP, DeFabo EC. Immunosuppression by ultraviolet B radiation: initiation by urocanic acid. *Immunol. Today* 1992;13(7):250–254.
19. Leitenberger J, Jacobe HT, et al. Photoimmunology—illuminating the immune system through photobiology. *Semin. Immunopathol.* 2007;29:65–70.
20. Vink AA, Roza L. Biological consequences of cyclobutane pyrimidine dimers. *J. Photochem. Photobiol. B: Biol.* 2001;65:101–104.

21. de Gruijl FR. UV-induced immunosuppression in the balance. *Photochem. Photobiol.* 2008;84:2–9.
22. Halliday GM, Rana S. Waveband and dose dependency of sunlight-induced immunomodulation and cellular changes. *Photochem. Photobiol.* 2008;84;35–46.
23. Norval M. The mechanisms and consequences of ultraviolet-induced immunosuppression. *Prog. Biophys. Mol. Biol.* 2006;92:108–118.
24. Shreedhar V, Giese T, et al. A cytokine cascade including prostaglandin E$_2$, IL-4, and IL-10 is responsible for UV-induced systemic immune suppression. *J. Immunol.* 1998;160:3783–3789.
25. Metz M, Maurer M. Mast cells: key effector cells in immune response. *Trends Immunol.* 2007;28: 234–241.
26. Tharp, MD. Skin mast cells. In: Freinkel RK, Woodley DT, editors. *The Biology of the Skin.* Pearl River: Parthenon, 2001; pp. 265–279.
27. Hart PH, Grimbaldeston MA, et al. A critical role for dermal mast cells in *cis*-urocanic acid-induced systemic suppression of contact hypersensitivity responses in mice. *Photochem. Photobiol.* 1999;70:807–812.
28. Hart PH, Grimbaldeston MA, et al. Mast cells in UV-B-induced immunosuppression. *J. Photochem. Photobiol. B: Biol.* 2000;55:81–87.
29. Byrne SN, Limón-Flores AY, et al. Mast cell migration from the skin to the draining lymph nodes upon UV-irradiation represents a key step in the induction of immune suppression. *J. Immunol.* 2008;180:4648–4655.
30. Gordon S. The macrophage: past, present and future. *Eur. J. Immunol.* 2007; *37* (Suppl. 1): S9–S17.
31. Hawk JL, Murphy GM, et al. The presence of neutrophils in human cutaneous ultraviolet-B inflammation. *Br. J. Dermatol.* 1988;118:27–30.
32. Lee PL, van Weelden H, et al. Neutrophil infiltration in normal human skin after exposure to different ultraviolet radiation sources. *Photochem. Photobiol.* 2008;84:1528–1534.
33. Rijken F, Kiekens RCM, et al. Skin-infiltrating neutrophils following exposure to solar-simulated radiation could play an important role in photoageing of human skin. *Br. J. Dermatol.* 2005;152: 321–328.
34. Rijken F, Kiekens RCM, et al. Pathophysiology of photoaging of human skin: focus on neutrophils. *Photochem. Photobiol. Sci.* 2006;5:184–189.
35. Fisher GJ, Datta SC, et al. Molecular basis of sun-induced premature skin ageing and retinoid antagonism. *Nature* 1996;379:335–339.
36. Fisher GJ, Wang ZQ, et al. Pathophysiology of premature skin aging induced by ultraviolet light. *N. Engl. J. Med.* 1997;337:1419–1428.
37. Quan T, Qin Z, et al. Matrix-degrading metalloproteinases in photoaging. *J. Invest. Derm. Symp. Proc.* 2009;14:20–24.
38. Rittié L, Fisher GJ. UV-light-induced signal cascades and skin aging. *Ageing Res. Rev.* 2002;1:705–720.
39. Romani N, Holzmann S, et al. Langerhans cells—dendritic cells of the epidermis. *APMIS* 2003;111:725–740.
40. Aubin F. Mechanisms involved in ultraviolet light-induced immunosuppression. *Eur. J. Dermatol.* 2003;13:515–523.
41. Schwarz T. Mechanisms of UV-induced immunosuppression. *Keio J. Med.* 2005;54:165–171.
42. Dvorak AM. Histamine content and secretion in basophils and mast cells. *Prog. Histochem. Cytochem.* 1998;33:169–320.
43. Krönauer C, Eberlein-König B, et al. Inhibition of histamine release of human basophils and mast cells *in vitro* by ultraviolet A (UVA) irradiation. *Inflamm. Res.* 2001;*50* (Suppl. 2): S44–S46.
44. Krönauer C, Eberlein-König B, et al. Influence of UVB, UVA and UVA1 irradiation on histamine release from human basophils and mast cells *in vitro* in the presence and absence of antioxidants. *Photochem. Photobiol.* 2003;77:531–534.
45. Monfrecola G, de Paulis A, et al. *In vitro* effects of ultraviolet A on histamine release from human basophils. *J. Eur. Acad. Dermatol. Venereol.* 2005;19:389–390.
46. Byrne SN, Halliday GM. B cells activated in lymph nodes in response to ultraviolet irradiation or by interleukin-10 inhibit dendritic cell induction of immunity. *J. Invest. Derm.* 2005;124:570–578.
47. Rana S, Byrne SN, et al. Ultraviolet B suppresses immunity by inhibiting effector and memory T cells. *Am. J. Pathol.* 2008;172:993–1004.

48. Jensen J. The involvement of antigen-presenting cells and suppressor cells in the ultraviolet radiation-induced inhibition of secondary cytotoxic T cell sensitization. *J. Immunol.* 1983;130:2071–2074.

49. Schwarz T. 25 years of UV-induced immunosuppression mediated by T cells—from disregarded T suppressor cells to highly respected regulatory T cells. *Photochem. Photobiol.* 2008;84:10–18.

50. Moodycliffe AM, Nghiem DX, et al. Immune suppression and skin cancer developments: regulation by NKT cells. *Nat. Immunol.* 2000;1:521–525.

51. Norval M, McLoone P, et al. The effect of chronic ultraviolet radiation on the human immune system. *Photochem. Photobiol.* 2008;84:19–28.

52. Allen Black C. Delayed type hypersensitivity: current theories with an historic perspective. *Derm. Online J.* 1999;5(1):7.

53. Cruz PD, Jr., Basic science answers to questions in clinical contact dermatitis. *Am. J. Contact Dermat.* 1996;7:47–52.

54. el-Ghorr AA, Norval M. The role of interleukin-4 in ultraviolet B light-induced immunosuppression. *Immunology* 1997;92:26–32.

55. Yokoyama WM. Contact hypersensitivity: not just T cells! *Nat. Immunol.* 2006;7:437–439.

56. Ullrich SE, Schmitt DA. Dissection of immunosuppressive effects of ultraviolet radiation. In: Nickoloff BJ,editor. *Melanoma Techniques and Protocols*, vol. 61 Totowa, NJ: Humana Press Inc., 2001; pp. 85–97.

57. Kim T-H, Ananthaswamy HN, et al. Advantages of using hairless mice versus haired mice to test sunscreen efficacy against photoimmune suppression. *Photochem. Photobiol.* 2003;78:37–42.

PART V

INNATE IMMUNITY MICROBIAL CHALLENGES

DERANGED ANTIMICROBIAL BARRIER IN ATOPIC DERMATITIS: ROLES OF SPHINGOSINE, HEXADECENOIC ACID, AND BETA-DEFENSIN-2

Genji Imokawa

School of Bioscience and Biotechnology, Tokyo University of Technology
Tokyo, Japan

15.1 INTRODUCTION

The stratum corneum of the skin of patients with atopic dermatitis (AD) is highly susceptible to colonization by various bacteria, including *Staphylococcus aureus*. Because, as described in Figure 15.1, the frequency of bacterial, especially of *S. aureus*, colonization, even in nonlesional skin of patients with AD, is significantly higher than that of other types of dermatitis [1,2], the defense system of the skin against bacterial invasion appears to be significantly disrupted in AD.

Little is known about the defense mechanisms involved, although a mechanism has been proposed for defense against bacteria for the increased incidence of *S. aureus* colonization in AD skin [3]. Thus, it has been suggested that the secretory form of IgA may play an essential role in the defense mechanism against *S. aureus* colonization as the first line of immunodefense both in the intestine and in the respiratory tract [3]. In another aspect, it has been speculated that the acidic pH existing in the normal stratum corneum plays an important role in protecting the skin from *S. aureus* colonization and that a disturbance leading to an alkaline pH results in vulnerability to increased bacterial colonization. However, such hypotheses are not based upon any substantial evidence as follows; although the reduction in IgA secretion through sweat in AD skin has been demonstrated, there is a lack of critical experiments to clarify the direct inhibitory effect of IgA isolated from AD patients or from healthy controls on *S. aureus* colonization. With respect to the change

Innate Immune System of Skin and Oral Mucosa: Properties and Impact in Pharmaceutics, Cosmetics, and Personal Care Products, First Edition. Nava Dayan and Philip W. Wertz.

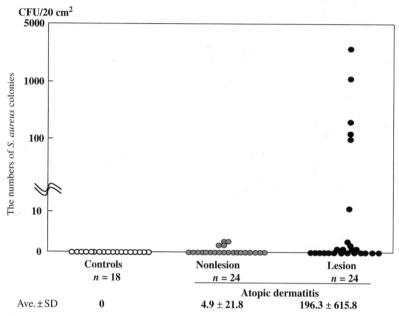

Figure 15.1 Comparison of the numbers of *S. aureus* colonies on the surface of the skin of healthy control subjects and patients with AD. The number of colonies were counted using the stamp technique and are expressed as the number per 20 cm². Control: healthy control subjects; NL: nonlesional skin of patients with AD; L: lesional skin of patients with AD.

toward an alkaline pH in AD skin [4], the change is not sufficient to allow bacteria to grow rapidly, showing only a slight change from an average pH of 5.0 in normal skin to an average pH of 5.5 in AD skin. Thus, collectively, it seems unlikely that a deficiency in IgA secretion or a slight alkalinization in AD skin is associated with increased frequency of *S. aureus* colonization. In contrast, although there is no direct evidence, the constitutive barrier disruption seen in the stratum corneum of patients with AD has been thought to be associated with their predisposition to *S. aureus* colonization.

An antimicrobial peptide, a skin fatty acid, and a sphingolipid metabolite— β-defensin-2 (BD-2) [5], *cis*-6-hexadecenoic acid (C16:1Δ6) [6], and sphingosine (SS) [7], respectively, which are present in abundance in the healthy stratum corneum—are known to exert an antimicrobial effect on *S. aureus* at physiological levels. Therefore, they may play a significant role in bacterial defense mechanisms of healthy normal skin and their abnormality may lead to deranged antimicrobial mechanisms in AD. In this chapter, to elucidate the mechanisms involved in *S. aureus* colonization in the AD stratum corneum, we evaluated the levels of these antimicrobial molecules in the upper stratum corneum from patients with AD and then compared those with the colonization levels of bacteria in the same subjects.

15.2 ROLE OF ONE OF THE SPHINGOLIPIDS: SPHINGOSINE

The general notion that the defective barrier function seen in the AD stratum corneum is indirectly linked to *S. aureus* colonization may lead to another important association between the sphingolipid metabolites and the defense mechanism against *S. aureus* colonization because the barrier disruption has been ascribed to decreased levels of ceramides [8] in the stratum corneum that appears to reflect possible altered sphingolipid metabolisms in the AD skin.

Such an altered sphingolipid metabolism in AD led us to assume that alterations in cellular levels of ceramide or its metabolite sphingosine may in part be involved in the vulnerability to *S. aureus* colonization. Indeed, one sphingolipid metabolite, sphingosine, but not ceramide, is well known to have potent antimicrobial effects on *S. aureus* at physiological levels [7,9]. Thus, it is conceivable that sphingosine may play a role, though not exclusively, in the bacterial defense mechanisms of healthy normal skin. It is therefore of particular interest to characterize the level of sphingosine in the stratum corneum of patients with AD. In this chapter, we have first evaluated the levels of sphingosine present in the upper stratum corneum of patients with AD and have compared that with the colonization levels of bacteria on the surface of the skin from the same subjects. The measurement of sphingosine (Figure 15.2) demonstrated that levels of sphingosine were significantly downregulated in uninvolved and in involved stratum corneum of patients with AD compared to healthy controls [2]. This decreased level of sphingosine was relevant to the increased numbers of bacteria including *S. aureus* present in the upper stratum corneum from the same subjects (Figure 15.3).

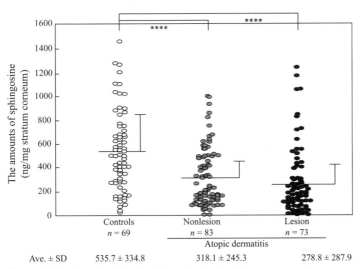

Figure 15.2   Quantitation of sphingosine levels in the upper stratum corneum of patients with AD or healthy controls. Sphingosine was quantified by radio-labeling with [^{14}C]-acetic anhydride, followed by separation using TLC. $****p < 0.001$.

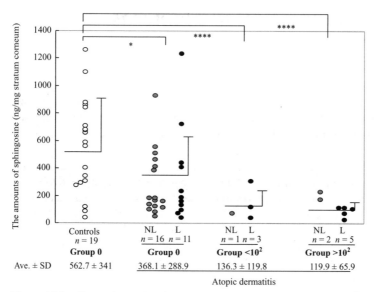

Figure 15.3 Comparison of sphingosine levels in AD groups according to different colony numbers of *S. aureus*. $^*p < 0.05$, $^{****}p < 0.001$.

This result suggests the possibility that the increased colonization of *S. aureus* found in patients with AD may result from a deficiency of sphingosine as a natural antimicrobial agent.

As sphingosine levels in the stratum corneum are believed to be exclusively regulated by at least two major factors, the hydrolysis of ceramide to sphingosine by ceramidases and the substrate pool for formation of sphingosine, namely, ceramide levels [10], it is also intriguing to evaluate ceramidase activity as a controlling factor for sphingosine levels in comparison with bacterial colonization and ceramide/sphingosine levels. Therefore, the activities of CDases in the upper stratum corneum were measured to compare with the colonization levels of bacteria and the sphingosine levels in the same subjects. Analysis of the activities of ceramidases, major sphingosine-producing enzymes, revealed that although the activity of alkaline ceramidase did not differ between patients with AD and healthy controls, the activity of acid ceramidase was significantly reduced in patients with AD and this had obvious relevance to the increased colonization of bacteria in those subjects (data not shown). Furthermore, there was a close correlation between the level of sphingosines and the acid ceramidase ($r = 0.65$, $p < 0.01$) (Figure 15.4) or ceramides ($r = 0.70$, $p < 0.01$) (Figure 15.5) in the upper stratum corneum from the same patients with AD.

Collectively, our results suggest the possibility that vulnerability to *S. aureus* colonization in the skin of patients with AD is associated with reduced levels of a natural antimicrobial agent, sphingosine, which results from decreased levels of ceramides as a substrate and from diminished activities of its metabolic enzyme, acid ceramidase.

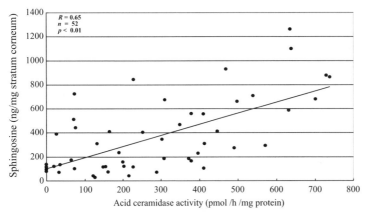

Figure 15.4   Correlation between levels of sphingosine and acid ceramidase activity in the upper stratum corneum. Lesional skin of AD patients: $n = 18$; nonlesional skin of AD patients: $n = 17$; healthy control skin: $n = 17$. Total $n = 52$, $r = 0.65$, $p < 0.01$.

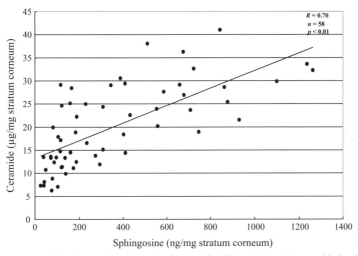

Figure 15.5   Correlation between levels of sphingosine and ceramide in the upper stratum corneum. Lesional skin of AD patients: $n = 19$; nonlesional skin of AD patients: $n = 20$; healthy control skin: $n = 19$. Total $n = 58$, $r = 0.70$, $p < 0.01$.

15.3   ROLE OF *CIS*-6-HEXADECENOIC ACID: ONE OF THE SEBACEOUS LIPIDS

It has been suggested that skin surface lipids (SSLs), the main source of which is the sebum secreted by sebaceous glands, contribute to the "self-sterilizing" properties of human skin [11,12]. In 1972, Aly et al. demonstrated that pathogenic microorganisms, such as *S. aureus* and *Streptococcus pyogenes*, increased their growth on the forearm skin following washing with acetone, which suggested the possible presence of antimicrobial substances in SSLs [12]. Since then, the nature of the antimicrobial species on the skin surface has been studied by many research groups. *cis*-6-Hexadecenoic acid (C16:1Δ6) [13] has been implicated as the most active antimicrobial lipid in SSLs. Because C16:1Δ6 is the most abundant fatty acid in SSLs [13] and is ubiquitous in human skin [14–16], it seems likely that it might play a specific role in innate defense mechanisms of healthy human skin against foreign bacteria such as *S. aureus*. However, little is known about the precise role of C16:1Δ6 in protection against the growth of *S. aureus* in healthy human skin because a selective depletion of C16:1Δ6 from sebum has not been experimentally attainable.

Because of the high susceptibility of AD skin to colonization by *S. aureus*, it would be intriguing to determine whether the content of free C16:1Δ6 in SSL and/or the composition of esterified fatty acids in sebum is significantly attenuated in AD skin compared to healthy control skin. In relation to this, Yamamoto et al. characterized the fatty acid composition of stratum corneum lipids of AD patients [17]. They reported that while there is a significant decrease in the C18:1 moiety of ceramide 1, the composition of other amide-linked or esterified fatty acids, including C16:1Δ6, in ceramide 1 or in wax esters, respectively, did not differ between AD and healthy controls [17] although there was no data available on the composition of fatty acids including C16:1Δ6 in the sebum of AD skin. We have characterized the composition of C16:1Δ6 both in sebum and in free fatty acids from AD skin and from healthy control skin, and compared the content of C16:1Δ6 with the colonization of *S. aureus* in AD skin.

Our study examined the role of C16:1Δ6, the major free fatty acid derived from the skin surface lipid in the colonization of *S. aureus* frequently seen in the skin of patients with AD. Because the major fatty acid in human SSL is C16:1Δ6 [14] and it has an active antimicrobial function [14], we first focused on the antimicrobial property of free C16:1Δ6. We hypothesized that free C16:1Δ6 plays a selective barrier function against the colonization of transient pathogens such as *S. aureus* on healthy human skin and that a deficiency in C16:1Δ6 may be responsible for the high susceptibility to *S. aureus* in AD skin. In support of our hypothesis, the antimicrobial analysis demonstrated that C16:1Δ6 has a preferential antimicrobial effect on *S. aureus* compared to *S. epidermidis*, one of the major residents in the normal skin flora (Figures 15.6). This effect of C16:1Δ6 on *S. aureus* was at a level similar to the other antimicrobials tested (Figure 15.6). While such a selective profile for bacterial species in the same genus (*Staphylococcus*) is unprecedented, this also implies that C16:1Δ6 has no detrimental effect on normal skin flora consisting mainly of *S. epidermis*, although it remains to be clarified how *S. epidermidis* is resistant to C16:1Δ6. This antimicrobial potential of C16:1Δ6 seems to support the hypothesis that healthy skin does not suffer from colonization by *S. aureus* due to the presence of free C16:1Δ6 on the surface at concentrations sufficient to exert its antimicrobial effect (log 5 reduction for 3 h at 100 ppm) on *S. aureus*. We estimate the concentration of free C16:Δ6 to average 2 μg/cm², nearly equal to 20,000 ppm in SSL assuming SSL to be 1 μm thick or 30,000 ppm and assuming the ratio of total free acids in SSL to be 25% [15].

This observed antimicrobial potential of C16:1Δ6 led us to determine whether the concentration of free C16:1Δ6 on the skin surface is downregulated in AD skin and is inversely correlated with the colonization by *S. aureus*. Thus, we hypothesized that the free fatty acid composition derived from sebum might be altered in AD skin, which

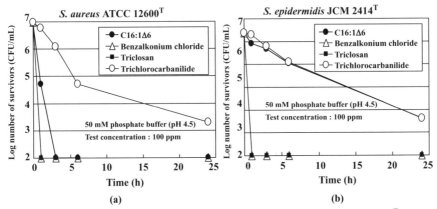

Figure 15.6   Comparison of antimicrobial effects against *S. aureus* ATCC 12600^T (a) and *S. epidermidis* JCM 2414^T (b). C16:1Δ6 or other antimicrobials at a final concentration of 100 mg/L in 50 mM phosphate buffer (pH 4.5) were compared.

would result in an insufficient level of the antimicrobial fatty acid, free C16:1Δ6, which would lead in turn to an abolished defense mechanism and a high susceptibility to colonization with *S aureus*. As expected, our analysis of the free fatty acid composition revealed that there is a significant decrease in free C16:1Δ6 on the skin surface of the majority of AD patients compared to healthy subjects (Figure 15.7).

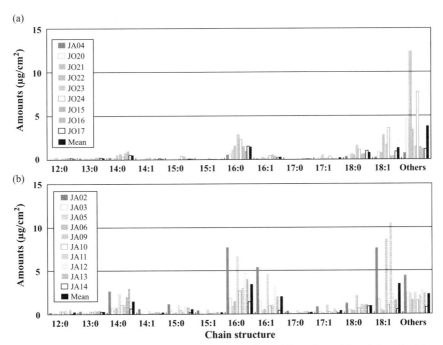

Figure 15.7   Amounts of free fatty acid in sebum from AD patients (a) and from healthy controls (b). Sebum was analyzed at the recovery level.

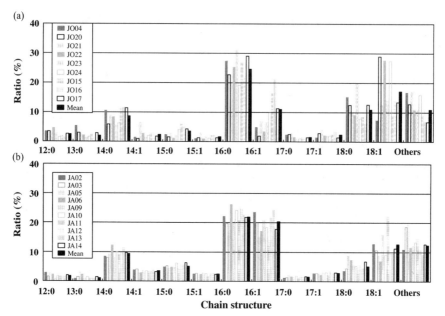

Figure 15.8   Ratios of total fatty acid in sebum from AD patients (a) and from healthy controls (b). Sebum was analyzed at the recovery level.

This decrease is also accompanied by a significant decrease in C16:1Δ6 in the total (free plus esterified) fatty acid composition of sebum (analyzed following hydrolysis) (Figure 15.8), which suggests that the decrease in free C16:1Δ6 can be ascribed to the decrease in C16:1Δ6 in the sebum. Regional differences in the concentration of C16:1Δ6 revealed that there is also a significant decrease in C16:1Δ6 at various body sites (e.g., the back) other than the region tested of AD patients. This suggests a systemic alteration in lipid metabolism in AD patients and is consistent with previous reports on the colonization of *S. aureus* not only in lesions but also in clinically normal (nonlesional) skin [18], and a significant decrease in ceramides [19] both in nonlesional skin and in lesional skin.

As for the metabolic mechanism(s) involved in the reduced content of free C16:1Δ6 in AD skin, it is interesting to note that Lan et al. [20] recently identified a Δ6 desaturase in human sebaceous glands that converts palmitate (C16:0) to C16:1Δ6. They speculated that the encoding gene was expressed in the environment of the sebaceous gland, but its expression was restricted in other organs. Based upon this evidence and the decreased content of C16:1Δ6 in AD sebum, it would be important to determine whether the expression of the Δ6 desaturase is significantly altered in AD skin. However, characterizing such enzymes in AD skin *in vivo* will present great challenges.

Comparison of free C16:1Δ6 levels with the colonization of *S. aureus* in AD patients reveals an inverse correlation between *S. aureus* colonization and levels of free C16:1Δ6 ($R^2 = 0.40998$, $p < 0.01$) (Figure 15.9), which implies that AD patients with lower levels of free C16:1Δ6 become susceptible to colonization by *S. aureus*.

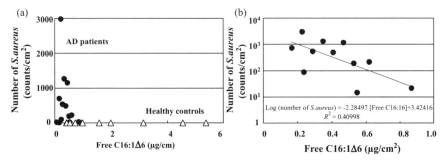

Figure 15.9   Relationship between free C16:1Δ6 and *S. aureus* in the skin. The amounts of free C16:1Δ6 in the sebum at the recovery level were analyzed, and colony counts for *S. aureus* were carried out by the "cup-scrub" method (16) at the adjacent area for collecting sebum for each volunteer. AD patients (●) and healthy controls (△).

It is, therefore, likely that free C16:1Δ6 plays a specific role in the antimicrobial barrier system through which healthy skin is defended against foreign microorganisms and that the observed deficiency of free C16:1Δ6 in AD skin triggers its susceptibility to colonization by *S. aureus*.

In order to strengthen the hypothesis for the role of C16:1Δ6 in *S. aureus* colonization, we determined whether supplementation of C16:1Δ6 to the skin of AD patients would lead to a reduced colonization by *S. aureus*. Through a pilot clinical trial using C16:1Δ6, we found that reduced numbers of colonies occurred in 75% (six out of eight) of AD patients tested, one of which was accompanied by a moderate improvement in clinical symptoms such as cutaneous inflammation (Figure 15.10). This clinical study reveals that the colonization by *S. aureus* seen frequently in AD skin is at least in part attributable to the deficiency in free C16:1Δ6, which is mainly derived from triglycerides via degradation by microbial lipases.

15.4   ROLE OF BETA-DEFENSIN-2: ANTIMICROBIAL PEPTIDE

Antimicrobial peptides such as defensins have recently been reported to serve key roles in host defense and in cutaneous innate immunity [21,22]. Consistently, human keratinocytes are stimulated to produce such antimicrobial peptides in response to bacteria, injury, or inflammatory stimuli [5,23,24]. Thus, it is plausible that if a significant alteration or deficiency of antimicrobial peptides occurs in the epidermis, which is the primary host defense system of the skin, skin diseases with a high vulnerability to infection by epidermidic bacteria, such as *S. aureus*, would develop. In this connection, Leung's group [25] recently reported that a deficiency in the expression of antimicrobial peptides may account for the susceptibility of patients with AD to skin infections with *S. aureus*. They based their observation on the evidence that the expression of β-defensin-2 is significantly downregulated in the AD epidermis at both the mRNA and the protein levels compared to psoriatic skin but not in healthy control skin. However, if one wishes to stress the role of antimicrobial peptides in the host defense mechanism against *S. aureus* infection, the situation in

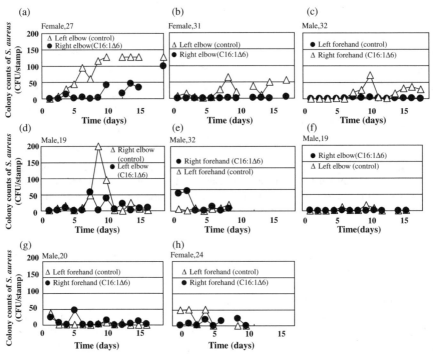

Figure 15.10   Time course of *S. aureus* counts during application of C16:1Δ6 lotion. Each volunteer applied the lotion with C16:1Δ6 to one side of the forearm and to the other side the lotion without C16:1Δ6. They were asked to apply the test lotion three times a day and to stamp with Food Stamp™ onto the region in order to detect *S. aureus* colonized on the skin once a day before bathing for 2 weeks of the test period.

healthy control skin, where there is no infection, should be compared with the skin of AD patients. A comparison between AD skin and psoriatic skin does not necessarily account for the host defensive role of antimicrobial peptides such as β-defensin-2 in the skin of healthy controls recognized as an uninfected site.

Although β-defensin-2 was reported to be downregulated at the mRNA and protein levels in the skin of AD patients compared to psoriatic patients but not healthy controls [25], little is known about its role in the colonization of *S. aureus* in the skin of AD patients. A precise evaluation of these peptides in the stratum corneum as an antimicrobial barrier against *S. aureus* colonization has not yet been performed, especially in comparison with healthy controls where no colonization of *S. aureus* exists. Since human β-defensin-2 peptides are localized in the Malpighian layer of the epidermis and/or in the stratum corneum [26] and are stored within lamellar bodies of keratinocytes in the spinous layer of the epidermis [27], it is likely that β-defensin-2 is primarily localized in intercellular lipid lamellar spaces of the stratum corneum. The antimicrobial functions of the stratum corneum play a key role in blocking the colonization of *S. aureus* in healthy skin. Therefore, a precise comparison of the level of β-defensin-2 with the colonization of *S. aureus* might provide a reasonable clue to the antimicrobial role of β-defensin-2 in the stratum corneum. Furthermore, previous studies were unable to precisely determine the levels of β-defensin-2 due to the nonspecific procedures used that consisted of direct immunoblotting or ion-exchange chromatography [28,29]. We developed a microanalytical technique to precisely measure β-defensin-2 in the stratum corneum using a combination of immunoprecipitation and Western blotting, and we used that method to compare β-defensin-2 levels in the skin of AD patients and healthy controls.

To determine whether the frequent colonization of bacteria on the skin of patients with AD is somehow related to the quantitative or qualitative alteration of the antimicrobial peptide, β-defensin-2, we measured levels of β-defensin-2 in the upper stratum corneum. Representative Western blots of stratum corneum extracts obtained from AD patients or from psoriasis patients are shown in Figure 15.11. Comparison of healthy control skin, nonlesional and lesional AD skin, and psoriatic skin revealed that the content of β-defensin-2 (expressed per μg stratum corneum protein) significantly increases in the lesional skin of AD patients and in psoriatic patients compared to that of the healthy controls (Figure 15.12). The content of β-defensin-2 in the lesional AD skin occurs at a significantly higher level than in the nonlesional skin. In contrast, there was no significant difference between healthy control skin and nonlesional AD skin (Figure 15.12).

To determine the distribution of β-defensin-2 through the stratum corneum layers, we measured levels of β-defensin-2 in 5 pools (each consisting of 3 successive

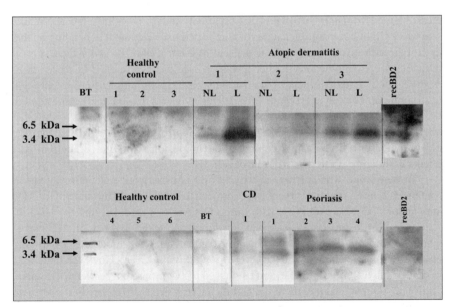

Figure 15.11   Immunoprecipitation/Western blotting of β-defensin-2 in the stratum corneum of patients with AD/psoriasis/contact dermatitis. BD2: β-defensin-2; CD: contact dermatitis; recBD2: recombinant BD2 (4.3 kDa); BT: blank tape; NL: nonlesion; L: lesion. Human β-defensin -2 was extracted from three tapes excluding the first strip with the extraction buffer. The extracts were subjected to immunoprecipitation followed by Western blotting in the text.

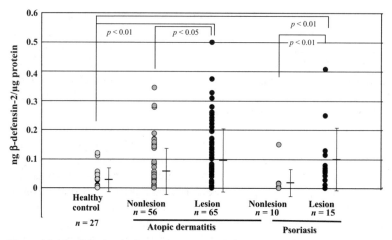

Figure 15.12 β-Defensin-2 content expressed per μg protein in the stratum corneum of AD/ psoriasis/healthy subjects. Each value represents the mean ± SD. Human β-defensin-2 was extracted from three tapes excluding the first strip with the extraction buffer. The extracts were subjected to immunoprecipitation followed by Western blotting as described in the text. β-Defensin-2 content was determined using the standard curve and expressed per μg protein after quantitation of stratum corneum protein.

tape strips through the stratum corneum layers, a total of 15 layers, excluding the first layer) obtained from uninvolved skin of AD patients and from healthy controls. While there was a slight but insignificant increase in β-defensin-2 content depending on the depth of the stratum corneum layers in the healthy control skin, the nonlesional skin of AD patients had significantly higher levels of β-defensin-2 in each of three strips (except for pool 4) than the healthy control skin with no substantial difference through the stratum corneum layers (Figure 15.13). This indicates that there is no substantial difference in the depth-dependent distribution of β-defensin-2 content within the stratum corneum layers of AD skin and of healthy control skin and strongly suggests a distinct increase in β-defensin-2 content in the nonlesional stratum corneum of AD patients compared to the healthy control skin.

To determine whether the severity of AD is associated with the content of β-defensin-2 in the stratum corneum, we compared its levels with the severity of AD. Comparisons between AD skins with different severities revealed that the level of β-defensin-2 in lesional skin increases in proportion to the severity of AD with a significant difference between the healthy controls and the moderate group and between the healthy controls and the severe group (Figure 15.14). However, there was no significant difference in the nonlesional skin. Comparison between the same severity of AD revealed that there is a significant or a slight difference in the level of β-defensin-2 between the lesional and the nonlesional skin in the moderate or the severe AD groups. This suggests that the disease severity predominantly triggers the defense mechanism by stimulating the production of β-defensin-2 in the epidermis.

Since the increased level of β-defensin-2 in the stratum corneum is associated with inflammation and/or the disease severity, it is plausible that the production of

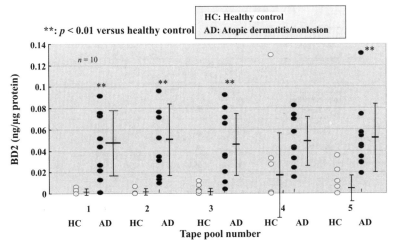

Figure 15.13   Distribution of β-defensin-2 through the stratum corneum layers of nonlesional AD skin and of healthy control skin. Each value represents the mean ± SD. BD2: β-defensin-2; Pool 1: $p = 0.0013$ between AD and healthy control; Pool 2: $p = 0.0015$; Pool 3: $p = 0.0020$; Pool 4: $p = 0.0553$; Pool 5: $p = 0.0018$. Numbers 1–5 represent each of the 5 tape pools that consist of 3 successive tape strips through the stratum corneum layers, a total of 15 strips, excluding the first strip.

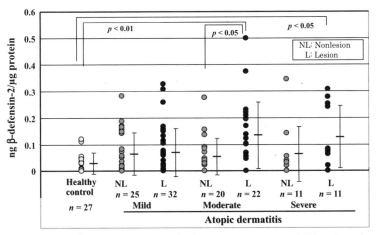

Figure 15.14   β-Defensin-2 content in the stratum corneum of AD patients in relation to AD severity. Each value represents the mean ± SD. The severity of AD was evaluated by the criteria reported by Rajka et al. and was classified into mild, moderate, or severe.

β-defensin-2 is primarily triggered by the colonization of *S. aureus* to be secondarily stimulated, rather than by an innate mechanism against *S. aureus*. When AD groups were classified according to different colony numbers, there was a weak correlation between increased levels of β-defensin-2 and increased numbers of *S. aureus* on the

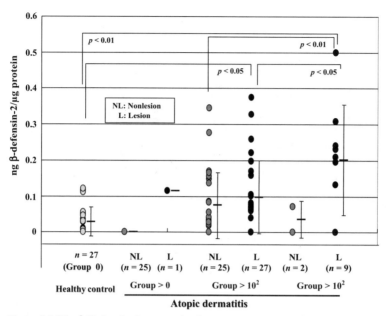

Figure 15.15 β-Defensin-2 content in the stratum corneum of AD patients in relation to *S. aureus* colonization. Each value represents the mean ± SD. Numbers of *S. aureus* colonies were counted, expressed as CFU per 20 cm², and were then classified into one of the following three groups: group 0: skin sites with no colonies; group <10²: skin sites with less than 100 colonies; or group >10²: skin sites with more than 100 colonies.

skin surface (Figure 15.15). Comparison of the increased colonization and the increased β-defensin-2 levels revealed a distinct correlation between these two parameters in both the lesional and the nonlesional skin (Figure 15.16a, $n = 67$, $r = 0.342$, $p = 0.004$) and only in the lesional skin (Figure 15.16b, $n = 38$, $r = 0.427$, $p = 0.006$) of the same AD patients. This close association of upregulated production of β-defensin-2 with increased colonization of the skin by *S. aureus*, which is significantly higher in the AD skin compared to healthy control skin, indicates the possibility that the colonization of AD skin by *S. aureus* directly triggers the increased level of β-defensin-2 because it is known that *S. aureus* itself induces the expression of human β-defensin [29]. In contrast to the report by Leung's group [25], which focused on the host defense mechanism against bacterial infection but not against colonization in AD skin, the observed abundance of β-defensin-2 in the present study may not account for the high incidence of *S. aureus* colonization seen on the AD skin. Therefore, the increased levels of β-defensin-2 and its relevance for increased colonization of AD skin suggests that β-defensin-2 does not play any significant role as an innate defense mechanism against the proliferation of *S. aureus* in the stratum corneum of healthy control skin.

Direct contact of cells with *S. aureus* or primary inflammatory cytokines such as interleukin-1 has been reported to stimulate the production of antimicrobial peptides, including β-defensin-2, via Toll-like receptors by various epithelial cells, including keratinocytes [30]. Beta-defensin-2 by itself induces IL-18 secretion through p38 and

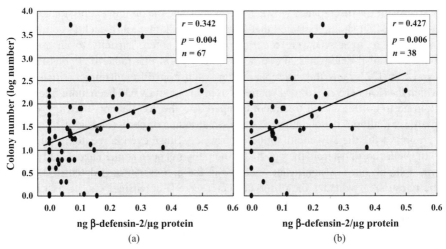

Figure 15.16   Relationship between β-defensin-2 content in the stratum corneum (three strips) of AD patients and *S. aureus* colonization. (a) Lesion + nonlesion; (b) lesion. Human β-defensin-2 was extracted from three tapes excluding the first strip with the extraction buffer. The extracts were subjected to immunoprecipitation followed by Western blotting as described in the text. β-Defensin-2 content was determined using the standard curve and expressed per µg protein after quantitation of stratum corneum protein as described in the text. Semiquantitation of *S. aureus* was carried out by the contact-plate method as described in the text. Numbers of colonies counted were expressed as CFU per $20\,cm^2$.

ERK MAPK activation in primary human keratinocytes [31]. Based on such evidence, a close positive correlation between the content of β-defensin-2 and the colonization of *S. aureus* in the upper stratum corneum, as observed in this study, suggests that the *S. aureus* colonization primarily occurs due to the lack of defense mechanisms other than a β-defensin-2 deficiency. It is likely that the *S. aureus* colonization itself results in the stimulation of β-defensin-2 production in living epidermal keratinocytes, which in turn reflects the increased content of β-defensin-2 in the stratum corneum. Analysis using RT-PCR has already revealed that although the expression level of mRNA encoding β-defensin-2 in the lesional skin of AD patients is significantly diminished compared to the skin of psoriasis patients, there is no significant difference in the faint levels of immunostaining between AD patients and healthy controls [25]. Our finding that the content of β-defensin-2 in the lesional stratum corneum of AD patients is significantly increased to a level similar to that of psoriatic skin compared to healthy control skin is not in agreement with Leungs' data [25] on the gene expression described above. In their study, the protein expression of β-defensin-2 was analyzed by immunohistochemistry or direct blotting using an antibody to β-defensin-2. Thus, their methods are not reliable for a precise detection of β-defensin-2. Therefore, there had been no precise way to determine the protein level of β-defensin-2 in AD skin. Our combined method using immunoprecipitation and Western blotting allows us to determine the precise protein level of β-defensin-2 in the stratum corneum for the first time.

As for the discrepancy between the mRNA and the protein expression levels of β-defensin-2, it should be noted that frequently available drugs, such as corticosteroids, used to treat AD were reported to have a potent capacity to enhance the expression of β-defensin-2 in contrast to cyclosporin that rather downregulates its expression [32]. Thus, this discrepancy may result from different clinical situations in which the skin derived from AD patients used in our study had been more frequently exposed to corticosteroid treatment compared to the AD patients used in Leung's study [25], although a quantitative study on amounts of corticosteroid used and the duration of the therapy could not be determined. Since even in the nonlesional AD skin, where corticosteroid therapy had principally not been applied in our study, there was a slight, but not significant, increase in the expression of β-defensin-2. Thus, the question of whether the observed increase in β-defensin-2 can be ascribed to corticosteroid treatment remains unresolved.

In summary, in the involved and uninvolved stratum corneum of AD patients, β-defensin-2 levels are not downregulated but are rather upregulated compared to healthy controls. Furthermore, *S. aureus* colonization is not inversely correlated with levels of β-defensin-2 in the involved stratum corneum of AD skin. These findings suggest that β-defensin-2 is induced in response to bacteria, injury, or inflammatory stimuli and is not associated with the vulnerability to *S. aureus* colonization in the skin of patients with AD.

REFERENCES

1. Akiyama H, Ueda M, Toi Y, Kanzaki H, Tada J, Arata J. Comparison of the severity of atopic dermatitis lesions and the density of *Staphylococcus aureus* on the lesions after antistaphylococcal treatment. *J. Infect. Chemother.* 1996;2:70.
2. Arikawa J, Ishibashi M, Kawashima M, et al. Decreased levels of sphingosine, a natural anti-microbial agent, may be associated with vulnerability of the stratum corneum from patients with atopic dermatitis to colonization by *Staphylococcus aureus*. *J. Invest. Dermatol.* 2002;119:433–439.
3. Imayama S, Shiimozono Y, Hoashi M, Hoashi M, Yasumoto S, Ohta S, Yoneyama K, Hori Y. Reduced secretion of IgA to skin surface of patients with atopic dermatitis. *J. Allergy Clin. Immunol.* 1994;94 (2Pt 1): 195–200.
4. Imokawa G. Skin moisturizers: development and clinical use of ceramides. In: M. Loden,editor. *Dry Skin and Moisturizers*, 1999. CRC Press. pp. 269–299.
5. Harder J, Bartels J, Christophers E, et al. A peptide antibiotic from human skin [letter]. *Nature* 1997;387:861.
6. Takigawa H, Nakagawa H, Kuzukawa M, Mori H, Imokawa G. Deficient production of hesadecenoic acid in the skin is associated in part with the vulnerability of atopic dermatitis patients to colonization by *Staphylococcus aureus*. *Dermatology* 2005;211(3):240–248.
7. Bibel DJ, Raza A, Shinefield HR. Antimicrobial activity of sphingosines. *J. Invest. Dermatol.* 1992;98: 269–268.
8. Imokawa G, Abe A, Jin K, Higaki Y, Kawashima M, Hidano A. Decreased level of ceramides in stratum corneum of atopic dermatitis: an etiologic factor in atopic dry skin? *J. Invest. Dermatol.* 1991;96: 523–526.
9. Bibel DJ, Aly RA, Shah S, Shinefield HR. Sphingosines: antimicrobial barriers of the skin. *Acta Derm. Venereol. (Stockh.)* 1993;73:407–411.
10. Hara J, Higuchi K, Okamoto R, Kawashima M, Imokawa G. High-expression of sphingomyelin deacylase is an important determinant of ceramide deficiency leading to barrier disruption in atopic dermatitis. *J. Invest. Dermatol.* 2000;115(3):406–413.

11. Ricketts CR, Squire JR, Topley E. Human skin lipids with particular reference to the self-sterilizing powder of the skin. *Clin. Sci.* 1951;10:89.

12. Aly R, Maibach HI, Shinefield HR, Strauss WG. Survival of pathogenic microorganisms on human skin. *J. Invest. Dermatol.* 1972;58:205–210.

13. Wille JJ, Drake D, Wertz PW. Identification of *cis*-palmitoleic acid as the active antimicrobial in human skin sebum. *J. Invest. Dermatol.* 1997;108:677.

14. Nicolaides N, Fu HC, Ansari MNA, Rice GR. The fatty acids of wax esters and sterol esters from vernix caseosa and from human skin surface lipid. *Lipids* 1972;7:506–517.

15. Nicolaides N. Skin lipids: their biochemical uniqueness. *Science* 1974;186:19–26.

16. Randall W, Lee T. Occurrence of unusual hexadecenoate fatty acid in hepatoma lipids. *Lipids* 1980;15:876–879.

17. Yamamoto A, Serizawa S, Ito M, Sato Y. Stratum corneum lipid abnormalities in atopic dermatitis. *Arch. Dermatol. Res.* 1991;283:219–223.

18. Leyden JJ, Marples RR, Kligman AM. *Staphylococcus aureus* in the lesions of atopic dermatitis. *Brit. J. Dermat.* 1974;90:525–530.

19. Imokawa G, Abe A, Jin K. Decreased level of ceramide in stratum corneum of atopic dermatitis: an etiologic factor in atopic dry skin? *J. Invest. Dermatol.* 1991;96:523–526.

20. Lan Ge, Gordon JS, Hsuan C, Stenn K, Prouty SM. Identification of the Δ-6 desaturase of human sebaceous glands: expression and enzyme activity. *J. Invest. Dermatol.* 2003;120:707–714.

21. Yang D, Chetrov O, Bykovskaia SN, et al. Beta-defensins: linking innate and adaptive immunity through dendritic and T cell CCR6. *Science* 1999;286:525–528.

22. Huttner KM, Bevins CL. Antimicrobial peptides as mediators of epithelial host defence. *Pediatr. Res.* 1999;45:785–7894.

23. Frohm Nilsson M, Sandstedt B, Sorensen O, et al. The human cationic antimicrobial protein (hCAP18), a peptide antibiotic, is widely expressed in human squamous epithelia and colocalizes with interleukin-6. *Infect. Immun.* 1999;67:2561–2566.

24. Frohm M, Agerbath B, Ahangari G, et al. The expression of the gene encoding for the antibacterial peptide LL-37 is induced in human keratinocytes during inflammatory disorders. *J. Biol. Chem.* 1997;272:15258–15263.

25. Ong PY, Ohtake T, Brandt C, et al. Endogenous antimicrobial peptides and skin infections in atopic dermatitis. *N. Engl. J. Med.* 2002;347:1151–1160.

26. Ali RS, Falconer A, Ikram M, et al. Expression of the peptide antibiotics human beta defensin-1 and human beta defensin-2 in normal human skin. *J. Invest. Dermatol.* 2001;117:106–111.

27. Oren A, Ganz T, Liu L, et al. In human epidermis, beta-defensin 2 is packed in lamellar bodies. *Invest. Ophthalmol. Vis. Sci.* 2003;44:1859–1865.

28. Huh WK, Oono T, Shirafuji Y, et al. Dynamic alteration of human beta-defensin 2 localization from cytoplasm to intercellular space in psoriatic skin. *J. Mol. Med.* 2002;80:678–684.

29. Dinulos JG, Mentele L, Fredericks LP, et al. Keratinocyte expression of human beta-defensin 2 following bacterial infection: role in cutaneous host defense. *Clin. Diagn. Lab. Immunol.* 2003;10:161–166.

30. Lui AY, Destoumieux D, Wong AV, et al. Human beta-defensin-2 production in keratinocytes is regulated by interleukin-1, bacteria, and the state of differentiation. *J. Invest. Dermatol.* 2002;118:275–281.

31. Niyonsaba F, Ushio H, Nagaoka I, et al. The human beta-defensins (-1, -2, -3, -4) and cathelicidin LL-37 induce IL-18 secretion through p38 and ERK MAPK activation in primary human keratinocytes. *J. Immunol.* 2005;175:1776–1784.

32. Terai K, Sano Y, Kawasaki S, et al. Effects of dexamethasone and cyclosporin A on human beta-defensin in corneal epithelial cells. *Exp. Eye Res.* 2004;79:175–180.

CHAPTER 16

RESIDENT MICROFLORA OF THE SKIN AND ORAL MUCOSA

David R. Drake

Dows Institute for Dental Research, University of Iowa, Iowa City, IA

16.1 INTRODUCTION

It is well known that the surfaces of the human body are colonized by a large number of bacteria. It is compelling that there are more bacteria than host cells, which for many creates an interesting picture. We are host to a very complex, dynamic microflora that is, for the most part, in a state of shared beneficence. This homeostasis can be perturbed by many external and environmental factors, which can lead to normally benign organisms causing disease in the human host—the appropriately named opportunistic pathogens. What are these bacteria? What are considered normal microflora on the skin surface and the oral mucosa? Are these microflora more similar in number and composition than different? This chapter explores what we know about the normal flora of these two important surfaces of the human body and how our new molecular biology approaches are providing a fascinating look at the complex bacterial world that grows and colonizes our surfaces.

16.2 MICROFLORA OF THE SKIN

The microflora on the skin can be roughly divided into two major groups: the "normal" flora colonizing the skin that is in homeostasis and transient flora that may initially establish themselves on the skin, but do not become permanent colonizers [1,2]. This characterization is common for all flora in the human body, but perhaps nowhere more prominently than the skin, being an outer surface in constant contact with the environment. There is a third group that some have characterized apart from the transient group or as a subset of this group and it includes organisms that colonize some individuals for periods of time longer than most transients. This group of organisms has been called "associate flora" because of apparent dependence on other, well-established flora for their longer survival and colonization. It is not clear how this varies across different populations, age groups, ethnicity, gender, and so on.

Innate Immune System of Skin and Oral Mucosa: Properties and Impact in Pharmaceutics, Cosmetics, and Personal Care Products, First Edition. Nava Dayan and Philip W. Wertz.

Some would see individuals with this group of organisms to be classified as "carriers," a status to imply that not all people would have this organism on their skin surfaces [1,3].

Apart from classifying organisms on the basis of their permanence versus transience, the flora of the skin can be classified into three major groups of organisms: (a) the coryneforms, (b) the micrococci, and (c) the yeasts [1,2,4,5]. The coryneforms are sometimes referred to as the "diphtheroids" because of the resemblance of these club-shaped bacteria to *Corynebacterium diphtheriae*. These organisms are Gram positive and exhibit a spectrum of atmospheric requirements from being aerobic to aerotolerant to anaerobic. An additional subdivision that has been used for the coryneforms is on the basis of their being lipophilic or nonlipophilic. Bacteria in the lipophilic group are commonly found in the more moist areas of the human body, and are represented by the species *C. jeikeium*, *C. striatum*, and *C. bovis*. A very prominent member of what used to be called the anaerobic diphtheroids is *Propionibacterium acnes*. This organism has been strongly associated with the development of acne in puberty and has been extensively studied [2,6]. A recent study using real-time PCR showed that people with hair follicles containing *P. acnes* are not at more risk for acne development, except for young teenagers [7].

The two major species within the micrococci group are *Staphylococcus aureus* and *S. epidermidis*. The latter comprises approximately 90% of the normal flora on some parts of the skin. While part of the normal flora, these species have been implicated in skin diseases and are potent opportunistic pathogens. More will be discussed in later sections as to their involvement in skin diseases and other infections in the body.

16.3   THE STAPHYLOCOCCI AND STREPTOCOCCI: PROMINENT OPPORTUNISTIC PATHOGENS

These two genera are common inhabitants of the skin and, depending on the site of the body, normally dominate the microflora. While considered as part of the normal flora of the skin in general, certain species within these genera are bold and successful opportunistic pathogens and have been implicated in a myriad list of diseases, from meningitis, necrotizing skin infections, to food poisoning [1,2,5]. Organisms within these genera have an array of virulence factors that allow them to compete and readily establish themselves as part of the permanent flora of the skin, and actively combat and evade host defense mechanisms. Two prominent species that have achieved considerable notoriety are *S. aureus* and *S. epidermidis*.

16.4   *STAPHYLOCOCCUS EPIDERMIDIS*

This organism is considered as a part of the normal skin flora and, in some cases, can comprise up to 90% of the cultivable flora [1,2,8]. They are sometimes referred to as the coagulase-negative staphylococci. While seemingly innocuous, it has been implicated in several infections of the skin and other parts of the body as a very successful opportunist. It accounts for most of nosocomial infections, particularly involving indwelling medical devices. However, in immunocompetent individuals, these infections are more low grade and chronic as this organism does not produce the wide array of virulence factors that the more pathogenic *S. aureus* does. It is a different story for immunocompromised individuals as these organisms can develop into severely life-threatening infections. This is exacerbated by the fact that these organisms are highly resistant to antibiotics and form biofilms relentlessly on surfaces of medical devices [9].

The emerging picture is of an organism that dominates the normal skin flora but is incredibly versatile in responding to its environment. Recent molecular analyses have revealed an organism that readily generates multiple phenotypic and genotypic variants [10]. The former occurs in rapid response to changing environments, with different phenotypes that exhibit the ability to form tenacious biofilms rapidly and resist host innate immune factors. Multilocus sequencing has shown that *S. epidermidis* readily acquires mobile genetic elements and therefore evolves easily and rapidly through recombination. A distinct set of genotypes has been identified in hospital settings worldwide that carry various gene cassettes that confer methicillin resistance and pronounced biofilm formation [10]. A key finding is how versatile these organisms are in changing expression of an array of virulence genes even within a course of infection. This ability to change and adapt so quickly has led to this organism becoming a serious opportunistic infection in hospitals and one exceedingly difficult to treat. A recent study has also found that *S. epidermidis* that produces the serine protease Esp inhibits biofilm formation and nasal colonization by *S. aureus* [11]. If one finds this particular subset of *S. epidermidis*, a striking absence of *S. aureus* in the nasal cavity will also be found. A novel mechanism of growth inhibition and rendering biofilms of *S. aureus* more susceptible to innate immune components occurs [11].

16.5   *STAPHYLOCOCCUS AUREUS*

While not as prevalent and not considered as a dominant member of the normal skin flora, this organism can be found mainly in the nose and perineum of individuals, ranging from 10% to 40% of subject carriage [1,2,12]. It appears to be found more readily in infants than adults. It is readily found on the skin of subjects that have atopic dermatitis with carriage ranging from 80% to 100%. This species has a large array of virulence factors that also allow it to be a successful opportunistic pathogen and in most cases it is considered more pathogenic than *S. epidermidis*. It has been implicated in infections ranging from localized abscesses to impetigo to scalded skin syndrome. While not exhibiting the same level of biofilm forming ability as its cousin, *S. epidermidis*, there too have been reports of high resistance to antibiotics in hospital settings [13–15]. In a current study looking at the potential importance of colonization sites in children, it was found that children that experience serious skin abscesses caused by methicillin-resistant and -sensitive *S. aureus* had nasal and rectal colonization rates of these organisms significantly higher than control children [12]. However, the key site appears to be rectal colonization as community-associated staphylococcal diseases are strongly associated with carriage at this site.

One of the greatest dangers occurring today in terms of life-threatening skin infections are infections caused by methicillin-resistant *S. aureus* (MRSA) [13–15]. These multidrug-resistant strains are highly aggressive colonizers, able to compete with normal skin flora, and cause significant morbidity and mortality in subjects. There are two major groups: (a) hospital-acquired MRSA (HA-MRSA) and (b) community-acquired MRSA (CA-MRSA). The former group establishes itself in hospitals worldwide and in the midst of high levels of antimicrobial usage. CA-MRSA is a rapidly growing problem in the United States and many countries around the world. The reader is referred to a recent, comprehensive review of CA-MRSA for a more in-depth analysis of this very troubling threat [15]. HA-MRSA has been known and extensively studied with untold hundreds to thousands of references readily available. There have been several worldwide and regional distinctive genotypes of *S. aureus* identified that differ in toxin, colonization factors, and antibiotic resistance profiles [4,13]. These organisms comprise some of the most serious nosocomial pathogens and are the scourge of hospital-acquired infections.

CA-MRSA normally occurs in healthy children and young athletes, with many stories of infections spreading within locker rooms. These organisms spread readily within families and any group where close contact can occur. There have been reports that infection "cores" can occur in public transportation and reinfection following treatment can readily occur. Therefore, there is strong consensus that considerable effort on the part of public health officials be employed to actively determine the location of infection cores for elimination. It has also been reported that CA-MRSA infections appear to heighten in influenza season. Finally, there is a particularly virulent genotype that originated in the United States (USA300) and is growing not only as a CA-MRSA but also as a HA-MRSA worldwide. CA-MRSA is a serious threat that is drawing attention from clinicians and researchers around the world to design active surveillance and rapid community response to infection cores [15].

16.6   MICROFLORA OF THE ORAL MUCOSA

Most of what we know about the microflora in the human mouth has come as a result of studies on polymicrobial biofilms on the teeth, both supragingival and sub-gingival communities of organisms. However, approximately 80% of the surface area of the human mouth is not hard tissue but rather keratinized and nonkeratinized soft tissues. What type of microorganisms do we find on these surfaces? When and how do we acquire these organisms? This section focuses on the spectrum of organisms we find on oral soft tissues and their role as commensals and sometimes opportunistic pathogens.

The microflora of the oral cavity in humans is exceedingly varied and complex, with different surfaces available for colonization [16–18]. Children acquire organisms soon after birth, with the majority of initial colonizers coming from their mothers in repeated vertical transmission events [16,19–24]. It is well known that oral bacteria exhibit considerable tropisms toward different surfaces in the oral cavity [16,25]. Thus, bacteria that possess specific adhesins for antigens found in the acquired pellicle on teeth will demonstrate a predilection for colonizing tooth surfaces. Likewise, organisms with the ability to adhere to surface antigens found on the dorsum of the tongue or oral mucosa will be found in higher numbers and perhaps dominate the microbial communities at these sites. There are many environmental and host factors that affect the establishment of bacterial biofilms on surfaces of the oral cavity, but it is readily apparent that differences in profiles of bacteria at different sites are initially governed strongly by the specific bacterial adhesion mechanisms [16].

In a study conducted by Mager et al. at Forsyth, it was found that bacterial profiles differed considerably from site to site, and also from person to person [26]. Using a checkerboard DNA–DNA hybridization approach, they looked at 40 different species. Differences were marked across the different sites in the oral cavity. Proportions of *Veillonella parvula* and *Prevotella melaninogenica* were higher on the dorsum of the tongue and in saliva. In contrast, *Streptococcus mitis* and *S. oralis* were found in significantly lower proportions on the dorsal surface of the tongue and in saliva. Comprehensive analyses of the data revealed different cluster groups of organisms that differed amongst the sites. Not only did different species of different genera show differences within these clusters, but species within a genus, such as *Streptococcus*, also differed considerably. Adding to the complexity of defining microbial profiles on various oral surfaces was the finding that these clusters differed remarkably across subjects. Major conclusions from this investigation were that the microflora found in saliva was highly similar to the microbiota found on dorsal and lateral surfaces of the tongue, and microbial profiles of oral soft tissues were more similar than those from both supragingival and subgingival plaque colonizing tooth surfaces [26].

The microflora found on the tongue has always been of interest as it is generally thought of as a reservoir of organisms that can reinfect treated subgingival tissues. In addition, halitosis is commonly associated with certain organisms found on the dorsal surface of the tongue that produce volatile sulfur compounds. An interesting investigation using molecular biology techniques to define the flora of the tongue in healthy subjects versus those with pronounced halitosis revealed a distinctively different flora associated with halitosis [27]. Microorganisms mostly associated with health include *Streptococcus salivarius*, *Rothia mucilaginosa*, and an uncharacterized *Eubacterium* species. *S. salivarius* was the dominant species, comprising up to 40% of the total clones analyzed from all healthy subjects in the study. Bacteria associated with halitosis were *Atopobium parvulum*, a specific *Dialister* phylotype, some uncharacterized streptococci, and *Solobacterium moorei*. A further important observation was that *S. salivarius*, a normally dominant species in health, was absent from the dorsum of the tongue in subjects with halitosis [27].

A comprehensive analysis of the normal bacterial flora of the oral cavity using molecular techniques revealed a fascinating glimpse of the complexity of the flora in this part of the human body [16]. More than 700 bacterial species of phylotypes have been identified, and there is growing evidence that this number will continue to increase as additional analyses are conducted. Over 60% of the bacterial flora is still represented by organisms that we cannot culture. The importance of this cannot be understated as essentially all of our analyses of organisms associated with major oral diseases are based on cultivable flora. No evidence exists indicating the lesser importance of the uncultivable components of the microbial communities.

A look at the complex profiles generated in this study shows the following general conclusions. First, there is a distinct flora associated with health. Second, there is considerable specificity at different sites in the oral cavity. These findings are in agreement with the previous comprehensive study reviewed here. Organisms dominating the flora of the hard palate include several streptococci species, particularly *S. mitis*, *Granulicatella elegans*, *G. haemolysans*, and *Neisseria subflava*. *S. mitis* dominated the soft palate, along with other cultivable streptococci, *G. adiacens*, and *G. haemolysans*. The most prominent groups of organisms found across all sites were species from the *Gemella*, *Streptococcus*, and *Veillonella*. But again, there were distinct microbial profiles/clusters at each site and these varied from person to person. But the trends were distinct—significant bacterial community profiles at various sites within the oral cavity [16].

16.7 SUMMARY

The normal flora of the skin and oral mucosa are distinctly different, yet there are similarities in how the microbial communities change in the face of environmental pressures. There are noteworthy opportunistic pathogens that reside on the skin, with one organism that for many years was considered to be benign—*S. epidermidis*. It is now a prominent opportunist that forms tenacious biofilms on indwelling medical devices and is exceedingly difficult to treat. Similarly, *S. aureus* has gained exceptional notoriety as a horrendous pathogen, the methicillin-resistant organisms that have become the scourge of hospitals, and now community-acquired outbreaks are growing and this threat will test our resolve to treat organisms that once were thought relatively easy to treat in the early penicillin days.

While our knowledge about the flora of the skin seems to be constant, with few major advances as to our understanding of this important flora, the exploration and definition of the oral flora is gaining by leaps and bounds. This is an exciting area of research, and with the increasing links of the oral flora with systemic health, there is little doubt that some great discoveries are pending on the very complex microbial communities that make up healthy oral flora ... and the shifts in communities of organisms that lead to oral diseases.

REFERENCES

1. Chiller K, Selkin BA, Murakawa GJ. Skin microflora and bacterial infections of the skin. *J. Invest. Dermatol. Symp. Proc.* 2001;6:170–174.
2. Roth RR, James WD. Microbiology of the skin: resident flora, ecology, infection. *J. Am. Acad. Dermatol.* 1989;20:367–390.
3. Aly R, Maibach HI, Shinefield HR, Strauss WG. Survival of pathogenic microorganisms on human skin. *J. Invest. Dermatol.* 1972;58:205–210.
4. Holland KT, Bojar RA. Cosmetics: what is their influence on the skin microflora? *Am. J. Clin. Dermatol.* 2002;3:445–449.
5. Soria X, Carrascosa JM. Normal cutaneous flora and secondary bacterial infection. *Actas Dermosifiliogr.* 2007;98 (Suppl. 1):15–21.

6. Till AE, Goulden V, Cunliffe WJ, Holland KT. The cutaneous microflora of adolescent, persistent and late-onset acne patients does not differ. *Br. J. Dermatol.* 2000;142:885–892.

7. Miura Y, Ishige I, Soejima N, Suzuki Y, Uchida K, Kawana S, Eishi Y. Quantitative PCR of *Propionibacterium acnes* DNA in samples aspirated from sebaceous follicles on the normal skin of subjects with or without acne. *J. Med. Dent. Sci.* 2010;57:65–74.

8. Greene JN. The microbiology of colonization, including techniques for assessing and measuring colonization. *Infect. Control Hosp. Epidemiol.* 1996;17:114–118.

9. Otto M. *Staphylococcus epidermidis*—the 'accidental' pathogen. *Nat. Rev. Microbiol.* 2009;7:555–567.

10. Schoenfelder SM, Lange C, Eckart M, Hennig S, Kozytska S, Ziebuhr W. Success through diversity—how *Staphylococcus epidermidis* establishes as a nosocomial pathogen. *Int. J. Med. Microbiol.* 2010;300:380–386.

11. Iwase T, Uehara Y, Shinji H, Tajima A, Seo H, Takada K, Agata T, Mizunoe Y. *Staphylococcus epidermidis* Esp inhibits *Staphylococcus aureus* biofilm formation and nasal colonization. *Nature* 2010;465:346–349.

12. Faden H, Lesse AJ, Trask J, Hill JA, Hess DJ, Dryja D, Lee YH. Importance of colonization site in the current epidemic of staphylococcal skin abscesses. *Pediatrics* 2010;125:e618–e624.

13. Higuchi W, Mimura S, Kurosawa Y, Takano T, Iwao Y, Yabe S, Razvina O, Nishiyama A, Ikeda-Dantsuji Y, Sakai F, Hanaki H, Yamamoto T. Emergence of the community-acquired methicillin-resistant *Staphylococcus aureus* USA300 clone in a Japanese child, demonstrating multiple divergent strains in Japan. *J. Infect. Chemother.* 2010;16:292–297.

14. Yabe S, Takano T, Higuchi W, Mimura S, Kurosawa Y, Yamamoto T. Spread of the community-acquired methicillin-resistant *Staphylococcus aureus* USA300 clone among family members in Japan. *J. Infect. Chemother.* 2010;16:372–374.

15. Yamamoto T, Nishiyama A, Takano T, Yabe S, Higuchi W, Razvina O, Shi D. Community-acquired methicillin-resistant *Staphylococcus aureus*: community transmission, pathogenesis, and drug resistance. *J. Infect. Chemother.* 2010;16:225–254.

16. Aas JA, Paster BJ, Stokes LN, Olsen I, Dewhirst FE. Defining the normal bacterial flora of the oral cavity. *J. Clin. Microbiol.* 2005;43:5721–5732.

17. Henderson B, Wilson M. Commensal communism and the oral cavity. *J. Dent. Res.* 1998;77:1674–1683.

18. Zou J, Zhou XD. Early colonization of normal microflora in oral cavity of children. *Zhonghua Er Ke Za Zhi* 2003;41:193–195.

19. Caufield PW. Dental caries: an infectious and transmissible disease. Where have we been and where are we going? *N. Y. State Dent. J.* 2005;71:23–27.

20. Lapirattanakul J, Nakano K, Nomura R, Hamada S, Nakagawa I, Ooshima T. Demonstration of mother-to-child transmission of *Streptococcus mutans* using multilocus sequence typing. *Caries Res.* 2008;42:466–474.

21. Li Y, Caufield PW. The fidelity of initial acquisition of mutans streptococci by infants from their mothers. *J. Dent. Res.* 1995;74:681–685.

22. Li Y, Caufield PW. Arbitrarily primed polymerase chain reaction fingerprinting for the genotypic identification of mutans streptococci from humans. *Oral Microbiol. Immunol.* 1998;13:17–22.

23. Li Y, Dasanayake AP, Caufield PW, Elliott RR, Butts, JT. 3rd, Characterization of maternal mutans streptococci transmission in an African American population. *Dent. Clin. North Am.* 2003;47:87–101.

24. Redmo Emanuelsson IM, Thornqvist E. Distribution of mutans streptococci in families: a longitudinal study. *Acta Odontol. Scand.* 2001;59:93–98.

25. Marsh PD, Percival RS. The oral microflora—friend or foe? Can we decide? *Int. Dent. J.* 2006;56:233–239.

26. Mager DL, Ximenez-Fyvie LA, Haffajee AD, Socransky SS. Distribution of selected bacterial species on intraoral surfaces. *J. Clin. Periodontol.* 2003;30:644–654.

27. Kazor CE, Mitchell PM, Lee AM, Stokes LN, Loesche WJ, Dewhirst FE, Paster BJ. Diversity of bacterial populations on the tongue dorsa of patients with halitosis and healthy patients. *J. Clin. Microbiol.* 2003;41:558–563.

CHAPTER 17

CORYNEBACTERIUM SPECIES AND THEIR ROLE IN THE GENERATION OF HUMAN MALODOR

Carol L. Bratt[1] and Nava Dayan[2]

[1]*Dows Institute, University of Iowa, Iowa City, IA*
[2]*Lipo Chemicals Inc., Paterson, NJ*

17.1 SWEAT

17.1.1 Why Do We Sweat?

Sweating is a physiological response to increasing core and skin temperatures during exposure to heat stresses such as those brought on by hot environmental conditions or metabolic heat production (such as that brought on by exercise). Under conditions that raise body temperatures above a very tightly regulated core temperature, heat balance is maintained by elevation of skin blood flow as well as evaporative heat loss through sweating. Emotional stress can also induce sweating, but this is generally confined to the palms, soles, axillae, and forehead, although some individuals sweat over their entire skin surface [1].

Axillary (armpit) sweat is produced by two types of glands: eccrine glands, which produce the largest volume of sweat and therefore contribute to the "wet" portion of axillary sweat, and apocrine glands, which produce a much smaller volume of sweat containing odiferous precursors that contribute to axillary malodor. Eccrine sweat glands respond to stimuli by immediate production and secretion of sweat, producing the response we normally think of as sweating [2]. In contrast, the response of apocrine glands was initially described by Shelley and Hurley as having a refractory period, meaning that after initial stimulation and consequent sweat response, no further response could be stimulated from the same gland for a number of hours [3]. Shelley and Levy later suggested that stimuli to apocrine glands do not result in immediate production of apocrine sweat, but only in the emptying of the

Innate Immune System of Skin and Oral Mucosa: Properties and Impact in Pharmaceutics, Cosmetics, and Personal Care Products, First Edition. Nava Dayan and Philip W. Wertz.

preformed contents of the glands, and production is a slow continual process uninfluenced by stimuli [2].

17.1.1.1 *Eccrine-Derived Sweat*
Thermal sweat is produced by an estimated 2–4 million eccrine sweat glands spread over most of the body's surface, but only about 5% of these glands are active at one time [4]. The primary function of the eccrine system is thermoregulation. Sweat rate is primarily influenced by elevation of core temperatures and secondarily by skin temperatures. Smiles et al. examined the influence of hypothalamic temperatures on sweating in rhesus monkeys and found that increased internal temperature is associated with increased hypothalamic temperature and sweat rate [5]. Furthermore, increase in internal temperature is approximately nine times more efficient at stimulating the sweat center than an increase in skin temperature [6]. Sweat gland size and density also play an important role [7,8]. Sweat gland size and density not only vary among different individuals but also vary in different skin regions within the same individual. Therefore, sweat rate is not uniform over the entire skin surface [9,10].

There are remarkable individual differences in levels of sweat responses to heat or exercise stresses. The maximum sweat rate occurs when rectal temperature reaches 39°C [11] and is also influenced by several factors such as age [12], gender [12], physical fitness [13], humidity [14], hydration levels [15,16], acclimation to heat [13,17,18], and work intensity [14,19]. During dynamic exercise in the heat, a person can lose between 1.0 and 2.5 L of sweat per hour and under severe heat stress, 10–15 L/day, depending on hydration levels [4]. Since thermoregulation of core temperatures relies heavily on the evaporation of sweat, environmental conditions are also very important determining factors. Humid conditions negatively affect the rate of evaporation and heat loss is minimal. However, heat acclimation induces a variety of physiological changes geared to reduction of physiological strain (decreased heart rate, decreased rectal and core body temperature, and increased plasma volume) resulting in an increased sweat rate and more effective thermoregulation [14].

In addition to regulation of the sweating response by an integration of skin and core temperatures, several nonthermal factors have also been suggested to regulate the eccrine sweat response. Van Beaumont and Bullard showed that sweating occurred immediately following dynamic exercise or isometric exercise in warm environments—even before a measurable change in body temperature—and suggested the possibility of nonthermal factors' influence on the sweat response [20,21]. Gisolfi and Robinson later examined cases of intermittent exercise and observed increased sweating independent of measurable changes in internal, muscle, or skin temperatures [22]. With the onset of either dynamic exercise or isometric exercise in a warm environment, sweat rate was shown to increase rapidly (within 1.5–2 s) and was initially independent of measurable core, skin, or muscle temperature increases. Later studies showed that two separate and distinct neural mechanisms—the muscle metaboreflex [23–25] and, to a lesser degree, muscle mechanoreceptors [26–29]—are capable of modulating sweat rate.

Eccrine sweat glands contain both adrenergic and cholinergic innervation [30] and respond to epinephrine and norepinephrine [31] but appear to be controlled primarily by cholinergic nerves. Therefore, eccrine sweat is primarily initiated by thermosensitive neurons in the preoptic area and anterior hypothalamus that receive integrated information from core and skin temperatures and initiate appropriate thermoregulatory responses [32]. Sweat glands actively secrete sweat when stimulated via nerve impulses through the sympathetic nervous system. Acetylcholine, released from the cholinergic sudomotor nerves, binds to muscarinic receptors on the gland, activating a complex exchange of electrolytes and creating sweat [33].

17.1.1.2 Apocrine-Derived Sweat

Apocrine sweat glands are found largely confined to the axillary and perineal regions [34]. These glands begin to function with the onset of puberty and in many species are thought to function as scent glands [1], although they do contribute to evaporative heat loss. Sweat produced by apocrine glands is much more viscous than that produced by eccrine glands and is without odor when first secreted [35]. However, upon bacterial action of resident coryneform bacteria on odiferous precursors within apocrine-derived sweat, a strong malodor is produced [36–38].

The quantity of sweat produced by apocrine glands is minute compared to the quantity of sweat produced by eccrine glands [3]. Apocrine sweat glands are primarily stimulated by adrenergic agents such as epinephrine or norepinephrine and apocrine sweat is primarily produced in response to emotional stressors such as pain and fear that stimulate sympathetic adrenergic nerves [3,31]. However, similar to eccrine glands, they also contain cholinergic innervation [30] and are suggested to be differentially controlled [31].

17.1.2 Composition of Sweat

Eccrine sweat is a dilute electrolyte solution containing some minerals and proteins. There is variation of sweat solute composition among individuals as well as solute concentration variations relating to age, gender, and sweat rate [9,39]. The concentration of some sweat components, such as sodium, chloride, lactate, and ammonia, depends on sweat rate. Table 17.1 lists concentrations of the major components of

TABLE 17.1 Composition of Eccrine Sweat [1,50]

	Concentration
NaCl	10–100 mM[a]
K^+	4–20 mM
HCO_3^-	10–20 mM
Lactate	10–40 mM[a]
Urea	15–25 mg/dL
Ammonia	0.5–8.0 mM[a,b]
Amino acids	5.5–154.0 mM
Proteins	15–25 mg/dL

[a] Concentration depends on sweat rate.
[b] Related to pH.

human eccrine sweat. In addition to the components listed in Table 17.1, other components present in eccrine sweat include proteolytic enzymes [40–42] and other organic compounds such as histamine [43], prostaglandin [44,45], vitamin K-like substances [46], amphetamine-like compounds [47], and glucose [48] as well as some orally ingested drugs [49].

Shelley and Hurley found that apocrine sweat is milky, without odor when first secreted, and dries to form a viscous, yellowish mass that fluoresces [3]. Determination of the composition of apocrine sweat is problematic because apocrine glands share a common opening with sebaceous glands. Therefore, obtaining apocrine sweat that is not mixed with both sebum and the much larger volume of eccrine sweat is difficult. The main detectable components were proteins, carbohydrates, ferric ions, ammonia, and sebum (due to common secretory opening with sebaceous glands). Since then, the secretions of apocrine glands have been shown to contain a complex mixture of steroid derivatives and fatty acids [51] and the odorless precursors of axillary malodor have been found within the water-soluble portion of apocrine sweat [37].

17.2   MALODOR

17.2.1   Role of Corynebacteria

The axilla is a region on the human body that is colonized with two types of bacteria: staphylococci and corynebacteria [52]. While there is a strong correlation between a high population of corynebacteria and strong axillary odor formation, such correlation is not found with staphylococci. Three main components were identified as malodorants. These were shown to be a result of conversion of malodor precursors by corynebacteria enzymes.

The first of these malodor precursors is a group of steroid derivatives, namely, 5-alpha-androst-16-en-3-one and 5-alpha-androst-16-en-3-alpha-ol. The second group is branched fatty acids with the major being (*E*)-3-methyl-2-hexenoic acid (E3M2H) and 3-hydroxy-3-methylhexanoic acid [53], and the third is a group of volatile sulfanylalkanols, with 3-methyl-3-sulfanylhexan-1-ol being the dominant one. Table 17.2 describes the different compounds released by corynebacteria enzymes. There is evidence suggesting that while the steroidal molecules produce more of a musky/urine scent, the fatty acids (branched, straight chain, and unsaturated) are increasingly being thought of as the cause of the more "traditional" axillary malodor [37,38,54].

17.2.2   Gender Differences

It is well known that gender, as well as ethnicity and emotional, physiological, and environmental factors, may influence both the quantity and quality of sweat [55]. Several factors may contribute to these differences. Differences in male versus female microflora have been reported with respect to the ratio of corynebacteria to staphylococci [56,57]. The size and number of sweat glands, as well as some odor-related

TABLE 17.2   Malodor Compounds Released in Axillary Sweat by Corynebacterial Secretions

Family of compounds	Main component(s)	Enzyme responsible for release	Corynebacteria responsible
Steroid derivatives	5-Alpha-androstenol and 5-alpha-androstenone	Beta-glucuronidase and aryl sulfatase	*C. striatum*
Branched fatty acids	(*E*)-3-Methyl-2-hexenoic acid and 3-hydroxy-3-methyl hexanoic acid	Zinc-dependent aminoacylase	*C. striatum*
Volatile sulfanylalkanols	3-Methyl 3-sulfanylhexan-1-ol	Dipeptidases: *N*-alpha acyl-GLN aminoacylase and beta lyase	*C. striatum*, *C. jeikeium*

compounds known to cause axillary malodor, vary among individuals and even among individuals of different ethnic groups [55,58–60].

Quantitative differences between the sexes have also been reported. Maximal sweat capacity has been shown to be lower for females than for males [14] and males are significantly more tolerant of heat stress than females [12]. Troccaz et al. showed that the average sweat yield for males was five times higher than that for females when axillary samples were obtained while taking a sauna [55]. Quantitative differences of axillary odor compounds between the sexes have been reported by Zeng et al. [60] and Penn et al. [61], while another study [62] showed no differences between the sexes. Penn et al. studied the composition of axillary sweat and using gas chromatography–mass spectrometry (GC–MS) showed differences in sweat profiles across different individuals, providing evidence for individual "axillary sweat" fingerprints [61]. In addition, although axillary sweat of men and women had very similar GC–MS profiles, they were able to statistically discriminate the sexes based on a few quantitative measurements of some specific compounds. These differences were based on a multivariate distribution of compounds and no unique gender-specific compounds were found. Zeng et al. also completed two separate GC–MS studies of male followed by female axillary secretions and found that men and women with similar axillary microflora are quantitatively similar in the array of volatiles produced [54,60]. Similar to Penn et al., they concluded that although the components of male sweat versus female sweat were very similar, the relative proportions of these components within axillary secretions were different.

Qualitative differences between male and female axillary malodor have also been recorded. According to Schleidt and Hold, after puberty, when the apocrine glands begin to function, discrimination between genders based on malodor becomes possible [63]. In general, male odor was more often classified as unpleasant and less often as pleasant, compared to female odor. Along the same lines, Doty showed that the stronger and more unpleasant the smell, the more likely it was to be assigned to the male gender while weaker or more pleasant odors were more likely to be assigned to the female gender, regardless of the true gender of the donors [64].

17.3   *CORYNEBACTERIUM* SPECIES: CHARACTERISTICS AND ABUNDANCE ON HUMAN SKIN

Corynebacterium species, aerobic Gram-positive rod diphtheroids, are widely spread in the environment and are part of the normal skin flora. They are found over the entire skin surface and in axillary sweat. In recent years, corynebacteria have attracted increased attention in the medical community because of the increasing number of immunocompromised patients harboring these species where they became pathogenic. Specifically, *C. amycolatum*, *C. jeikeium*, and *C. urealyticum* are currently recognized as important pathogens [65].

The morphological term "coryneform" replaced in the early 1990s the more familiar term "diphtheria." The coryneform group usually includes aerobic and anaerobic, nonacid-fast, pleomorphic, nonbranching rods that do not form spores [66]. The morphology of corynebacteria is straight to slightly curved rods with tapered ends, and sometimes club-shaped forms (Figure 17.1). Although some strains stain unevenly, they usually stain Gram positive. They are also characterized by the formation of metachromatic granules, lack of motility, facultative anaerobic growth (although some organisms are aerobic), and catalase production. When analyzing cell wall and lipid composition, the *Corynebacterium* genus is most closely related to the genera of *Mycobacterium*, *Nocardia*, *Rhodococcus*, and *Caseobacter*.

The prevalence of distribution of corynebacteria species on human skin varies between genders and is species related. For example, the rate of colonization of group D2 was found to be higher in females (43.3%) than in males (17.7%), but the JK species was isolated more often from males (32.1%) than from females (13.5%) [67]. Both groups of corynebacteria are commonly found on human skin and oral mucosa and are highly resistant to most antimicrobial agents.

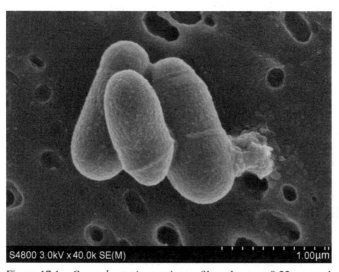

Figure 17.1   *Corynebacterium striatum* filtered onto a 0.22 μm nuclepore membrane.

Corynebacteria have been suggested to be a significant part of the axillary flora, accounting for up to 70% of the flora population. In fact, the human axilla provides an ideal environment for growth of corynebacteria and other microorganisms. Its anatomy secures a semiocclusive moist shelter that is rich in nutrients secreted from sweat and sebum, such as minerals, amino acids, and lipids.

Corynebacterium species were identified as an odor positive population while *Corynebacterium xerosis* was shown to be involved in the transformation of steroids to malodor molecules in the axilla [68]. They were shown to convert both androstadienone and androstadienol to androstenone and 3a-androstenol. Moreover, a variety of studies demonstrated a correlation between a decrease in axillary malodor and a decrease in corynebacteria population.

When incubated with corynebacteria, apocrine secretions isolated from axillary sweat were shown to produce (*E*)-3-methyl-2-hexenoic acid [59]. This C-7 branched unsaturated fatty acid was found in sweat of both Caucasians and Asians and is characterized by a strong malodor. In addition to E3M2H, compounds that were shown to produce malodor are volatile steroids (androstenol, androstenone, and androstadienone) as well as linear and branched saturated and unsaturated fatty acids. Two additional acids were identified as contributing to axillary odor: (*S*)-3-hydroxy-3-methylhexanoic acid and (*S*)-3-methyl-3-sulfanyl-hexan-1-ol. The natural precursor of these three acids was purified from nonhydrolyzed axilla secretions. These acids appear to be covalently linked to a glutamine residue. It is believed that a Zn^{2+}-dependent aminoacylase released from *C. striatum* cleaves the odor-generating acids from the odorless precursors [69]. After being cleaved from the glutamine residue, the acids might subsequently react, noncovalently, with apolipoprotein D. This noncovalent association may serve as a slow release mechanism of these volatiles from sweat. Moreover, while in the past it was thought that both corynebacteria and staphylococci may be responsible for the generation of malodor, it is now clear that nonodoriferous precursors must be transformed by bacterial enzymes present in corynebacteria and not in staphylococci. While the aminoacylase released from corynebacteria has strong selectivity for the glutamine residue, it has broad substrate specificity regarding the acyl part. This opens up the possibility that other potential glutamine-containing precursors in sweat will be cleaved by the same enzyme to generate additional volatile substances such as branched fatty acids.

17.3.1   Corynebacteria A and B

In researching the cause of malodor, scientists identified two classes of uncharacterized corynebacteria species that were classified as A and B [70]. While corynebacteria A was shown to be responsible for partial catabolism of methyl-branched long-chain fatty acids, the B class was proven incapable of growing on fatty acids. Short- and medium-chain (C2–C11) fatty acids, in particular, 3-methyl-2-hexenoic acid, serve as the primary cause of axillary malodor. In addition, 16-androstene steroids are also among the casual molecules leading to malodor. Since these fatty acids are initially conjugated to peptides, it was postulated that a corynebacterial aminoacylase is responsible for cleaving and releasing the fatty acid from its conjugate.

This Zn^{2+}-dependent enzyme was derived from *C. striatum* and its corresponding gene Ax20 was identified and cloned.

17.3.2 *Corynebacterium bovis*

C. bovis is a small Gram-positive rod with one end wider than the other. It is persistent in the environment, since it is lipophilic and survives well on skin flakes and other organic material. As a lipid-requiring bacterium, it is often isolated from milk of infected mammary glands of dairy cows [71]. Preliminary identification of *C. bovis* can be based on staining, oxidase, catalase, and growth on unsupplemented trypticase soy agar. Further identification can be based on the presence of small, white, nonhemolytic colonies on 5% bovine blood agar. It also has a tendency to grow on milk fat as it requires oleic acid.

17.3.3 *Corynebacterium striatum*

C. striatum was reported to be a normal inhabitant of the external part of the nostrils and skin and was only rarely recognized as a pathogen. It was mainly shown to be responsible for infections in immunocompromised patients, causing illnesses such as pneumonia and meningitis with relatively low mortality rates. Although usually susceptible to a wide range of antibiotics, particularly beta-lactams, strains that demonstrated resistance to multiple antibiotics have been described in nosocomial outbreaks. It was also shown to spread from patient to patient via the hands of attending personnel [72]. Nevertheless, its role as a human pathogen is not fully understood. In patients with immunocompromised skin, it was shown to act as a pathogenic opportunistic pathogen.

17.3.4 *Corynebacterium jeikeium*

The International Committee on Systematic Bacteriology defined in the early 1990s the CDC group JK of corynebacteria as *C. jeikeium*. Infections continue to be reported mainly in patients who are immunocompromised (especially by malignancies) and those with medical devices, particularly for patients that have been hospitalized for prolonged periods, have compromised body barriers, or have previously received broad-spectrum antimicrobial therapy. The prevalence of skin colonization with *C. jeikeium* was shown to be the highest in patients with malignancies or other severe immunocompromised conditions. Skin colonization is found in the inguinal, axillary, and rectal areas.

There is contradicting evidence with regard to the transmission of *C. jeikeium*. While some studies claim that the organism is spread within hospitals, presumably by the hand-to-hand route, others claim that patient-to-patient transmission did not occur. It is important to note that while Some analyses demonstrate that the plasmid provides evidence that the strain has a common origin, others demonstrate it does not [73].

Some strains of *C. jeikeium* were found to be fully susceptible to beta-lactam antibiotics, while others were only moderately resistant to these antibiotics but could be fully eradicated by combined penicillin and aminoglycoside therapy. The mechanism for the multiresistance to antibiotics in *C. jeikeium* strains is not fully understood, although repeat exposure to beta-lactams in cell cultures led to the development of moderately resistant strains [74].

It has been proposed that *C. jeikeium* can be identified on the basis of an absolute requirement for lipids, the production of catalase, resistance to multiple antibiotics, and production of acid from maltose. This species does not reduce nitrate, hydrolyze urea, or digest gelatin. It can also be identified on the basis of analysis of cell wall carbohydrates, amino acids, and mycolic acids as well as whole cell protein patterns and by DNA hybridization studies. It can grow on 0.03% tellurite agar and on bile salt agar. It can hydrolyze polysorbate 20 and 80 and produce acid from glucose and galactose. Some strains can also attack maltose.

17.4 ANTIMICROBIALS AND THEIR ROLE IN CONTROL OF MALODOR

17.4.1 Triclosan

Triclosan is known as an antibacterial agent, bactericide, disinfectant, and fungicide. The use of triclosan started in the 1970s when it was incorporated into soaps. While the uses of triclosan have risen dramatically in the past few years, it seems that the reason is more marketing-based rather than based on true need. It is now found in a variety of personal care products including hand soaps, deodorants and antiperspirants, cosmetics, hair products, and toothpastes. The use of triclosan is regulated by both the Food and Drug Administration (FDA) and the Environmental Protection Agency (EPA) (because of its use as a pesticide). The content of this compound in personal care products ranges from 0.1% to 1%.

The main concerns associated with the use of triclosan can be summarized as follows:

1. The medical community is not certain that triclosan is required for better protection against microbial inhabitation when compared to a simple effective wash with soap and water.

2. The extensive expanded use of triclosan in a variety of products may allow the development of resistant bacteria, not only to triclosan but also to other antimicrobials and antibiotics.

3. Possible toxicological concerns to human health that result from the accumulation of the compound in body tissues and insufficient clearance.

4. Harmful effects to the environment, and especially accumulation in water, that was shown to be toxic to aquatic life.

With regard to bioaccumulation, the Centers for Disease Control (CDC) issued a report on triclosan in November 2009 [75]. The report states that the health effects from exposure to low environmental levels of triclosan are unknown and therefore more research is required. The report further notes a study conducted by the National Health and Nutrition Examination Survey (NHANES) that detected triclosan in the urine of 2517 individuals in a study conducted during the years 2003–2004. The scientists detected the compound in nearly 75% of the individuals. Absorption of the compound to systemic circulation is thought to be via the skin or oral mucosa. The fact that measurable amounts of triclosan were found in the urine does not necessarily correlate with a toxicological effect. Another paper published in 2007 [76] notes that triclosan levels as high as 2000 µg/kg lipids were detected in human breast milk. Concentrations in human fluids such as milk and plasma correlate to levels of exposure.

It was demonstrated that bacteria can develop resistance to triclosan. The site of activity was identified as the enzyme enoyl reductase that is essential in fatty acid synthesis [77]. In the presence of triclosan, fatty acid biosynthesis is inhibited. Some bacteria do not carry the gene that encodes this enzyme and in the presence of triclosan, they will survive. They may therefore grow at the expense of the more sensitive bacteria. Following a few additional studies on the antimicrobial power of triclosan against resistant bacteria, Levy concluded that antimicrobial agents will have an impact on the environmental flora and on resistance emergence with cross-resistance to antibiotics.

A study that was published by Chang Ahn et al. in 2008 [78] reported the effects of triclosan and other antimicrobial agents on biochemical mechanisms utilizing a few *in vitro* cell-based bioassays. The group found that the compound exhibited antagonistic activity in the estrogen receptor-mediated bioassay as well as in the androgen assay. The scientists also point out that the phenolic structure of the compound resembles the structure of nonsteroidal estrogens such as diethylstilbestrol and bisphenol A.

As for environmental concerns, there is evidence that it is acutely and chronically toxic to aquatic organisms. It was shown to influence both structure and function of algal communities [79]. In addition, scientists found triclosan to accumulate in fish tissue. The concentration found in fish is a thousand times higher than the concentrations found in water [80]. Furthermore, triclosan can be transformed to a more lipophilic derivative upon methylation, that is, to methyl triclosan. This lipophilic derivative is likely to accumulate in biological fat tissues even more than triclosan itself. In a study conducted in lakes and rivers of Switzerland, scientists found significant amounts of methyl triclosan that was probably formed by biological methylation both in water and in the tissues of a variety of fish. The strength of the evidence suggested that it can be selected as a marker for aquatic contamination [81].

With relevancy to this chapter, when it comes to efficacy of triclosan against corynebacteria to eliminate or prevent generation of malodor, not much is published. A publication from 1987 summarizes a study testing the effect of triclosan on axillary flora and on malodor *in vivo* [82]. In this study, bacteria were recovered from the middle axillae region of subjects. The total bacteria count was obtained after body site treatment with an aerosol spray containing 0%, 0.05%, or 0.2% triclosan. In addition, an olfactory study was conducted where the use of triclosan was compared with a soap washing. The results indicated that when the axilla is washed with soap, the microbial count is initially reduced but the intermediate counts hours and days later show restoration of microbial growth, with full restoration at the fourth day. When treated with 0.2% triclosan, the microbial count reduction was maintained at low levels even 9 h after product application. These results show the advantage of triclosan as contributing to a prolonged effect of bacteria reduction and not necessarily to effectiveness upon application. The main bacteria detected in axillary sweat were corynebacteria. In the olfactory study, both sprays with and without triclosan produced odor score reductions but the spray containing 0.15% showed superiority. This advantage was clear especially when odor was assessed 12 h after application supporting the prolonged effect of triclosan on bacteria population recovery.

In a study conducted by Proctor & Gamble, scientists studied the effect of triclosan in commercial products on axillary microbial growth and corresponding malodor [83]. They concluded that while glycol-based products alone control odor-causing bacteria for at least 24 h, the inclusion of triclosan in the product dramatically improved its effectiveness.

The studies on triclosan clearly demonstrate a positive correlation between reduction of the amount of corynebacteria and assessment of malodor. The health and environmental issues it brings foster the development of a safer biodegradable antimicrobial agent.

17.4.2 Natural Antimicrobials

Historically, the combat of axillary malodors has been based on the topical addition of antimicrobials in order to nonspecifically decrease bacterial load on the skin. A number of natural antimicrobial systems also serve to provide antimicrobial defense and help to control bacterial numbers on the skin surface through a variety of mechanisms. These are primarily mediated through antimicrobial peptides (AMPs), iron-binding proteins, skin surface acidification, and skin lipids [83–86].

More than 20 individual cutaneous proteins (including defensins, cathelicidins, psoriasins, and dermcidins) have been shown to exhibit antimicrobial activity [85] and are sorted into families based on similarities in charge, sequence homology, functional similarity, and three-dimensional structure. These antimicrobial peptides are thought to trigger and coordinate multiple components of the innate and adaptive immune system [85,88] and are produced by many different cell types. Eccrine glands constitutively produce dermcidins [89,90] while defensins and cathelicidins are induced by damage to the skin [91,92].

Skin lipids of epidermal and sebaceous origin are another important class of inhibitory molecules [91]. Fatty acids and long-chain bases found at the skin surface have been shown to exhibit potent and broad-spectrum antimicrobial activity [93–98]. In our laboratory, we found strong antimicrobial effects of the long-chain base, phytosphingosine, against each of *C. bovis* and *C. striatum* (unpublished observations). When compared with the effects of triclosan, an approximately 16 times higher concentration of triclosan (250 µg/mL) was required to inhibit either *C. bovis* or

TABLE 17.3 Minimum Inhibitory Concentrations of Lipids That Will Inhibit Bacterial Growth By ≥50%

| Bacteria | Minimum inhibitory concentrations (µg/mL) (N = 3) | |
	Triclosan, mean (SD)	Phytosphingosine, mean (SD)
C. bovis	250 (0)	15.6 (0)
C. striatum	250 (0)	15.6 (0)

TABLE 17.4 Synergistic Activity Between Phytosphingosine and LAE

Bacteria	FIC	FBC
C. bovis	0.28	0.31
C. striatum	0.16	0.53

[a] FIC ≤0.5 indicates agents have synergistic activity (e.g., each agent at fourth of its MIC or less). FIC >0.5–4 indicates agents have additive activity (e.g., each agent at half of its MIC). FIC ≥4.0 indicates agents have antagonistic activity (e.g., each agent at twice MIC or higher) [97].

C. striatum growth than was required when treated with phytosphingosine (15.6 µg/mL) (Table 17.3).

We also discovered that two compounds, phytosphingosine and ethyl lauroyl arginate laurate (LAEL), exhibited synergistic and strong bactericidal effects against each of *C. bovis* (FIC = 0.28) and *C. striatum* (FIC = 0.16) (Table 17.4). Fractional inhibitory concentration (FIC) represents the lowest concentration of lipid concentrations that reduce growth by 50% while fractional bactericidal concentration (FBC) is the lowest concentration of lipid that exhibits bactericidal effects (no viable cells present). *C. bovis*, when treated simultaneously with phytosphingosine and LAEL, had an FIC of 0.28, meaning that bacterial inhibition was seen when LAEL was diluted to 1/4 of its minimum inhibitory concentration (MIC) and phytosphingosine was diluted to 1/31 of its MIC (31.25 and 0.5 µg/mL, respectively). *C. striatum*, when treated simultaneously with phytosphingosine and LAEL, had an FIC of 0.16, meaning that bacterial inhibition was seen when LAEL was diluted to 1/8 of its MIC and phytosphingosine was diluted to 1/31 of its MIC (15.6 and 0.5 µg/mL, respectively).

17.5 SUMMARY

The literature available on colonization of *Corynebacterium* species in human skin refers mostly to its harmful pathogenic potential and only anecdotally to the role of these species in the maintenance of healthy skin flora as part of the skin's innate immunity. While axillary sweat may contain different types of bacteria it is mainly populated with *Corynebacterium* species. This family of bacteria was shown to be the only one contributing to the generation of malodor compounds. Moreover, in the process of identifying the specific enzymes actively converting sweat components to malodor components, it is the *C. striatum* that was shown to release these enzymes. We are not sure if the reason is its ease of growth and cultivation when compared to the other strains or simply because it is the only one actively producing the effect. When reviewing market approaches to addressing undesired body odor with antimicrobials, it is clear that triclosan is the most popular antimicrobial used in deodorants and antiperspirants. Yet, in recent years, its use has been criticized by the medical community, toxicologists, environmentalists, and other nongovernmental organizations. Its use was demonstrated to be unnecessary and its accumulation in the body and the environment as well as its possible toxicity and buildup of bacterial resistance has raised a true concern. In the search for alternative natural and safe compounds to combat malodor, we found two antimicrobials that exhibited a synergistic effect in killing two strains of corynebacteria with the most potent effect in *C. striatum*. This combination exceeded by far the effect of triclosan on these strains.

REFERENCES

1. Sato K. Biology of the eccrine sweat gland. In: Fitzpatrick TB, Eisen AZ, Wolff K, Freedbrg IM, Austen KF, editors *Dermatology in General Medicine*, Vol. 1, 4th ed. McGraw-Hill, Inc., 1993.
2. Shelley WB, Levy EJ. Apocrine sweat retention in man. II. Fox-Fordyce disease (apocrine miliaria). *AMA Arch. Dermatol.* 1956;73(1):38–49.
3. Shelley WB, Hurley HJ. The physiology of the human axillary apocrine sweat gland. *J. Invest. Dermatol.* 1953;20(4):285–297.
4. Kenny GP, Journeay WS. Human thermoregulation: separating thermal and nonthermal effects on heat loss. *Front. Biosci.* 2010;15:259–290.
5. Smiles KA, Elizondo RS, Barney CC. Sweating responses during changes of hypothalamic temperature in the rhesus monkey. *J. Appl. Physiol.* 1976;40:653–657.
6. Nadel ER, Bullard RW, Stolwijk JA. Importance of skin temperature in the regulation of sweating. *J. Appl. Physiol.* 1971;31(1):80–87.
7. Sato K, Dobson RL. Regional and individual variations in the function of the human eccrine sweat gland. *J. Invest Dermatol.* 1970;54(6):443–449.
8. Sato K, Sato F. Individual variations in structure and function of human eccrine sweat gland. *Am. J. Physiol.* 1983;245:203–208.
9. Patterson MJ, Galloway SDR, Nimmo MA. Variations in regional sweat composition in normal human males. *Exp. Physiol.* 2000;85(6):869–875.
10. Groscurth P. Anatomy of a sweat gland. In: Kreyden O, Boni R, Burg G, editors. *Hyperhidrosis and Botulinum.* Basel: Karger, 2002.
11. Ogawa T. Evaporative heat loss. In: Nakayama T, editor. *Thermal Physiology.* Tokyo: Rikohgakusha, 1981. pp. 135–166.
12. McLellan TM. Sex-related differences in thermoregulatory responses while wearing protective clothing. *Eur. J. Appl. Physiol.* 1998;78:28–37.
13. Shvartz E, Bhattacharya A, Sperinde SJ, Brock PJ, Sciaraffa D, Van Beaumont W. Sweating responses during heat acclimation and moderate conditioning. *J. Appl. Physiol.* 1979;46(4):675–680.
14. Torii M. Maximal sweating rate in humans. *J. Hum. Ergol.* 1995;24:137–152.
15. Montain SJ, Latzka WA, Sawka MN. Control of thermoregulatory sweating is altered by hydration level and exercise intensity. *J. Appl. Physiol.* 1995;79:1434–1439.
16. Sawka MN, Young AJ, Francesconi RP, Muza SR, Pandolf KB. Thermoregulatory and blood responses during exercise at graded hypohydration levels. *J. Appl. Physiol.* 1985;59:1394–1401.

17. Hofler W. Changes in regional distribution of sweating during acclimatization to heat. *J. Appl. Physiol.* 1968;46(25):503–506.

18. Fox RH, Goldsmith R, Hampton IF, Lewis HE. The nature of the increase in sweating capacity produced by heat acclimatization. *J. Physiol.* 1964;171:368–376.

19. Kenny GP, Périard J, Journeay WS, Sigal RJ, Reardon FD. Effect of exercise on the postexercise sweating threshold. *J. Appl. Physiol.* 2003;95:2355–2360.

20. Van Beaumont W, Bullard RW. Sweating: its rapid response to muscular work. *Science* 1963;141:643–646.

21. Van Beaumont W, Bullard RW. Sweating exercise stimulation during circulatory arrest. *Science* 1966;152(728):1521–1523.

22. Gisolfi C, Robinson S. Central and peripheral stimuli regulating sweating during intermittent work in men. *J. Appl. Physiol.* 1970;29(6):761–768.

23. Shibasaki M, Kondo N, Crandall CG. Evidence for metaboreceptor stimulation of sweating in normothermic and heat-stressed humans. *J. Physiol.* 2001;534:605–611.

24. Eiken O, Mekjavic IB. Ischaemia in working muscles potentiates the exercise-induced sweating response in man. *Acta Physiol. Scand.* 2004;181:305–311.

25. Kacin A, Golja P, Eiken O, Tipton MJ, Gorjanc J, Mekjavic IB. Human temperature regulation during cycling with moderate leg ischaemia. *Eur. J. Appl. Physiol.* 2005;95:213–220.

26. Journeay WS, Reardon FD, Martin CR, Kenny GP. Control of cutaneous vascular conductance and sweating during recovery from dynamic exercise in humans. *J. Appl. Physiol.* 2004;96:2207–2212.

27. Kondo N, Tominaga H, Shiojiri T, Shibasaki M, Aoki K, Takano S, Koga S, Nishiyasu T. Sweating responses to passive and active limb movements. *J. Therm. Biol.* 1997;22:351–356.

28. Shibasaki M, Sakai M, Oda M, Crandall CG. Muscle mechanoreceptor modulation of sweat rate during recovery from moderate exercise. *J. Appl. Physiol.* 2004;96:2115–2119.

29. Mitchell JH. Neural control of the circulation during exercise. *Med. Sci. Sports Exerc.* 1990;22:141–154.

30. Uno H. Sympathetic innervations of the sweat glands and piloerector muscle of macaques and human beings. *J. Invest. Dermatol.* 1977;69:112–130.

31. Robertshaw D. Neural and humoral control of apocrine glands. *J. Invest. Dermatol.* 1974;63:160–167.

32. Boulant JA. Hypothalamic mechanisms in thermoregulation. *Fed. Proc.* 1981;40:2843–3850.

33. Torres NE, Zollman PJ, Low PA. Characterization of muscarinic receptor subtype of rat eccrine sweat gland by autoradiography. *Brain Res.* 1991;550(1):129–132.

34. Robertshaw D. Apocrine sweat glands. In: Goldsmith LA, editor. *Biochemistry and Molecular Biology of the Skin.* Oxford: Oxford University Press, 1991. p. 763.

35. Shelley WB, Hurley HJ, Nichols AC. Axillary odor: experimental study of the role of bacteria, apocrine sweat, and deodorants. *Arch. Derm. Syphilol.* 1953;68(4):430–446.

36. Shehadeh N, Kligman AM. The bacteria responsible for apocrine odor, II. *J. Invest. Dermatol.* 1963;41:1–5.

37. Zeng X-N, Leyden JJ, Brand JG, Spielman AI, McGinley KJ, Preti G. An investigation of human apocrine gland secretion for axillary odor precursors. *J. Chem. Ecol.* 1992;18:1039–1055.

38. Zeng C, Spielman AI, Vowels BR, Leyden JJ, Biemann K, Preti G. A human axillary odorant is carried by apolipoprotein D. *Proc. Natl. Acad. Sci. USA* 1996;93:6626–6630.

39. Meyer F, Laitano O, Bar-Or O, McDougall D, Heigenhauser GJ. Effect of age and gender on sweat lactate and ammonia concentrations during exercise in the heat. *Braz. J. Med. Biol. Res.* 2007; 40(1):135–143.

40. Horie N, Yokozeki H, Sato K. Proteolytic enzymes in human eccrine sweat: a screening study. *Am. J. Physiol.* 1986;250(4Pt 2):R691–R698.

41. Yokozeki J, Hibino T, Sato K. Partial purification and characterization of cysteine proteinases in eccrine sweat. *Am. J. Physiol.* 1987;252(6):R1119–R1129.

42. Yokozeki J, Hibino T, Takemura T, Sato K. Cysteine protease inhibitor in eccrine sweat is derived from the sweat gland. *Am. J. Physiol.* 1991;260(2):R314–R320.

43. Garden JW. Plasma and sweat histamine concentration after heat exposure and physical exercise. *J. Appl. Physiol.* 1966;21:631.

44. Frewin DB, Eakins KE, Downey JA, Bhattacherjee F. Prostaglandin-like activity in human eccrine sweat. *Aust. J. Exp. Biol. Med. Sci.* 1973;51(5):701–702.

45. Förström L, Goldyne ME, Winkelmann RK. Prostaglandin activity in human eccrine sweat. *Prostaglandins* 1974;7(6):459–464.

46. Seutter E, Sutorius AHM. The vitamin K derivatives of some skin-mucins. 1. Properties and vitamin K origin. *Int. J. Vitam. Nutr. Res.* 1971;41:57.

47. Vree TB, Muskens AT, van Rossum JM. Excretion of amphetamines in human sweat. *Arch. Int. Pharmacodyn. Ther.* 1972;199(2):311–317.

48. Kuno Y. *Human Perspiration.* Springfield, IL: Thomas, 1956.

49. Sato K. The physiology, pharmacology, and biochemistry of the eccrine sweat gland. *Rev. Physiol. Biochem. Pharmacol.* 1977;79:51.

50. Sato K, Kang WH, Sato F. Eccrine sweat glands. In: Goldsmith LA, editor. *Physiology, Biochemistry, and Molecular Biology of the Skin*, 2nd ed. New York: Oxford University Press, 1991. pp. 741–762.

51. Gower DB, Nixon A, Jackman PJH, Mallett AI. Transformation of steroids by axillary coryneform bacteria. *Int. J. Cosmet. Sci.* 1986;8:149–158.

52. Emter R, Natsch A. The sequential action of dipeptidase and beta lyase is required for the release of the human body odorant 3-methyl-3 sulfanylhexan-1-ol from secreted Cys-Gly-(S) conjugate by corynebacteria. *J. Biol. Chem.* 2008;283(30):20645–20652.

53. Natsch A, Gfeller H, Gygax P, Schmid J. Isolation of a bacterial enzyme releasing axillary malodor and its use as a screening target for novel deodorant formulations. *Int. J. Cosmet. Sci.* 2005;27:115–122.

54. Zeng X, Leyden JJ, Lawley HJ, Sawano K, Nohara I, Preti G. Analysis of characteristic odors from human male axillae. *J. Chem. Ecol.* 1991;17(7):1469–1492.

55. Troccaz M, Borchard G, Vuilleumier C, Raviot-Derrien S, Niclass Y, Beccucci S, Starkenmann C. Gender-specific differences between the concentrations of nonvolatile (*R*)/(*S*)-3-methyl-3-sulfanylhexan-1-ol and (*R*)/(*S*)-3-hydroxy-3-methyl-hexanoic acid odor precursors in axillary secretions. *Chem. Senses* 2009;34:203–210.

56. Labows JN, McGinley KJ, Kligman AM. Perspectives on axillary odor. *J. Soc. Cosmet. Chem.* 1982;34:193–202.

57. Jackman PJH, Noble WC. Normal axillary skin microflora in various populations. *Clin. Exp. Dermatol.* 1983;8:259–268.

58. Ikeda S, Arata J, Nishikawa T, Takigawa M. *Standard Dermatology*, Tokyo: Igakushoin, 2001.

59. Akutsu T, Sekiguchi K, Ohmori T, Sakurada K. Individual comparisons of the levels of (*E*)-3-methyl-2-hexanoic acid, an axillary odor-related compound. *Chem. Senses* 2006;31:557–563 (in Japanese).

60. Zeng X, Leyden JJ, Spielman AI, Preti G. Analysis of characteristic human female axillary odors: qualitative comparison to males. *J. Chem. Ecol.* 1996;22(2):237–257.

61. Penn DJ, Oberzaucher E, Grammer K, Fisher G, Soini HA, Wiesler D, Novotny MV, Dixon SJ, Xu Y, Brereton RG. Individual and gender fingerprints in human body odour. *J. R. Soc. Interface* 2007;4:331–340.

62. Asano KG, Bayne CK, Horsman KM, Buchanan MV. Chemical composition of fingerprints for gender determination. *J. Forensic Sci.* 2002;47:805–807.

63. Schleidt M, Hold B. Human odour and identity. In: Breipohl W, editor. *Olfaction and Endocrine Regulation.* London: IRL Press, Ltd, 1982. pp. 181–194.

64. Doty R. Olfactory communication in humans. *Chem. Senses* 1981;6:351.

65. Superti SV, Martins DS, Caierao J, Soares F, Prochnow T, Cantarelli VV, Zavascki AP. *Corynebacterium striatum* infecting a malignant cutaneous lesion: the emergence of opportunistic pathogen. *Rev. Inst. Med. Trop. São Paulo* 2009;51(2):115–116.

66. Coyle MB, Lipsky BA. Coryneform bacteria is infectious diseases: clinical and laboratory aspects. *Clin. Microbiol. Rev.* 1990;3(3):227–246.

67. Soriano F, Rodrigez-Tudela JL, Fernandez-Roblas R, Aguado JM, Santamaria M. Skin colonization by *Corynebacterium* groups D2 and JK in hospitalized patients. *J. Clin. Microbiol.* 1988;26(9): 1878–1880.

68. Labows J, Reilly J, Leyden J, Preti G. Axillary odor determination, formation and control. In: Laden K, editor. Antiperspirants and Deodorants, 2nd ed. *Cosmetic Science and Technology Series*, Vol. 20 New York: Marcel Dekker Inc., 1999. pp. 59–82.

69. Natsch A, Gfeller H, Gygax P, Schmid J, Acuna G. A specific bacterial aminoacylase cleaves odorant precursors secreted in the human axilla. *J. Biol. Chem.* 2003;287(8):5718–5727.

70. James AG, Casey J, Hyliards D, Mycock G. Fatty acid metabolism by cutaneous bacteria and its role in axillary malodor. *World J. Microbiol. Biotechnol* 2004;20:787–793.

71. Watts JL, Lowery DE, Teel JF, Rossbach S. Identification of *Corynebacterium bovis* and other coryneforms isolated from bovine mammary glands. *J. Dairy Sci.* 2000;83(10):2373–2379.

72. Brandenburg AH, Van Belkum A, Van Pelt C, Bruining HA, Mouton JW, Verburg HA. Patient to patient spread of single strain of *Corynebacterium striatum* causing infections in a surgical intensive care unit. *J. Clin. Microbiol.* 1996;34(9):2089–2094.

73. Charles PC, Stock F, Kruczak-Filipov PM, Gill VJ. Rapid method for presumptive identification of *Corynebacterium jeikeium. J. Clin. Microbiol.* 1993;31(12):3320–3322.

74. Riegel P, Briel DD, Prevost FJ, Monteil H. Genomic diversity among *Corynebacterium jeikeium* strains and comparison with biochemical characteristics and antimicrobial susceptibilities. *J. Clin. Microbiol.* 1994;32(8):1860–1865.

75. Centers for Disease Control and Prevention (CDC) report on triclosan issued in November 2009. http://origin.cdc.gov/exposurereport/Triclosan_FactSheet.html.

76. Dayan AD. Risk assessment of triclosan in human breast milk. *Food Chem. Toxicol.* 2007;45:125–129.

77. Levy SB. Antibacterial household products: cause and concern. *Emerg. Infect. Dis.* 2001;7 (3 Suppl.): 512–515.

78. Chang Ahn K, Zhao B, Chen J, Cheredinchenko G, Sanmarti E, Dension MS, Lasley B, Pessah IN, Kultz D, Chang DPY, Gee SJ, Hammock B. *In vitro* biologic activities of the antimicrobials triclocarban, its analogs, and triclosan in bioassay screens: receptor-based bioassay screens. *Environ. Health Perspect.* 2008;116(9):1203–1210.

79. Ky N. Antibacterial soap: unnecessary and harmful. A report prepared for the San Diego Oceans Foundation, October 2005.

80. Samsoe-Peterson L, Winther-Nielsen M, Madsen T. Fate and effects of triclosan. Environmental Project 861, Danish Environmental Protection Agency, 2003.

81. Balmer ME, Poiger T, Droz C, Romanin K, Bergqvist PA, Muller MD, Buser HR. Occurrence of methyl triclosan, a transformation product of the bactericide triclosan in fish from various lakes in Switzerland. *Environ. Sci. Technol.* 2004;38(2):390–395.

82. Cox AR. Efficacy of the antimicrobial agent triclosan in topical deodorant products: recent developments *in vivo. J. Soc. Cosmet. Chem.* 1987;38:223–231.

83. Lanzalanco AC, Rocchetta HL, Chabi G. Clinical effect of three-day application of a commercial deodorant on axilla malodor intensity, microbial population level and longevity of fragrance expression. In: *American Academy of Dermatology Meeting,* San Diego, CA, 2004.

84. Bowdish DM, Davidson DJ, Hancock RE. A re-evaluation of the role of host defense peptides in mammalian immunity. *Curr. Protein Pept. Sci.* 2005;6:35–51.

85. Braff MH, Bardan A, Nizet V, Gallo RL. Cutaneous defense mechanisms by antimicrobial peptides. *J. Invest. Dermatol.* 2005;125:9–13.

86. Lee SH, Jeong SK, Ahn SK. An update of the defensive barrier function of skin. *Yonsei Med. J.* 2006; 47(3):293–306.

87. Schauber J, Gallo RL. Update review: antimicrobial peptides and the skin immune defense system. *J. Allergy Clin. Immunol.* 2008;122(2):261–266.

88. Schauber J, Gallo RL. Expanding the roles of antimicrobial peptides in skin: alarming and arming keratinocytes. *J. Invest. Dermatol.* 2007;127(3):510–512.

89. Murakami M, Ohtake T, Dorschner RA, Schittek B, Garbe C, Gallo RL. Cathelicidin anti-microbial peptide expression in sweat, an innate defense system for the skin. *J. Invest. Dermatol.* 2002;119:1090–1095.

90. Rieg S, Seeber S, Seffen H, Humenv A, Kalbacher H, Stevanovic S, Kimura A, Garbe C, Schittek B. Generation of multiple stable dermcidin-derived antimicrobial peptides in sweat of different body sites. *J. Invest. Dermatol.* 2006;126(2):354–365.

91. Murakami M, Lopez-Garcia B, Braff M, Dorschner RA, Gallo RL. Postsecretory processing generates multiple cathelicidins for enhanced topical antimicrobial response. *J. Immunol.* 2004;172:3070–3077.

92. Harder J, Bartels J, Christophers E, Schroder JM. A peptide antibiotic from human skin (letter). *Nature* 1997;387:861.

93. Drake DR, Brogden KA, Dawson DV, Wertz PW. Thematic review series: skin lipids. Antimicrobial lipids at the skin surface. *J. Lipid Res.* 2008;49(1):49–11.

94. Bibel DJ, Aly R, Shah S, Shinefield HR. Antimicrobial activity of sphingosines. *J. Invest. Dermatol.* 1992;98:269–273.

95. Bibel DJ, Aly R, Shah S, Shinefield HR. Sphingosines: antimicrobial barriers of the skin. *Acta Derm Venereol.* 1993;73:407–411.

96. Gell G, Drake DR, Wertz PW. Peridex and lauric acid exhibit a synergistic effect on *Streptococcus mutans*. *J. Dent. Res.* 1995;74:76.

97. Gell G, Drake D, Wertz P. Antimicrobial effects of epithelial lipids. *J. Dent. Res.* 1993;72:399.

98. Payne CD, Ray TL, Downing DT. Cholesterol sulfate protects *Candida albicans* from inhibition by sphingosine *in vitro*. *J. Invest. Dermatol.* 1996;106:549–552.

99. Gradelski E, Kolek B, Bonner DP, Valera L, Minassian B, Fung-Tomc J. Activity of gatifloxacin and ciprofloxacin in combination with other antimicrobial agents. *Int. J. Antimicrob. Agents* 2001; 17(2):103–107.

INDEX

Innate Immune System of Skin and Oral Mucosa: Properties and Impact in Pharmaceutics,
Cosmetics, and Personal Care Products, First Edition. Nava Dayan and Philip W. Wertz.
© 2011 John Wiley & Sons, Inc. Published 2011 by John Wiley & Sons, Inc.